Traditional Herbal Medicines for Modern Times

Bupleurum Species

Scientific Evaluation and Clinical Applications

Traditional Herbal Medicines for Modern Times

Each volume in this series provides academia, health sciences, and the herbal medicines industry with in-depth coverage of the herbal remedies for infectious diseases, certain medical conditions, or the plant medicines of a particular country.

Edited by Dr. Roland Hardman

Traditional Herbal Medicines for Modern Times

Bupleurum Species

Scientific Evaluation and Clinical Applications

Edited by
Sheng-Li Pan

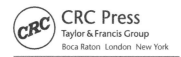

CRC Press
Taylor & Francis Group
Boca Raton London New York

CRC Press is an imprint of the
Taylor & Francis Group, an **informa** business

A TAYLOR & FRANCIS BOOK

CRC Press
Taylor & Francis Group
6000 Broken Sound Parkway NW, Suite 300
Boca Raton, FL 33487-2742

© 2006 by Taylor & Francis Group, LLC
CRC Press is an imprint of Taylor & Francis Group, an Informa business

First issued in paperback 2019

No claim to original U.S. Government works

ISBN 13: 978-0-367-45366-4 (pbk)
ISBN 13: 978-0-8493-9265-8 (hbk)

Library of Congress Card Number 2005035151

Library of Congress Cataloging-in-Publication Data

Bupleurum species : scientific evaluation and clinical applications / edited by Sheng-Li Pan.
    p. ; cm. -- (Traditional herbal medicines for modern times ; v. 7)
  Includes bibliographical references and index.
  ISBN-13: 978-0-8493-9265-8 (hardcover : alk. paper)
  ISBN-10: 0-8493-9265-9 (hardcover : alk. paper)
  1. Bupleurum--Therapeutic use. 2. Herbs--Therapeutic use--China. 3. Herbs--Therapeutic use--Japan.
  [DNLM: 1. Bupleurum. 2. Medicine, Chinese Traditional. 3. Medicine, Kampo. 4. Phytotherapy. 5.
Plant Preparations--therapeutic use. 6. Saponins--pharmacology. QV 766 B944 2006] I. Pan, Sheng-Li. II.
Series.

RM666.B855B87 2006
615'.321--dc22   2005035151

**Visit the Taylor & Francis Web site at
http://www.taylorandfrancis.com**

**and the CRC Press Web site at
http://www.crcpress.com**

Series Preface

Global warming and global travel are among the factors resulting in the spread of such infectious diseases as malaria, tuberculosis, hepatitis B, and HIV. All these are not well controlled by the present drug regimes. Antibiotics, too, are failing because of bacterial resistance. Formerly less well-known tropical diseases are reaching new shores. A whole range of illnesses, for example cancer, occurs worldwide. Advances in molecular biology, including methods of *in vitro* testing for a required medical activity, give new opportunities to draw judiciously upon the use and research of traditional herbal remedies from around the world. The re-examining of the herbal medicines must be done in a multidisciplinary manner.

Since 1997, 42 volumes have been published in the book series Medicinal and Aromatic Plants — Industrial Profiles. The series continues and is characterised by a single plant genus per volume. With the same series editor, this new series, Traditional Herbal Medicines for Modern Times, covers multiple genera per volume. It accommodates, for example, the traditional Chinese medicines (TCM), the Japanese Kampo versions of this, and the Ayurvedic formulations of India. Collections of plants are also brought together because they have been re-evaluated for the treatment of specific diseases such as malaria and diabetes. Yet other collections are of the most recent investigations of the endemic medicinal plants of a particular country, e.g., India, South Africa, Mexico, Brazil (with its vast flora), and Malaysia with its rainforests, said to be the oldest in the world.

Each volume reports on the latest developments and discusses key topics relevant to interdisciplinary health science research by ethnobiologists, taxonomists, conservationists, agronomists, chemists, pharmacologists, clinicians, and toxicologists. The series is relevant to all these scientists and will enable them to guide business, government agencies, and commerce in the complexities of these matters. The background to the subject is outlined below.

Over many centuries, the safety and limitations of herbal medicines have been established by their empirical use by the "healers" who also took a holistic approach. The healers are aware of the infrequent adverse effects and know how to correct these when they occur. Consequently and ideally, the pre-clinical and clinical studies of a herbal medicine need to be carried out with the full cooperation of the traditional healer. The plant composition of the medicine, the stage of the development of the plant material, when it is to be collected from the wild or when from cultivation, its post-harvest treatment, the preparation of the medicine, the dosage and frequency, and much other essential information are required. A consideration of the intellectual property rights and appropriate models of benefit sharing may also be necessary.

Wherever the medicine is being prepared, the first requirement is a well-documented reference collection of dried plant material. Such collections are encouraged by organisations like the World Health Organisation and the United Nations Industrial Development Organisation. The Royal Botanic Gardens at Kew in the UK is building up its collection of traditional Chinese dried plant material relevant to its purchase and use by those who sell or prescribe TCM in the United Kingdom.

In any country, the control of the quality of plant raw material, of its efficacy, and of its safety in use is essential. The work requires sophisticated laboratory equipment and highly trained personnel. This kind of "control" cannot be applied to the locally produced herbal medicines in the rural areas of many countries, on which millions of people depend. Local traditional knowledge of the "healers" has to suffice.

Conservation and protection of plant habitats are required and breeding for biological diversity is important. Gene systems are being studied for medicinal exploitation. There can never be too many seed conservation "banks" to conserve genetic diversity. Unfortunately, such banks are usually dominated by agricultural and horticultural crops with little space for medicinal plants. Developments such as random amplified polymorphic DNA enable the genetic variability of a species to be checked. This can be helpful in deciding whether specimens of close genetic similarity warrant storage.

From ancient times, a great deal of information concerning diagnosis and the use of traditional herbal medicines has been documented in the scripts of China, India, and elsewhere. Today, modern formulations of these medicines exist in the form of, e.g., powders, granules, capsules, and tablets. They are prepared in various institutions, e.g., government hospitals in China and Korea, and by companies such as Tsumura Co. of Japan, with good quality control. Similarly, products are produced by many other companies in India, the USA, and elsewhere with a varying degree of quality control. In the USA, the Dietary Supplement and Health Education Act of 1994 recognised the class of physiotherapeutic agents derived from medicinal and aromatic plants. Furthermore, under public pressure, the USA Congress set up an Office of Alternative Medicine, and this office in 1994 assisted in the filing of several Investigational New Drug (IND) applications, required for clinical trials of some Chinese herbal preparations. The significance of these applications was that each Chinese preparation involved several plants and yet was handled as a *single* IND. A demonstration of the contribution to efficacy, of *each* ingredient of *each* plant, was not required. This was a major step forward towards more sensible regulations with regard to phytomedicines.

Something on the subject of Western herbal medicines is now being taught again to medical students in Germany and Canada. Throughout Europe, the USA, Australia, and other countries, pharmacy and health-related schools are increasingly offering training in phytotherapy. TCM clinics are now common outside of China. An Ayurvedic hospital now exists in London with a B.Sc.Hons. degree course in Ayurveda available: Prof. Dr. Shrikala Warrier, Resistrar/Dean, MAYUR, The Ayurvedic University of Europe, 81 Wimpole Street, London, WIG 9RF, Tel +44207 224 6070, e-mail sw@unifiedherbal.com. This is a joint venture with a university in Manipal, India.

The term "integrated medicine" is now being used, which selectively combines traditional herbal medicine with "modern medicine." In Germany there is now a hospital in which TCM is integrated with Western medicine. Such co-medication has become common in China, Japan, India, and North America by those educated in both systems. Benefits claimed include improved efficacy, reduction in toxicity and the period of medication, as well as a reduction in the cost of the treatment. New terms such as adjunct therapy, supportive therapy, and supplementary medicine now appear as a consequence of such co-medication. Either medicine may be described as an adjunct to the other depending on the communicator's view.

Great caution is necessary when traditional herbal medicines are used by doctors not trained in their use, and likewise when modern medicines are used by traditional herbal doctors. Possible dangers from drug interactions need to be stressed.

Dr. Roland Hardman, B.Pharm., B.Sc., Ph.D., F.R.Pharm.S.
Reader and Head of Pharmacognosy (Retired)
University of Bath, United Kingdom

Preface

The editor and a number of the chapter contributors are affiliated with Fudan University, founded in Shanghai in 1905. This book is one of its centennial publications.

The Japanese equivalent of Traditional Chinese Medicine (TCM), which arrived in Japan from China in the 16th century, is known as Kampo medicine. Typically, these traditional medicines contain three to six different dried plant materials derived from different species of plants in the prescription. These are dispensed as individually weighed-out crude, dried drugs, which are put together into one package sufficient for the doses for a single day's treatment and as many such lots as are prescribed by the medical practitioner. The patient would then boil one lot with water for a defined time and, after straining the liquid from the plant material, would divide the decoction into portions, i.e., doses, taking one of these once, twice, or three times a day as recommended in the treatment. This procedure is still followed by many patients in rural and other areas.

Today, modern formulations such as dripping pills, granules, or powders are available from large-scale quality-controlled production. These provide a single oral dose with boiling water (like making instant coffee) and are available for patients attending some hospitals and for those able to afford privately such convenient medication.

Examples of companies producing such modern formulations in China are Shanghai No. 1 TCM Factory (products: Chaihu Injection, Chaihu Oral Liquid, etc.), Tasly Group (products: Bupleuri Dripping Pill etc.), Xiamen TCM Co. (products: Xiaoyao-Wan, Buzhong-Yiqi-Wan, etc.), and more than 100 other factories. In Japan, Tsumura & Co. is a notable manufacturer.

Today, at least 66% of *all* the formulations/prescriptions of TCM and Kampo contain *Bupleurum* spp., usually in the form of the dried root. The *Bupleurum* spp. used in China and Japan are different: the Chinese root may be from *B. chinense* DC. or *B. scorzonerifolium* Willd., whereas in Japan *B. falcatum* L. is used. Furthermore, the aerial parts of some Chinese species, e.g., *B. polyclonum* Y. Li et S.L. Pan, *B. scorzonerifolium* Willd. f. *pauciflorum* Shan et Y. Li, *B. marginatum* Wall. ex DC. var. *stenophyllum* Shan et Y. Li, and 16 other species, or their essential oils, are used in Chinese formulations but not in Japanese formulations.

In this volume, the important *Bupleurum* spp. are covered: their botany, including detailed descriptions of the plant parts used in medicine; their constituents; quality control; pharmacology; and clinical usage with named/defined polyherbal formulations. This book will appeal to botanists, pharmacognosists, phytochemists, pharmacologists, pharmacists, clinicians, and other health care professionals.

Medicinal *Bupleurum* spp. and the plant parts are listed in the pharmacopoeias of China and Japan. Because of their medicinal properties, these plant parts are important to a wider clinical audience and are freely available in the U.S. in the form of "dietary supplements" under Dietary Supplement Health & Education Act (DSHEA) legislation, and similarly in other countries.

The demand for the root of the official *B. falcatum* in Japan is so great that it is now contract-grown in Korea. In Japan in 2002, the gross proceeds of manufactured prescription medicines containing this root amounted to 27 billion yen, which was 26% of the total sales of Kampo clinical medicines covered under Japan's health insurance payment scheme.

The worldwide distributions of *Bupleurum* spp. are discussed. For example, in China 44 species are found, 17 varieties, and 7 forms; in Spain, 23 species; and Italy, 15 species.

Medicinally, the saikosaponins of the oleanane series are very important. They are comprehensively dealt with — for instance, there are 113, in 5 different chemical classes, in 23 *Bupleurum* spp. found in China. The structural transformation of saikosaponins in gastric juice and in the intestinal contents is described.

The 222 different constituents of essential oils are tabulated from 19 *Bupleurum* spp. and 2 varieties with their geographical distributions. Other constituents described in detail are lignans, flavonoides, coumarins, polyacetylenes, phenyl propanides, and polysaccharides (these with anti-ulcer, antitumor, and immunomodulating properties).

In Spain, 7 *Bupleurum* spp. have received detailed study, notably yielding 20 new lignans (some with activity against the potato cyst nematode) in addition to all the usual constituents. *Bupleurum salicifolium* has demonstrated activity against *Staphylococcus aureus* ATCC 6538. The constituents and biological activities of Italian species have been similarly reported.

My thanks go to all the contributors for their work, especially Dr. Roland Hardman for his enthusiastic and continuous support throughout the preparation of this book.

Professor Sheng-Li Pan

The Editor

Sheng-Li Pan is a professor in the Department of Pharmacognosy, School of Pharmacy, Fudan University, Shanghai, People's Republic of China. He studies aspects of Traditional Chinese Medicine (TCM), including identification of components, chemical constituents, pharmacological effects, and mechanism of action. He has discovered and published six new species in the genus *Bupleurum*. He received the Academic Award from Shanghai Health Bureau in 1985, the Academic Award from Chinese TCM Ministry in 1996, and the Advanced Award on Science and Technology from the Scientific and Technical Ministry of China in 1997.

The Contributors

Byung-Zun Ahn
College of Pharmacy
Chungnam National University
Taejon, Republic of Korea

Pilar Arteaga
Departamento de Química Orgánica
Facultad de Ciencias
Universidad de Granada
Campus de Fuentenueva
Granada, Spain

Alejandro F. Barrero
Departamento de Química Orgánica
Facultad de Ciencias
Universidad de Granada
Campus de Fuentenueva
Granada, Spain

Hae-Gon Chung
Division of Industrial Crop
National Crop Experiment Station
Kwonsunku Seodun-dong Suwon,
  Republic of Korea

Xiao-Min Du
Pharmaceutical Industrial Institute of Shandong
Jinan, People's Republic of China

M. Mar Herrador
Departamento de Química Orgánica
Facultad de Ciencias
Universidad de Granada
Campus de Fuentenueva
Granada, Spain

Osamu Iida
Tsukuba Medicinal Plant Research Station
National Institute of Health Sciences
Ibaraki, Japan

Yun Kang
School of Pharmacy
Fudan University
Shanghai, People's Republic of China

Kwan-Su Kim
Department of Medicinal Plant Resources
School of Biotechnology & Resources
Mokpo National University
Muan, Republic of Korea

Eiji Miki
Kampo and Pharmacognosy Laboratory
Tsumura & Co.
Ibaraki, Japan

Naohito Ohno
Laboratory for Immunopharmacology of
  Microbial Products
School of Pharmacy
Tokyo University of Pharmacy and
  Life Science
Tokyo, Japan

Shigeki Ohta
Science and Art Section
Shinwa Pharmaceutical Co. Ltd.
Tokyo, Japan

Sheng-Li Pan
School of Pharmacy
Fudan University
Shanghai, People's Republic of China

Luisa Pistelli
Dipartimento di Chimica Bioorganica e
  Biofarmacia
Università di Pisa
Pisa, Italy

José F. Quílez
Departamento de Química Orgánica
Facultad de Ciencias
Universidad de Granada
Campus de Fuentenueva
Granada, Spain

Shuhei Sakaguchi
First Department of Hygienic Chemistry
Tohoku Pharmaceutical University
Sendai, Japan

Nak-Sul Seong
Division of Industrial Crop
National Crop Experiment Station
Kwonsunku Seodun-dong Suwon,
  Republic of Korea

Ichiro Shimizu
Department of Digestive and Cardiovascular
  Medicine
Tokushima University School of Medicine
Tokushima, Japan

Dai-Eun Sok
College of Pharmacy
Chungnam National University
Taejon, Republic of Korea

Jun Wang
School of Pharmacy
Fudan University
Shanghai, People's Republic of China

Hui Xie
School of Pharmacy
Fudan University
Shanghai, People's Republic of China

Toshiro Yadomae
Laboratory for Immunopharmacology of
  Microbial Products
School of Pharmacy
Tokyo University of Pharmacy and Life Science
Tokyo, Japan

Bai-Can Yang
Shanghai University of Traditional Chinese
  Medicine
Shanghai, People's Republic of China

Chang-Qi Yuan
Botanical Institute of Jiangsu Province and
  Chinese Academy of Science
Nanjing, China

You-Chang Zhu
Heilongjiang Institute of Natural Resources
  Research
Harbin, China

Contents

SECTION IV   Pharmacology

SECTION V   Clinical Application

SECTION VI   Patents

1 Introduction

Sheng-Li Pan

Bupleurum is a genus of family Umbelliferae (Apiaceae), comprising about 200 species and primarily located in the Northern Hemisphere, Eurasia, and North Africa. The anatomy of the more important species and their geographical distribution are given in Chapters 2 and 3. The chromosomes are considered in relation to classification and cross-breeding in Chapter 4.

Under the name of Chaihu (Saiko in Japanese and Shiho in Korean), the roots of several species from the genus have been frequently used in the prescriptions of Oriental traditional medicine for the treatment of common cold with fever, influenza, inflammation, hepatitis, malaria, and also menopausal syndrome in China for 2000 years. Chaihu was first recorded in *Shen-Nong's Herbal*, a pharmaceutical book published 2000 years ago in China. In it, Chaihu was described as the best medicine to treat diseases with fever. In 1058 A.D., an atlas of materia medica, *Bencao Tu-jing*, was published, which contained five illustrations of Chaihu (Figure 1.1): Zizhou Chaihu, Danzhou Chaihu, Shouzhou Chaihu, Jiangningfu Chaihu, and Xiangzhou Chaihu. According to the figures and descriptions, four (Zizhou Chaihu, Danzhou Chaihu, Jiangningfu Chaihu, and Xiangzhou Chaihu) belong to the *Bupleurum* genus.

The requirement of *Bupleurum* radix for prescriptions and exports is about 8 million kg every year in China. This is met chiefly from wild plants, but nowadays *B. falcatum* and *B. chinense* are extensively cultivated in China, Japan, Korea, and in some regions of Europe (Figure 1.2 and Figure 1.3). In some districts of China (especially in Yunnan Province), other species, *B. polyclonum, B. marginatum* var. *stenophyllum, B. rockii*, are also cultivated (Figure 1.4). Their seasonal variations in growth and content of saikosaponins are reported in Chapters 5 and 6.

About 50 species from the genus (e.g., *B. falcatum, B. chinense, B. fruticosum, B. salicifolium, B. scorzonerifolium, B. gibraltaricum, B. polyclonum, B. marginatum* var. *stenophyllum, B. kunmingense,* etc.) have been studied chemically (Chapters 7, 8, and 9) resulting in the isolation of approximately 120 derivatives of saikosaponins, more than 50 lignans, as well as a number of

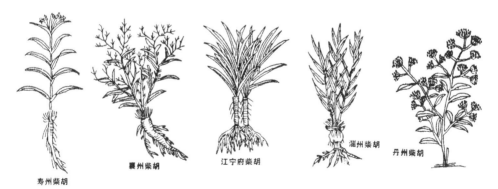

寿州柴胡   襄州柴胡   江宁府柴胡   淄州柴胡   丹州柴胡

FIGURE 1.1 Five illustrations of Chaihu in *Bencao Tu-jing,* left to right: Zizhou Chaihu; Danzhou Chaihu; Jiangningfu Chaihu; Xiangzhou Chaihu; Shouzhou Chaihu.

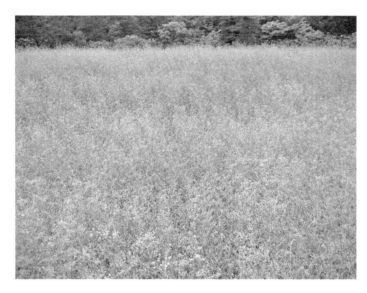

FIGURE 1.2 *Bupleurum chinense* DC. cultivated in Gansu Province of China.

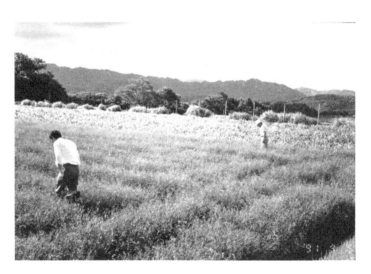

FIGURE 1.3 *Bupleurum falcatum* L. cultivated in Nagasaki, Japan.

coumarins, flavonoids, polyacetylenes, polysaccharides, sterols, phenylpropanoids, and organic acids. Moreover, the essential oils of genus *Bupleurum* have been investigated, and more than 220 compounds in these essential oils have been identified.

Saikosaponins, the principal ingredients from *Bupleurum* root, exhibit the pharmacological activity (Chapters 10, 11, and 12): anti-inflammatory, antivirus, hepatoprotective, antipyretic, anodynic, sedative, antidepressive, and anticancer. The aglycones of the chief saikosaponins (i.e., saikosaponin-a, -c, and -d) are 13β, 28-epoxyolean-11-ene-16-ol. The content of saikosaponin-a, -c, and -d in most species is 1 to 2%, but in *B. polyclonum,* it is up to 7% (Pan et al., 2000a, 2000b).

Numerous lignans are described from *B. salicifolium* (an endemic species in the Canary Islands of Spain). Some lignans (e.g., actigenin, trachelogenin) show the inhibitory effect of topo-isomerase II, an enzyme associated with the replication of HIV-1 virus responsible for AIDS (Eich et al., 1990). Bursehenin and matairesinol from the same plant inhibit the hatching of the nematodes

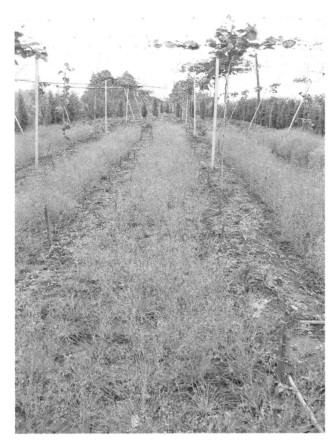

FIGURE 1.4 *Bupleurum polyclonum* Y. Li et S.L. Pan cultivated in Yunnan Province of China.

Globodera pallida and *G. rostochiensis* (Gonzalez et al., 1994). Both compounds are the first natural products known to affect the hatching of *G. pallida* and the first lignans ever reported to have an effect on a phytoparasitic nematode. The essential oils of *B. chinense, B. fruticosum,* and *B. gibraltaricum,* etc. demonstrate marked anti-inflammatory effects. The polysaccharides of *B. falcatum, B. chinense,* and *B. kunmingense* possess immunomodulatory activity, and their antiulcer and B-cell proliferation activities have also been reported (see Chapter 12).

Prescriptions and their clinical applications (Chapters 10, 11, and 12), including Chaihu Oral Liquid (containing small amounts of saikosaponins and essential oils of Bupleuri radix) and Chaihu Injection (distillate of Bupleuri radix), are used for the treatment of influenza and common cold in China. Xiao-Chaihu-Tang (Sho-Saiko-To in Japanese), an extract made from *Bupleurum* root, *Pinellia* tuber, *Scutellaria* root, jujube fruit, ginseng root, *Glycyrrhiza* root, and ginger rhizome, is widely used for the treatment of chronic disease, such as hepatitis, asthma, nephrotic syndrome, and cancer. Other prescriptions containing Bupleurum radix, such as Da-Chaihu-Tang (Dai-Saiko-To in Japanese), Chaihu-Guizhi-Tang (Saiko-Keishi-To in Japanese), are also extensively used in China and Japan. They can induce an increase in the levels of tumor necrosis factor-alpha (Yamashiki et al., 1994), stimulate natural killer cell–mediated cytotoxic activity (Kaneko et al., 1994), and enhance immunomodulation.

To date, the published patents containing *Bupleurum* number more than 500 (Chapter 16).

REFERENCES

Eich, E., Schulz, J., Trumm, S., Sarin, P.S., Maidhof, A., Merz, H., Schroder, H.C., and Miller, W.E.G. (1990) Lignanolides: novel *in vitro* anti-HIV active agents, *Planta Med.*, 56, 506.

Gonzalez, J.A., Estevez-Braun, A., Estevez-Reyes, R., and Ravelo, A.G. (1994) Inhibition of potato cyst nematode hatch by lignans from *Bupleurum salicifolium* (Umbelliferae), *J. Chem. Ecol.*, 20, 517–524.

Kaneko, M., Kawakita, T., Tauchi, Y., Saito, Y., Suzuki, A., and Nomoto, K. (1994) Augmentation of NK activity after oral administration of a traditional Chinese medicine, Xiao-Chaihu-Tang (Sho-Saiko-To). *Immunopharmacol. Immunotoxicol.*, 16, 41–53.

Pan, S.L., Wang, Z.H., Hong, X.K., Lin, D.H., Mao, R.G., and Ohashi, H. (2000a) Determination on saiko-saponin-a, -c and -d in 23 species of *Bupleurum* by HPLC, *J. Jpn. Med. Bot.*, 23, 35–39.

Pan, S.L., Wang, Z.H., Hong, X.K., Lin, D.H., Mao, R.G., and Ohashi, H. (2000b) Determination on saiko-saponin-a, -c and -d by HPLC in *Bupleurum* from different districts of China, *J. Jpn. Med. Bot.*, 23, 40–44.

Yamashiki, M., Nishimura, A., Nomoto, M., Nakano, T., Sato, T., Suzuki, H., Zheng, Q.X., Klapproth, J.M., James, S.P., and Kosaka, Y. (1994) Effects of Japanese herbal medicine "Sho-Saiko-To" on *in vitro* production of tumor necrosis factor-alpha on peripheral blood mononuclear cells, *Drug Dev. Res.*, 31, 170–174.

Section I

Botany

2 Macroscopical Characters of the Medicinal Species of *Bupleurum* and Their Distribution in China

Sheng-Li Pan and Yun Kang

CONTENTS

2.1 INTRODUCTION

Bupleurum genus, which was named by Linnaeus in 1735, belongs to Umbelliferae, Apioideae, Ammineae. Approximately 200 species occur in the world (Su et al., 1998), primarily located in the Northern Hemisphere, Eurasia, and North Africa. In China, 44 species, 17 varieties, and 7 forms have been reported (Li and She, 1979; Pan et al., 2002). Under the name Chaihu (Saiko in Japanese), the roots of several species from *Bupleurum* genus frequently occurred in the prescriptions of Oriental Traditional Medicine. They have been utilized to treat common cold with fever, influenza, hepatitis, malaria, and menoxenia for more than 2000 years. The *Pharmacopoeia of the People's Republic of China* (2000) states that *B. chinense* DC. and *B. scorzonerifolium* Willd. were officially regarded as the standard medical plants. But according to the investigations in all provinces of China, it has been discovered that there were many more species used as medicine in different districts and markets (Song, 1981; Li, 1989; Li et al., 1993; Pan, 1996; Pan and Ohashi, 1996).

2.2 CHARACTERISTICS OF *BUPLEURUM* GENUS

2.2.1 GENERAL DESCRIPTION

A perennial rarely annual or biennial, glabrous, often rather glaucous herb, with a stout, woody stock. Stems solid or hollow, striate. Leaves simple, alternate, entire, with parallel veins, sometimes with cartilaginous margin. Basal leaves petiolated, cauline leaves amplexcaule at base. Compound umbel loose. Bracts leaf-like, 1 to 5, unequal. Bracteoles 3 to 10, linear, lanceolate, ovate, obovate, or orbicular; green, yellow, or purplish. Flowers bisexual; calyx teeth absent; petals 5, yellow, rarely purplish; stamens 5, yellow; stylopodium broadly conical. Cremocarps oblong or ovate, slightly compressed laterally, mericarps subterete, somewhat prominently 5 ribbed.

2.2.2 MAIN MEDICINAL SPECIES OF *BUPLEURUM* IN CHINA

Distributions of the main medicinal species in China are detailed in Table 2.1, and the commercial samples in Table 2.2. The microscopical characters of the following species are given in Chapter 3.

2.2.2.1 *Bupleurum chinense* DC. (Figure 2.1)

A glabrous perennial with a stout, woody stock. Root straight or curved with 2 to 3 branch roots, gray to brown at surface. Stems up to 150 cm high, solid, striate. Leaves simple, the basal 5 to 10 cm long, 0.8 to 1.2 cm wide, oblanceolate or linear-elliptic, long petiolate, with 7 to 9 parallel veins, cauline oblanceolate to long elliptic-lanceolate, 5 to 16 cm long and 0.6 to 2.5 cm wide, acuminate to obtuse-acute at apex, long attenuate and semi-amplexicaule at base. Umbellules 5- to 12-flowered, 3 to 9 per umbel. Bracts 2 to 4, narrowly lanceolate, unequal, 1 to 5 mm long and 0.5 to 1 mm wide; bracteoles 5, lanceolate, 2.5 to 4 mm long, 0.5 to 1 mm wide. Fruit ellipsoid, 2.5 to 3.5 mm long, 1.5 to 2 mm wide. Vitta 3 at vallecula and 4 at commissure. This is the most common species growing in the north and middle of China.

TABLE 2.1
Distribution and Resources of Medicinal *Bupleurum* in China

Name	Distribution (Province of China)	Resources
B. chinense	Hebei Shanxi Shaanxi Gansu Heilongjiang Jilin Henan Shandong Hubei Jiangsu Jiangxi	++++
B. scorzonerifolium	Hebei, Shaanxi, Jiangsu, Henan, Liaoning Jilin, Heilongjiang, Neimenggu Zhejiang	++
B. scorzonerifolium f. pauciflorum	Anhui Jiangsu	++
B. smithii var. *parvifolium*	Neimenggu, Qinghai Gansu, Ningxia Shanxi, Shaanxi, Heilongjiang, Liaoning	++++
B. smithii	Hebei, Shanxi, Shaanxi, Gansu, Qinghai, Neimenggu	+
B. marginatum var. *stenophyllum*	Xizhang Yunnan Guizhou Sichuan, Gansu, Hubei, Hunan	++++
B. marginatum	Sichuan, Yunnan, Guizhou, Gansu, Shaanxi	+
B. yinchowense	Shaanxi, Ningxia, Gansu, Neimenggu	++
B. bicaule	Neimenggu, Ningxia, Liaoning, Heilongjiang	++
B. angustissimum	Hebei, Ningxia, Shaanxi, Gansu, Liaoning	++
B. polyclonum	Yunnan	++
B. kunmingense	Yunnan	+
B. luxiense	Yunnan	+
B. rockii	Yunnan, Sichuan, Xizhang	++
B. sibiricum	Hebei, Heilongjing, Liaoning, Neimenggu	+
B. sichuanense	Sichuan	+
B. wenchuanense	Sichuan	++
B. chaishoui	Sichuan	++
B. malconense	Sichuan	++
B. longiradiatum	Heilongjiang, Liaoning, Jilin, Shaanxi, Gansu, Zhejiang	++++
B. komarovianum	Jilin, Heilongjiang, Liaoning	+
B. euphorbioides	Jilin	+
B. krylovianum	Xinjiang	++
B. densiflorum	Xinjiang, Qinghai	+
B. exaltatum	Xinjiang	+
B. aureum	Xinjiang	+
B. commelynoideum var. *flaviflorum*	Gansu, Qinghai, Sichuan	++
B. hamiltonii	Yunnan, Guizhou, Sichuan, Xizhang, Hubei	+++
B. candollei	Yunnan, Sichuan	++
B. longicaule var. *franchetii*	Sichuan, Yunnan, Guizhou, Hubei	++
B. longicaule var. *giraldii*	Yunnan	+
B. petiolulatum var. *tenerum*	Yunnan, Sichuan, Xizhang	+

2.2.2.2 *Bupleurum scorzonerifolium* Willd. (Figure 2.2)

Perennial, 30 to 80 cm high. Root brown reddish at surface, with many brushlike fibers in the base of stem. Leaves lanceolate to linear-lanceolate 6 to 16 cm long, 3 to 8 mm wide. 5- to 7-veined. Umbellules 7- to 12-flowered, 4 to 10 per umbel. Bracts 2 to 4, narrowly lanceolate, unequal; bracteoles 5, linear-lanceolate, 3 to 4 mm long and 0.5 to 1 mm wide. Fruit ovoid, 2 to 3 mm long, 2 mm wide. Vitta 3 at vallecula and 4 at commissure.

2.2.2.2.1 *Bupleurum scorzonerifolium* Willd. f. *pauciflorum* Shan et Y. Li

Similar to *B. scorzonerifolium* Willd., from which it differs in that the rays of umbel are only 2 to 3, and the umbellules have 4 to 6 flowers. Distributed in Jiangsu and Anhui; 30- to 50-cm-high seedling used as Spring Chaihu.

TABLE 2.2
Identification of 110 Commercial Samples of Chaihu

Commodity Name	Markets (City or County in China)	Identification Result
	Qingan Shenyang Beijing Tianjin Shijiazhuang Chengde Zhanhuang Taiyuan Xi'an Lueyang Kangxian Luoyang Zhengzhou Wuhan Fuyang Yushan Gao'an Pingxiang Lin'an Shaoxing Ningbo Fuzhou Xiamen Quanzhou Liuzhou	*B. chinense* (root) (25 samples)
	Kangxian Wulian Huaibei Guilin Fuzhou	*B. chinense* (aerial part) (5)
	Shenyang Fuyang Yinchuan Ankang Xining Datong Guiling Shanghai	*B. smithii* var. *parvifolium* (root) (8)
	Fuyang Suzhou Fuzhou	*B. scorzonerifolium* (aerial part) (3)
Chaihu	Tianjin Xilinhaote Hulunbeier	*B. bicaule* (root) (3)
	Wuzhong Heshui Zhenning	*B. yinchowense* (root) (3)
	Wulumuqi Aertai	*B. krylovianum* (root) (2)
	Guangzhou Nanning	*B. marginatum* var. *stenophyllum* (root) (2)
	Xinglong	*B. sibiricum* (root) (1)
	Shanghai (from Gansu)	*B. angustissimum* (root) (1)
	Antu	*B. komarovianum* (root and rhizome) (1)
	Wulumuqi	*B. densiflorum* (root) (1)
	Huangzhong	*B. commelynoideum* var. *flaviflorum* (root) (1)
	Tianjin Jinhua	*B. scorzonerifolium* (root) (2)
Red Chaihu	Tongxin Lanzhou	*B. bicaule* (root) (2)
	Guyang	*B. angustissimum* (root) (1)
	Yuzhong	*B. yinchowense* (root) (1)
Bamboo-leaf Chaihu	Liuzhou Lipu Guiyang Chengdu Lezhi Dali Kunming Deqin, Mile Huize Xishuangbanna Dianbai	*B. marginatum* var. *stenophyllum* (aerial part) (12)
	Kunming Chuxiong Huize Lijiang	*B. hamiltonii* (aerial part) (4)
	Kunming Huize Wenshan	*B. polyclonum* (aerial part) (3)
	Kunming Lijiang	*B. rockii* (aerial part) (2)
	Luxi Jianshui	*B. luxiense* (aerial part) (2)
	Kunming Bijie	*B. longicaule* var. *franchetii* (aerial part) (2)
	Wenchuan Maoxian	*B. wenchuanense* (aerial part) (2)
	Wenchuan Maoxian	*B. malconense* (aerial part) (2)
	Kunming	*B. kunmingense* (aerial part) (1)
	Wenchuan	*B. sichuanense* (aerial part) (1)
	Wenchuan	*B. chaishoui* (aerial part) (1)
Black Chaihu	Yinchuan Tongxin Kangxian Tianshui Lanzhou Yuzhong Tianzhu Baotou	*B. smithii* var. *parvifolium* (root) (8)
Large-leaf Chaihu	Shangzhi Tonghua	*B. longiradiatum* (rhizome and root) (2)
Chaishou	Aba	*B. wenchuanense* (root) (1)
	Maerkang	*B. chaishoui* (root) (1)
Spring Chaihu	Chuzhou Fengyang Nanjing Xuzhou	*B. scorzonerifolium* f. *pauciflorum* (seedling) (4)

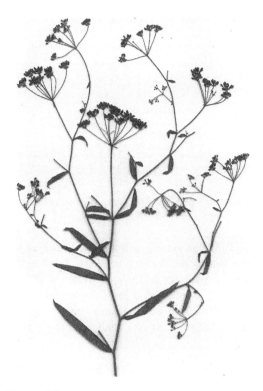

FIGURE 2.1 *Bupleurum chinense* DC.

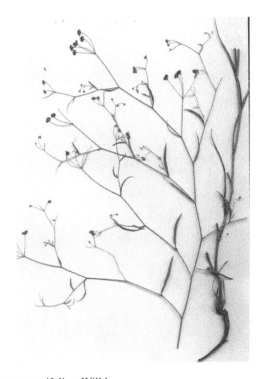

FIGURE 2.2 *Bupleurum scorzonerifolium* Willd.

2.2.2.3 *Bupleurum smithii* Wolff var. *parvifolium* Shan et Y. Li (Figure 2.3)

Perennial, 10 to 30 cm high. Root brown black at surface. Leaves elliptic or oblong-lanceolate, 4 to 11 cm long, 0.3 to 1 cm wide. Umbellules 10- to 18-flowered, 4 to 9 per umbel. Bracts 1 to 2 or 0; bracteoles 5 to 8, ovate, 3.5 to 8 mm long, 2.5 to 3.5 mm wide. Fruit ellipsoid, 2.5 to 3.5 mm long, 1.5 to 2 mm wide. Vitta 3 at vallecula and 4 at commissure.

A common species distributed in the north of China.

2.2.2.3.1 Bupleurum smithii Wolff

Similar to *B. smithii* Wolff var. *parvifolium* Shan et Y. Li, from which it differs in the leaves greater, 10 to 20 cm long, 1 to 2 cm wide.

2.2.2.4 *Bupleurum marginatum* Wall. ex DC. var. *stenophyllum* Shan et Y. Li (Figure 2.4)

Perennial, 60 to 100 cm high. Rhizome very long, sometimes reached 80 cm, and hardly differentiated from root. Leaves linear-lanceolate to oblanceolate, with whitish cartilaginous margin, 6 to 10 cm long, 3 to 5 mm wide. Umbellules 6- to 14-flowered, 4 to 7 per umbel. Bracts 3 to 5, lanceolate; bracteoles 5, lanceolate, 1 to 2.5 mm long, 0.4 to 0.6 mm wide. Fruit oblong, 2.5 to 3.5 mm long, 1.5 to 2 mm wide. Vitta 3 at vallecula and 4 at commissure.

A common species distributed in southern and southwestern China.

2.2.2.4.1 Bupleurum marginatum Wall. ex DC.

Similar to *B. marginatum* Wall. ex DC. var. *stenophyllum* Shan et Y. Li, from which it differs in that the leaves are wider.

2.2.2.5 *Bupleurum yenchowense* Shan et Y. Li

Perennial, 20 to 50 cm high. Main roots long and straight, grayish at surface. Leaves oblanceolate 5 to 8 cm long, 2 to 5 mm wide, acute at apex. Umbellules 6- to 12-flowered, 4 to 8 per umbel.

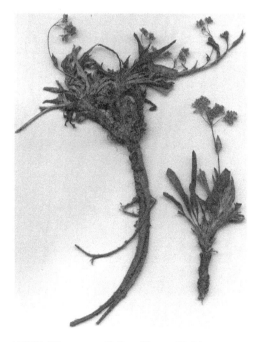

FIGURE 2.3 *Bupleurum smithii* Wolff var. *parvifolium* Shan et Y. Li.

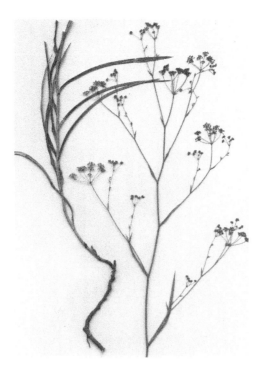

FIGURE 2.4 *Bupleurum marginatum* Wall. ex DC. var. *stenophyllum* Shan et Y. Li.

Bracts 1 to 3 or 0, narrowly lanceolate, unequal; bracteoles 5, linear, 1 to 2 mm long and 0.2 mm wide. Fruit ovoid, 2.5 to 3 mm long, 2 mm wide. Vitta 3 at vallecula and 4 at commissure.

2.2.2.6 *Bupleurum bicaule* Helm. (Figure 2.5)

Perennial, 5 to 20 cm high. Root with many brushlike fibers in the base of stem, and many obvious nodes at surface. Leaves linear, 6 to 16 cm long, 1 to 3 mm wide, 3- to 5-veined, upper cauline tapered, 1 to 4 cm long, 0.5 to 2.5 mm wide, 5- to 7-veined. Umbellules 7- to 13-flowered, 4 to 7 per umbel. Bracts 1 to 3; unequal, bracteoles 5, linear-lanceolate, 2 to 2.5 mm long and 0.6 to 0.8 mm wide. Fruit ellipsoid, 2.5 to 3 mm long, 1.5 to 2 mm wide. Vitta 3 at vallecula and 3 to 4 at commissure.

2.2.2.7 *Bupleurum angustissimum* (Franch.) Kitagawa

Perennial, 15 to 80 cm high. Root with many brushlike fibers in the base of stem. Leaves linear, 6 to 18 cm long, 0.8 to 1 mm wide. Umbellules 6- to 12-flowered, 5 to 7 per umbel. Bracts 1 to 3, lanceolate, 1 to 3 mm long, 1 mm wide; bracteoles 5, lanceolate, 2 to 2.5 mm long and 0.6 to 0.8 mm wide. Fruit ovoid, 2 mm long, 1 to 1.5 mm wide. Vitta 3 at vallecula and 4 at commissure.

2.2.2.8 *Bupleurum polyclonum* Y. Li et S.L. Pan (Figure 2.6) (Pan et al., 1984)

Perennial, 15 to 60 cm high. Root soft, grayish at surface. Stem with many branchlets. Leaves basal and lower cauline linear, 10 to 20 cm long, 2 to 3 mm wide; 3- to 7-veined, upper cauline tapered. Umbellules 7- to 15-flowered, 3 to 7 per umbel. Bracts 4 to 5, unequal, elliptic to obovate; 2 to 8 mm long, 1.5 to 3 mm wide, semi-amplexicaule; bracteoles 5, obovate, 3 to 4 mm long, 2 to 3 mm wide. Fruit oblong, 2 to 3 mm long, 1.2 to 1.8 mm wide. Vitta 3 at vallecula and 4 at commissure.

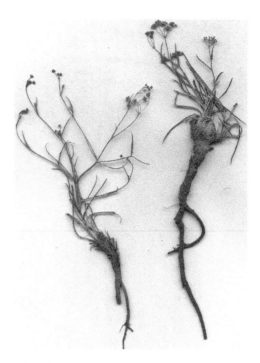

FIGURE 2.5 *Bupleurum bicaule* Helm.

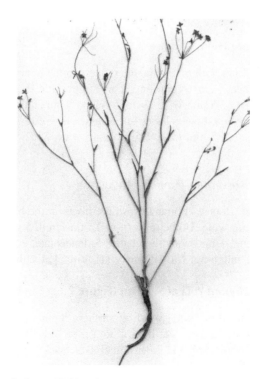

FIGURE 2.6 *Bupleurum polyclonum* Y. Li et S.L. Pan.

This is a new species that author Pan discovered in Yunnan Province and published in 1984. Its content of saikosaponin-a, -c, and -d reaches 6 to 7% — the highest content in the genus (Pan et al., 2000a, 2000b).

2.2.2.9   *Bupleurum kunmingense* Y. Li et S.L. Pan (Figure 2.7) (Li et al., 1984)

Perennial, 60 to 100 cm high. Root with long rhizome, dark brown at surface. Leaves linear or lanceolate, papery, basal linear 10 to 15 cm long, 3 to 5 mm wide; cauline lanceolate to narrowly lanceolate, 0.8 to 10 cm long, 1.5 to 5 mm wide, 3- to 5-veined. Umbellules 8- to 14-flowered, 4 to 11 per umbel. Bracts 5 to 8, unequal, narrowly elliptic; bracteoles 5, obovate, 2.5 to 3.5 mm long, 1 to 2 mm wide. Fruit oblong, 2 to 3 mm long, 2 mm wide. Vitta 3 at vallecula and 4 at commissure.

2.2.2.10   *Bupleurum luxiense* Y. Li et S.L. Pan (Li et al., 1986)

Perennial, 55 to 125 cm high. Root hard, short, and dark brown at surface. Leaves lanceolate, 10 to 20 cm long, 1.5 to 3 cm wide, leathery. Umbellules 7- to 12-flowered, 4 to 9 per umbel. Bracts 5, unequal, obovate, 4 to 7 mm long, 3 to 4 mm wide; bracteoles 5, obovate, 4 to 6 mm long, 2 to 3 mm wide. Fruit oblong, 2 to 3.5 mm long, 1 to 2 mm wide. Vitta 3 at vallecula and 4 at commissure.

2.2.2.11   *Bupleurum rockii* Wolff (Figure 2.8)

Perennial, 40 to 60 cm high. Rhizome straight, brown black at surface. Leaves basal oblong, 8 to 12 cm long, 1 to 1.2 cm wide; cauline ovate to elliptic, amplexicaule at base, 2 to 7 cm long, 1.2 to 2 cm wide, sometimes with broad reddish margin, 9- to 19-veined. Umbellules 11- to 14-flowered,

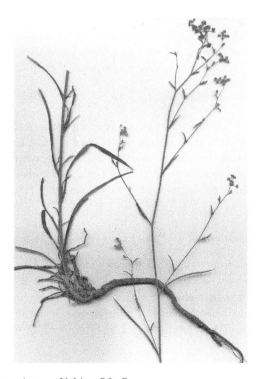

FIGURE 2.7 *Bupleurum kunmingense* Y. Li et S.L. Pan.

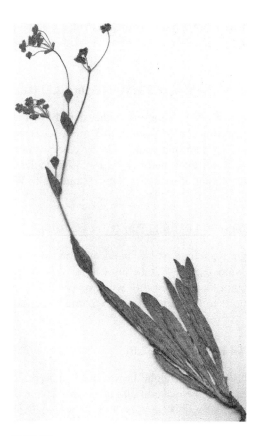

FIGURE 2.8 *Bupleurum rockii* Wollf.

6 to 10 per umbel. Bracts 1 to 3, unequal, broadly ovate, 6 to 20 mm long, 5 to 12 mm wide; 9- to 15-veined, bracteoles 5 to 6, obovate, 4 to 5 mm long, 3 to 4 mm wide, 5- to 7-veined. Fruit ovoid, 3 to 4 mm long, 2 to 2.5 mm wide. Vitta 3 at vallecula and 4 at commissure.

2.2.2.12   *Bupleurum sibiricum* Vest (Figure 2.9)

Perennial, 30 to 80 cm high. Root straight, brown to gray at surface. Leaves basal linear-lanceolate 10 to 25 cm long, 0.5 to 1.5 cm wide, attenuate to petiolate at base; cauline narrowly lanceolate, 5 to 12 cm long, 0.6 to 1 cm wide, acuminate to obtuse-acute at apex, attenuate at base. Umbellules 10- to 22-flowered, 5 to 14 per umbel. Bracts 1 to 2, unequal; bracteoles 7 to 12, elliptic-lanceolate, 5 to 7 mm long, 1.5 to 3 mm wide. Fruit ovoid, 3 to 3.5 mm long, 1.5 to 2.5 mm wide. Vitta 3 at vallecula and 4 at commissure.

2.2.2.13   *Bupleurum sichuanense* S.L. Pan et Hsu (Pan and Hsu, 1992)

Perennial, 40 to 100 cm high. Root straight, dark brown at surface. Leaves basal and lower cauline linear, 5 to 10 cm long, 1 to 5 mm wide; 7-veined, middle and upper cauline linear, 2 to 8 cm long, 2 to 5 mm wide, 5- to 7-veined, acuminate at apex, cuneate at base. Umbellules 5- to 11-flowered, 4 to 8 per umbel. Bracts 1 to 3, linear, unequal; bracteoles 5, lanceolate, 1 to 2 mm long, 0.2 to 0.8 mm wide. Fruit ellipsoid, 2 to 3 mm long, 1.2 to 1.5 mm wide. Vitta 3 at vallecula and 4 at commissure.

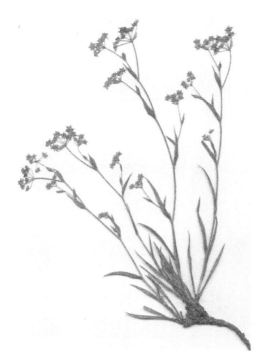

FIGURE 2.9 *Bupleurum sibiricum* Vest.

2.2.2.14   *Bupleurum wenchuanense* Shan et Y. Li (Figure 2.10)

Perennial, 40 to 90 cm high. Root with 2 to 3 branch roots, sometimes swell at the middle of taproot. Stem with many branchlets. Leaves basal linear, 5 to 12 cm long, 2 to 4 mm wide; 3- to 5-veined, lower cauline linear 1.5 to 3 cm long, 1.5 to 2.5 mm wide; middle and upper cauline tapered. Umbellules 1- to 4-flowered, 2 to 3 per umbel. Bracts 2 to 3, tapered; bracteoles 5 to 6, obovate, 0.6 to 1 mm long, 0.3 to 0.5 mm wide, 3-veined. Fruit ovoid, 2 mm long, 1.5 mm wide. Vitta 2 to 3 at vallecula and 3 to 4 at commissure.

2.2.2.15   *Bupleurum chaishoui* Shan et Sheh

Perennial, 80 to 120 cm high. Root dark brown at surface, with several fingerlike branches at the top. Leaves elliptic-lanceolate to oblong-elliptic, sometimes with different size in the near nodes, always reflexed, 1.5 to 9 cm long, 0.3 to 1.2 cm wide. Umbellules 6- to 12-flowered, 4 to 6 per umbel. Bracts 2 to 4, linear, unequal; bracteoles 5, lanceolate to obovate, 1.2 to 2.8 mm long, 0.5 to 0.8 mm wide. Fruit ellipsoid, 3 to 3.5 mm long, 2 mm wide. Vitta 3 at vallecula and 4 at commissure.

2.2.2.16   *Bupleurum malconense* Shan et Y. Li

Perennial, 40 to 80 cm high. Root dark brown at surface. Leaves linear, 4 to 15 cm long, 2.5 to 5 mm wide, 5- to 7-veined. Bracts 2 to 3, linear; bracteoles 5, lanceolate, 2 to 2.5 mm long, 0.5 to 0.8 mm wide. Fruit ellipsoid, 2.5 to 3 mm long, 1.5 to 1.8 mm wide. Vitta 3 at vallecula and 4 at commissure.

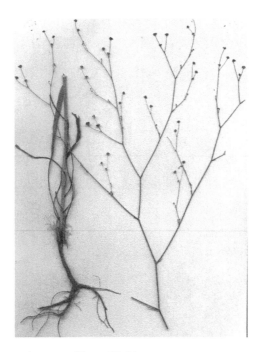

FIGURE 2.10 *Bupleurum wenchuanense* Shan et Y. Li.

2.2.2.17 *Bupleurum longiradiatum* Turcz. (Figure 2.11)

Perennial, 80 to 160 cm high, with short creeping rhizome. Main roots not obvious. Leaves large, 8 to 17 cm long, 2.5 to 6 cm wide, auriculately amplexicaul at base. Umbellules 5- to 16-flowered, 3 to 9 per umbel. Bracts 3 to 5, unequal, lanceolate 2 to 8 mm long, 1 to 1.5 mm wide; bracteoles 5 to 6, lanceolate-obovate, 2 to 5 mm long, 1 to 2 mm wide. Fruit oblong-ellipsoid, 3 to 6 mm long, 2 to 2.5 mm wide. Vitta 3 to 4 at vallecula and 4 to 6 at commissure.

The roots and rhizomes contained toxic constituents — bupleurotoxin and acetyl-bupleurotoxin (Zhao et al., 1987).

2.2.2.18 *Bupleurum komarovianum* Lincz.

Perennial, 70 to 140 cm high. Main roots not obvious. Leaves large, 15 to 20 cm long, 2 to 3 cm wide, 7- to 9-veined, cuneate at base. Umbellules 6- to 20 flowered, 4 to 9 per umbel. Bracts 1 to 3, unequal, lanceolate to linear, 1 to 4 mm long, 0.5 to 2 mm wide; bracteoles 5, narrowly lanceolate, 2 to 3 mm long, 0.5 to 1 mm wide. Fruit ovoid, 2.5 to 3.5 mm long, 1.5 to 2 mm wide. Vitta 4 to 5 at vallecula and 6 to 8 at commissure.

2.2.2.19 *Bupleurum euphorbioides* Nakai (Figure 2.12)

Annual to biennial, 10 to 60 cm high. Roots slender. Leaves basal linear, 7 to 15 cm long, 1 to 3 cm wide, attenuate to petiolate at base; lower cauline narrowly lanceolate to linear, upper cauline broadly lanceolate to ovate, 2.5 to 9 cm long, 0.8 to 1.5 mm wide, long acuminate at apex, cordate-amplexicaule at base. Umbellules 16- to 24-flowered, 4 to 12 per umbel. Bracts 2 to 5, unequal; bracteoles 5 to 7, elliptic to obvate, 4 to 9 mm long, 2 to 5 mm wide. Fruit ovoid, 3 to 3.5 mm long, 2 to 2.5 mm wide. Vitta 3 at vallecula and 4 at commissure.

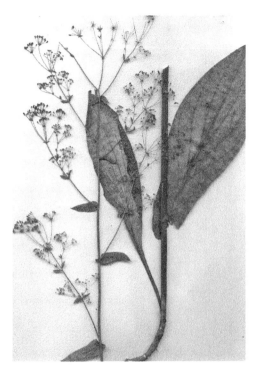

FIGURE 2.11 *Bupleurum longiradiatum* Turcz.

2.2.2.20   *Bupleurum krylovianum* Schisch K. ex Kryl.

Perennial, 40 to 100 cm high. Root brown yellowy at surface, with several fingerlike branches at the top. Leaves basal narrowly lanceolate, 10 to 20 cm long, 1 to 2 cm wide, attenuate to petiolate at base; lower cauline lanceolate, 4 to 17 mm long, 0.7 to 1.5 mm wide, acute at apex, cuneate at base; upper cauline smaller. Umbellules 16- to 22-flowered, 10 to 20 per umbel. Bracts 4 to 8, unequal, 4 to 12 mm long, 0.5 to 3 mm wide; bracteoles 5, ovate-lanceolate, 3 to 4 mm long, 1 to 1.5 mm wide. Fruit oblong-ellipsoid, 3.5 to 4 mm long, 1.5 to 2 mm wide. Vitta 1 at vallecula and 2 at commissure.

2.2.2.21   Bupleurum densiflorum Rupr.

Perennial, 10 to 30 cm high. Root short, dark brown at surface. Leaves basal narrowly lanceolate to linear, 6 to 15 cm long, 3 to 8 mm wide, obtuse-acute at apex, attenuate and anplexicaule at base; cauline 1 to 3, lanceolate, acuminate at apex, amplexicaule at base. Umbellules 10- to 20-flowered, 2 to 3 per umbel. Bracts 1 to 3, unequal, lanceolate to ovate, 5 to 15 mm long, 3 to 5 mm wide; bracteoles 5 to 6, ovate to broadly obovate, 5 to 8 mm long, 3 to 7 mm wide. Fruit oblong-ellipsoid, 3 to 4 mm long, 1.5 to 2.5 mm wide. Vitta 1 at vallecula and 2 at commissure.

2.2.2.22   *Bupleurum exaltatum* Marsch.-Bieb.

Perennial, 40 to 80 cm high. Root brown yellowy at surface, with several fingerlike branches at the top. Leaves basal narrowly linear, 8 to 12 cm long, 2 to 4 mm wide, attenuate to amplexicaule at base; lower cauline lanceolate to tapered, up to 9 cm long, 3 mm wide, 3- to 5-veined, upper cauline tapered, 5 mm long and 1 mm wide, 1- to 3-veined. Umbellules 5- to 10-flowered, 3 to 5 per umbel. Bracts 2 to 3, narrowly lanceolate, 1 to 6 mm long, 0.5 to 1 mm wide; bracteoles 5,

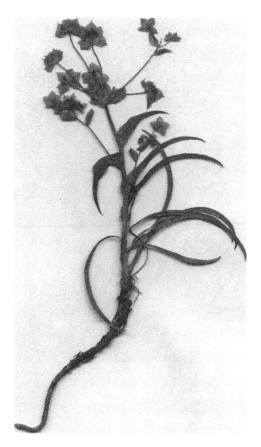

FIGURE 2.12 *Bupleurum euphorbioides* Nakai.

oblong-lanceolate, 1 to 1.8 mm long, 0.5 mm wide. Fruit oblong-ellipsoid, 3.5 to 4.5 mm long, 1.5 to 2 mm wide. Vitta 1 at vallecula and 2 at commissure.

2.2.2.23 *Bupleurum aureum* Fisch.

Perennial, 50 to 120 cm high, with short creeping rhizome. Main roots not obvious. Leaves large, broadly ovate or wide elliptical, basal and lower cauline with long petiole, 8 to 17 cm long, 2.5 to 6 cm wide, upper cauline 12 to 20 cm long, 3 to 3.5 cm wide, auriculately amplexicaul or perfoliate at base, 9- to 13-veined. Umbellules 15- to 20-flowered, 6 to 10 per umbel. Bracts 3 to 5, unequal, bracteoles 5 to 7, broadly ovate to obovate, 5 to 12 mm long, 7 to 9 mm wide. Fruit oblong or ellipsoid, 4 to 6 mm long, 2.5 to 3 mm wide. Vitta 3 at vallecula and 4 at commissure.

2.2.2.24 *Bupleurum commelynoideum* de Boiss. var. *flaviflorum* Shan et Y. Li

Perennial, 30 to 50 cm high. Root slender, dark brown at surface. Leaves basal linear, 10 to 18 cm long, 3 to 5 mm wide; lower cauline lanceolate to oblanceolate, upper cauline ovate-lanceolate, amplexicaule at base. Umbellules 12- to 20-flowered, 5 to 11 per umbel. Bracts 1 to 3, unequal; bracteoles 7 to 9, ovate, 5 to 7 mm long, 3 to 4 mm wide. Fruit ovoid, 2 to 2.5 mm long, 1.2 to 1.6 mm wide. Vitta 3 at vallecula and 4 at commissure.

2.2.2.25　*Bupleurum hamiltonii* Balak

Biennial, 25 to 80 cm high. Root slender, highly lignified. Leaves papery, linear, 3 to 8 cm long, 3 to 6 mm wide, 7- to 9-veined. Umbellules 3- to 5-flowered, 3 to 4 per umbel. Bracts 3 to 4, lanceolate, 3 to 6 mm long, 1 to 2 mm wide; bracteoles 5, lanceolate, 4 to 5 mm long, 0.8 to 1.2 mm wide. Fruit ovoid, 2 to 2.5 mm long, 0.6 to 1 mm wide. Vitta 1 at vallecula and 2 at commissure.

2.2.2.26　*Bupleurum candollei* Wall ex DC.

Perennial, 80 to 150 cm high. Root hard, lignous highly, grayish at surface. Leaves basal and lower cauline linear lanceolate or oblong-elliptic, 12 to 15 cm long, 5 to 8 mm wide, attenuate at base; 11- to 13-veined, middle and upper cauline flatted, oblong, 1.5 to 4 cm long, 0.8 to 1 cm wide, obtuse-acute at apex, cuneate at base, semi-amplexicaule, 15 to 19-veined. Umbellules 10- to 15-flowered, 4 to 8 per umbel. Bracts 3 to 5, ovate, unequal, 3 to 20 mm long, 2 to 10 mm wide; 7- to 17-veined, bracteoles 5, elliptic, 5 to 8 mm long, 2 to 5 mm wide. Fruit ellipsoid, 2 to 5 mm long, 1.8 to 2 mm wide. Vitta 3 at vallecula and 4 at commissure.

2.2.2.27　*Bupleurum longicaule* Wall ex DC. var. *franchetii* de Boiss.

Perennial, 80 to 130 cm high. Root hard, with 2 to 3 branch roots, grayish at surface. Stem hollowed, usually sparingly branched. Leaves oblong, papery, 5 to 10 cm long, 1 to 1.8 cm wide, 5- to 13-veined. Umbellules 9- to 15-flowered, 8 to 14 per umbel. Bracts 4 to 5, ovate, unequal; bracteoles 5, obovate to elliptic, 2 to 5 mm long, 1.5 to 2 mm wide. Fruit ellipsoid, 2 to 4 mm long, 1 to 2 mm wide. Vitta 3 at vallecula and 4 at commissure.

2.2.2.28　*Bupleurum longicaule* Wall ex DC. var. *giraldii* Wolff

Perennial, 20 to 50 cm high. Root slender, grayish at surface. Stem hollowed, usually sparingly branched. Leaves basal and lower cauline linear to oblanceolate, papery, 6 to 12 cm long, 0.8 to 1.2 cm wide, cuneate at base; upper cauline lanceolate to ovate, 1.5 to 5 cm long, 1 to 2 cm wide, auriculate amplexicaule at base. Umbellules 10- to 16-flowered, 4 to 9 per umbel. Bracts 3 to 4, ovate, unequal; bracteoles 5 to 6, elliptic-lanceolate to ovate, 3 to 4 mm long, 1.5 to 3 mm wide. Fruit ellipsoid, 3 to 4 mm long, 2 to 2.5 mm wide. Vitta 3 at vallecula and 4 at commissure.

2.2.2.29　*Bupleurum petiolulatum* Franch. var. *tenerum* Shan et Y. Li

Perennial, 40 to 80 cm high. Root brown yellowy at surface. Stem slender, hollowed. Leaves basal and lower cauline linear, 10 to 20 cm long, 2 to 3 mm wide; middle and upper cauline lanceolate, 2 to 10 cm long, 0.6 to 1 cm wide, petiolate, acuminate at apex. Umbellules 9- to 19-flowered, 8 to 14 per umbel. Bracts 5 to 6, ovate, unequal, 5 to 10 mm long, 2 to 5 mm wide; bracteoles 5, narrowly ovate, 3 to 5 mm long, 1.5 to 2 mm wide. Fruit ellipsoid, 3 to 5 mm long, 1.6 to 2 mm wide. Vitta 3 at vallecula and 4 at commissure.

2.3　DISTRIBUTION AND RESOURCES OF MEDICINAL *BUPLEURUM* IN CHINA

The plants of genus *Bupleurum* L. are distributed throughout the temperate region of the Northern Hemisphere. In China, they are distributed in all provinces except Hainan. More species occur in the south than in the north, especially in Yunnan and Sichuan provinces. Sometimes four to five species of *Bupleurum* grow on the same mountain.

The distribution and resources of medicinal *Bupleurum* in China are given in Table 2.1.

2.4 USAGE OF MEDICINAL *BUPLEURUM* IN CHINA (PAN, 1998)

The commodities (commercial material) of Chaihu (Table 2.2) can be mainly divided into three major types: (1) Chaihu (or North Chaihu), (2) Red Chaihu (or South Chaihu), and (3) Bamboo-leaf Chaihu. In a few regions, the commodity names of Black Chaihu, Large-leaf Chaihu, Spring Chaihu and Chaishou are also used. The utilized parts of North Chaihu and Red Chaihu are roots. But the part used of Bamboo-leaf Chaihu is the total herb, i.e., aerial parts. In the north or central sections of China, the *Bupleurum* part used is the root, whereas in the southwest of China, the total herb is used. The root is used to treat hepatitis, influenza, and menoxenia, and the aerial part for fever. During 1997–98 110 commercial samples from more than 80 country markets in 27 provinces of China were collected. Among them, 66 samples were root (60%), and 44 samples were aerial part (40%). The results of identification of the species of these samples are given in Table 2.2.

REFERENCES

Li, G.M. (1989) The original plants of "Chaihu" (*Bupleurum*) in Shaanxi, Gansu, Ningxia, Qinghai and Xinjiang Province of China, *Zhongguo Zhongyao Zazhi*, 14, 262–267.

Li, Y. and She, M.L. (1979) *Bupleurum, Flora Republicae Popularis Sin.*, 55(1), 215–295.

Li, Y., Pan, S.L., and Luo, S.Q. (1984) Two new species of the genus *Bupleurum* (Umbelliferae) from China, *Acta Phytotaxon. Sin.*, 22, 131–138.

Li, Y., Pan, S.L., and Luo, S.Q. (1986) A new species of the genus *Bupleurum* (Umbelliferae) from China, *Acta Phytotaxon. Sin.*, 24, 150–155.

Li, Y., Guo, J.X., Pan, S.L., and Luo, S.Q. (1993) Investigation and exploitation of new medicinal resources of genus *Bupleurum* (Umbelliferae) in Qinghai Province and Xizhang (Tibet) Autonomous Region in China, *J. Chin. Pharm. Sci.*, 2, 39–44.

Pan, S.L. (1996) Investigation on resources of "Chaihu" (*Bupleurum*) and identification of its commodities, *J. Chin. Med. Mat.*, 19, 231–234.

Pan, S.L. (1998) Medicinal *Bupleurums* in China, *Proceeding of the 7th International Symposium on Traditional Medicine in Toyama*, 127–139.

Pan, S.L. and Hsu, P.S. (1992) A new *Bupleurum* (Umbelliferae) from central China, *SIDA*, 15, 91–93.

Pan, S.L. and Ohashi, H. (1996) The medicinal species and distribution of *Bupleurum* genus in China, *J. Jpn. Med. Bot.*, 19, 1–17.

Pan, S.L., Li, Y., Dai, K.M., and Luo, S.Q. (1984) Studies on taxonomy and chemical constituents of medicinal plants "Chaihu" (genus *Bupleurum*) from Yunnan Province, *Acta Acad. Med. Prim. Shanghai*, 11, 1–13.

Pan, S.L., Wang, Z.H., Hong, X.K., Lin, D.H., Mao, R.G., and Ohashi, H. (2000a) Determination on saiko-saponin-a, -c and -d in 23 species of *Bupleurum* by HPLC, *J. Jpn. Med. Bot.*, 23, 35–39.

Pan, S.L., Wang, Z.H., Hong, X.K., Lin, D.H., Mao, R.G., and Ohashi, H. (2000b) Determination on saiko-saponin-a, -c and -d by HPLC in *Bupleurums* from different districts of China, *J. Jpn. Med. Bot.*, 23, 40–44.

Pan, S.L., Shun, Q.S., Bo, Q.M., and Bao, X.S. (2002) *The Coloured Atlas of Medicinal Plants from Genus Bupleurum in China*, Shanghai Sci. Tech. Doc. Publishing House, Shanghai, China.

Song, W.Z. (1981) Investigation of original plants of Chaihu, *Zhongyao TongBao*, 11–15.

State Pharmacopoeia Commission of the People's Republic of China. (2000) *Pharmacopoeia of the People's Republic of China, Volume I*, Chemical Industry Press, Beijing, China, pp. 163–164.

Su, P., Yuan, C.Q., She, M.L., Liu, Y.Z., Xian, B.R., and An, D.K. (1998) Numerical taxonomy of medicinal *Bupleurum* species in China, *Acta Bot. Boreal.-Occident. Sin.*, 18, 277–283.

Zhao, J.F., Guo, Y.Z., and Meng, X.S. (1987) The toxic principles of *Bupleurum longiradiatum*, *Acta Pharm. Sin.*, 22, 507–511.

3 Microscopical Characters of the Medicinal Species of *Bupleurum* in China

Sheng-Li Pan

CONTENTS

3.1 VEGETATIVE ORGANS

3.1.1 ROOT

The root of *Bupleurum* is covered by periderm composed of five to ten regularly arranged cork cell layers of quadrangular cells elongated periclinally (Figure 3.1). In some species, such as *B. bicaule, B. yinchowense*, cork cells are up to 20 to 22 cell layers. Under the periderm there are three to four cell layers of pericyclic parenchyma, the corners of which are usually slightly thickened. Several resin ducts occur in pericyclic parenchyma. Nagoshi and Odani (1976) discovered that these ducts are reticulately distributed in a single layer under the periderm. The primary phloem is at in the periphery of the phloem bundle. The sieve elements are collapsed and almost invisible. In secondary phloem, the sieves and the companion cells are arranged in groups and can be distinguished from parenchyma by their size and darker cytoplasm. Oil cavities are scattered in the pericyclic parenchyma, the secondary phloem, and phloem rays. The number of oil cavities varies in different species. In a few species, e.g., *B. polyclonum, B. marginatum* var. *stenophyllum, B. rockii,* and *B. wenchuanense,* oil cavities cannot be found in phloem and phloem rays. In some species, for example, *B. chinense, B. krylovianum*, the oil cavities in phloem and phloem rays are up to seven to eight layers. The transversally dilated cells of the phloem rays of some species, i.e., *B. marginatum* var. *stenophyllum, B. kunmingense, B. polyclonum,* and *B. longiradiatum,* are filled with starch grains 4 to 12 μm in diameter.

    The ring of cambium cells is not obvious. The secondary xylem holds the main part of the root. The vessels are varied in diameter and accompanied by parenchyma cells. Spiral vessels and reticulated vessels are the chief ones in the secondary xylem (Figure 3.2). Annular vessels can be

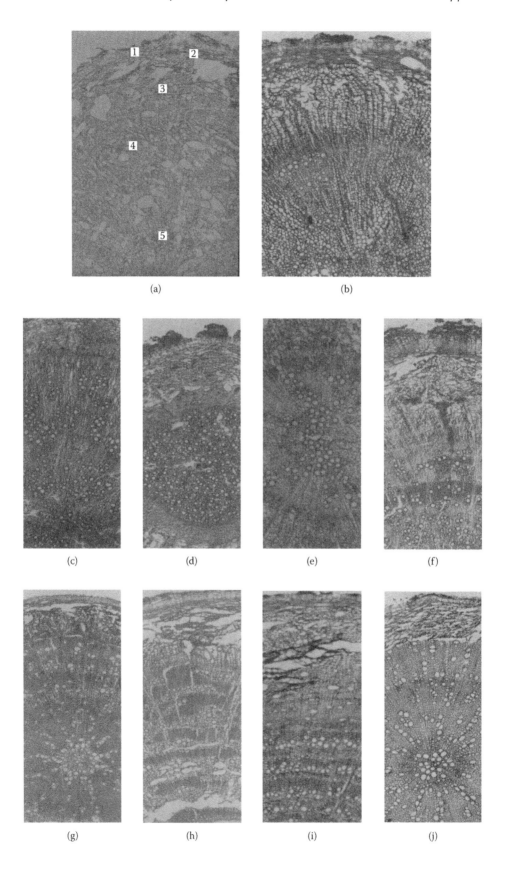

(a)　　　　(b)

(c)　　(d)　　(e)　　(f)

(g)　　(h)　　(i)　　(j)

FIGURE 3.1 (opposite page) Root cross section of *Bupleurum* genus (original magnification ×50). (a) *Bupleurum chinense* DC. 1, periderm; 2, pericyclic parenchyma; 3, oil duct; 4, vessel; 5, xylem fibers; (b) *B. polyclonum* Y. Li et S.L. Pan; (c) *B. scorzonerifolium* Willd.; (d) *B. sibiricum* Vest; (e) *B. marginatum* Wall. ex DC. var. *stenophyllum* Shan et Y. Li; (f) *B. yinchowense* Shan et Y. Li; (g) *B. petiolulatum* Franch. var. *tenerum* Shan et Y. Li; (h) *B. rockii* Wolff; (i) *B. krylovianum* Schischk. ex Kryl.; (j) B. *candollei* Wall. ex DC.

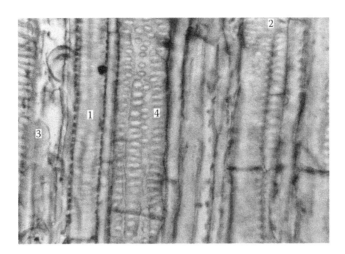

FIGURE 3.2 The vessels in radial section of *B. chinense* DC. (original magnification ×900). 1, spiral vessel; 2, reticulated vessel; 3, annular vessel; 4, pitted vessel.

found in the primary xylem, which otherwise is not obvious. Some species have pitted vessels in the secondary xylem, e.g., *B. chinense, B. smithii* var. *parvifolium, B. rockii, B. bicaule, B. angustissimum, B. sichuanense,* and *B. wenchuanense.* Fibers occur in secondary xylem of most species. The xylem fibers are arranged in one or two discontinuous rings. In very few species, the xylem fibers can be in up to five to seven rings, such as in *B. krylovianum* or *B. rockii.* Pan et al. (1996, 2002) observed the root transverse sections of 22 species from *Bupleurum* genus. Their differences are presented in Table 3.1.

3.1.2 STEM

The stems of most species in *Bupleurum* genus are ribbed in surface (Figure 3.3). In some species, e.g., *B. euphorbioides, B. scorzonerifolium,* and *B. hamiltonii,* the ribs become smaller or almost disappear (Figure 3.4). The stem is covered with one layer of epidermal cells, the outer tangential wall of which are slightly thicker and covered by cuticle. Under the epidermis there are 6 to 20 cell layers of cortex parenchyma, and collenchyma bundles occur in the ribs. Depending on the species, there are one or two collenchyma bundles between two folds in the cortex. Beneath the collenchyma bundles of a rib, there is one oil duct. The collateral vascular bundles comprise one wavy ring. The phloem is more or less hemispherical in shape. In most cases the oil cavities are near to the phloem. Cambial activity is not high. In the secondary part of the xylem the vessels are much smaller, surrounded and separated by fibers. The primary part of a vascular bundle comprises vessels of relatively wide diameter. The center part of the stem is a great pith composed of parenchyma cells. In some species, such as *B. euphorbioides, B. longiradiatum, B. longicaule* var. *franchetii,* and *B. petiolulatum* var. *tenerum,* the broken cells of pith form a pith cavity in the center of the stem. Sometimes, in the outer part of pith near the primary xylem, oil ducts occur as well.

TABLE 3.1
Anatomical Characters of Roots in *Bupleurum* Genus from China

Species	Cork Cell Layers	Oil Cavities	Starch Grains	Pitted Vessels	Xylem Fibers
B. chinense	6–10	+++		+	+++
B. smithii var. *parvifolium*	7–12	+++		+	+
B. scorzonerifolium	8–16	++++		−	±
B. marginatum var. *stenophyllum*	3–7	−	++++	−	+
B. yinchowense	12–20	++		−	++
B. bicaule	15–22	++++		+	−
B. angustissimum	8–15	++++		+	−
B. polyclonum	3–7	−		−	+
B. rockii	7–10	±		+	+++
B. longiradiatum	5–9	−	++++	−	++
B. komarovianum	4–7	±	+++	−	++
B longicaule var. *franchetii*	3–7	+	+	−	++
B. hamiltonii	2–4	−		−	++++
B. kunmingense	3–6	±		−	+
B. luxiense	3–5	−	++	−	±
B. sichuanense	10–16	±	+	+	++
B. wenchuanense	6–12	−		+	+
B. chaishoui	6–10	+		+	−
B. malconense	5–9	+	++	+	±
B. candollei	2–4	−		−	++++
B. commelynoideum var. *flaviflorum*	6–12	+++		+	+
B. petiolulatum var. *tenerum*	5–8	±	++	+	+++

3.1.3 LEAF

The leaf blade is thin, covered by epidermis and cuticle (Figure 3.5). The adaxial cells are larger than the abaxial cells. The leaves of *Bupleurum* are bifacial, usually with one layer of palisade parenchyma and five to eight cell layers of spongy parenchyma. A few species, e.g., *B. scorzonerifolium* (Figure 3.6), *B. chinense* (Figure 3.7), *B. petiolulatum* var. *tenerum*, have two or three layers of palisade parenchyma. Especially in *B. scorzonerifolium*, just under the abaxial cells there are two layers of palisade parenchyma as well. Anisocytic type stomata (Figure 3.8) mainly occur on the abaxial epidermis. The central vascular bundle of the leaves is in a rib. An oil duct is attached to the abaxial side of the collateral vascular bundle. Some species, such as *B. chinense* and *B. polyclonum*, have a smaller oil duct attached to the adaxial side of the vascular bundle as well (Figure 3.7). In a very few species, e.g., *B. scorzonerifolium*, fiber bundles occur on adaxial and abaxial side of the collateral vascular bundles (Figure 3.6).

3.2 GENERATIVE ORGANS

3.2.1 FRUIT

The number of oil ducts at the vallecula and commissure in the cremocarp is used in the classification of *Bupleurum* genus. Most species have three oil ducts at vallecula, and four at the commissure (Figure 3.9). Some species, e.g., *B. hamiltonii, B. krylovianum, B. densiflorum,* and *B. exaltatum,* have one oil duct at the vallecula and two at the commissure (Figure 3.10). The schizocarp is five ribbed. Under the epidermis, there is a collenchyma bundle in each rib. The exocarp has isodiametric

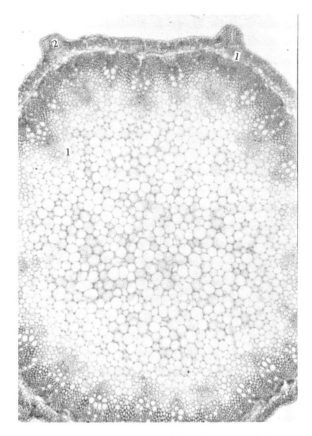

FIGURE 3.3 Stem cross section of *B. kunmingense* Y. Li et S.L. Pan (original magnification ×100). 1, oil duct; 2, collenchyma.

cells. The endocarp is unicellular, and consists of narrow cells with varied arrangement. In the center of the schizocarp is a great endosperm.

3.2.2 POLLEN GRAIN

The pollen grains of *Bupleurum* genus belong to tricolporate type (Figure 3.11). The exine ornamentation is coarsely reticulate or foveolate to brain-like (Figure 3.12). Some pollen grains are long (Figure 3.13) and some are nearly circular (Figure 3.14). Based on the shapes and aperture types, Wang and Fu (1995) observed 24 species, 7 varieties, and 2 forms of *Bupleurum* genus from China and other countries in Himalayan region, and divided the pollen grains of *Bupleurum* genus into three types:

1. Nearly rhomboidal goniotreme type — P (polar axis)/E (equatorial axis) = 1.1 to 1.5; sexine thicker than or equal to nexine, or both nearly equally thick; pores goniotreme or rectangular, rarely circular; the exine ornamentation reticulate or coarsely reticulate under light microscope (LM); subspilate or foveolate along the colpi and rugulose or striato-reticulate on the mesocolpium under scanning electron microscope (SEM). Examples are *B. euphorbioides*, *B. triradiatum*, *B. exaltatum*, *B. angustissimum*, *B. longiradiatum*, *B. scorzonerifolium*, and *B. chinense* f. *octoradiatum*.

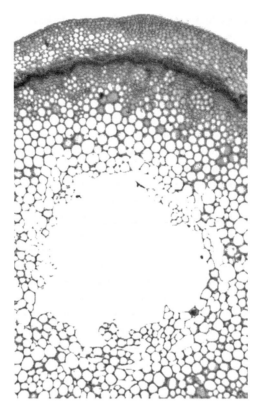

FIGURE 3.4 Stem cross section of *B. euphorbioides* Nakai (original magnification ×100).

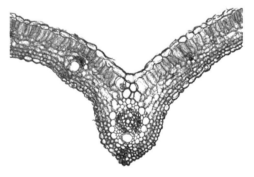

FIGURE 3.5 Leaf cross section of *B. sichuanense* S.L. Pan et Hsu (original magnification ×100).

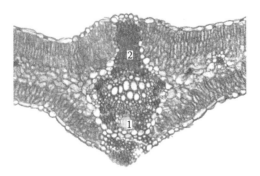

FIGURE 3.6 Leaf cross section of *B. scorzonerifolium* Willd. (original magnification ×100). 1, oil duct; 2, fibers.

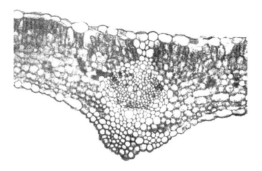

FIGURE 3.7 Leaf cross section of *B. chinense* DC. (original magnification ×100).

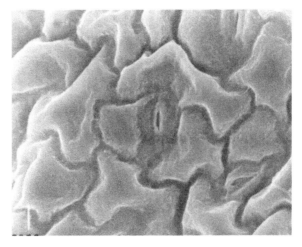

FIGURE 3.8 The anisocytic type stoma of *B. chinense* DC. (original magnification ×1000).

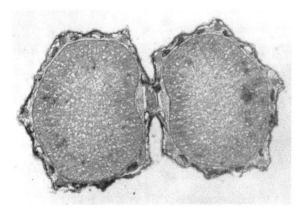

FIGURE 3.9 Cremocarp cross section of *B. marginatum* Wall. ex DC. var. *stenophyllum* Shan et Y. Li (original magnification ×40).

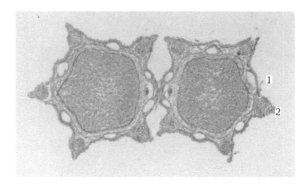

FIGURE 3.10 Cremocarp cross section of *B. hamiltonii* Balak (original magnification ×60). 1, oil duct; 2, collenchyma.

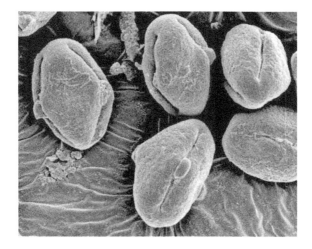

FIGURE 3.11 Pollen grains of *B. sichuanense* S.L. Pan et Hsu (original magnification ×1500).

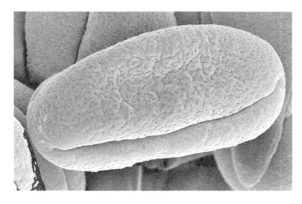

FIGURE 3.12 Pollen grains of *B. chinense* DC. (original magnification ×3000).

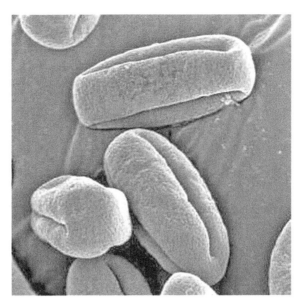

FIGURE 3.13 Pollen grains of *B. komarovianum* Lincz. (original magnification ×1800).

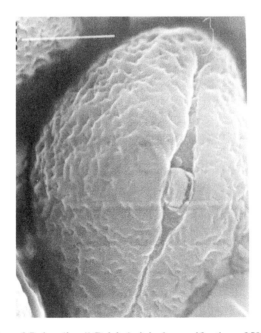

FIGURE 3.14 Pollen grains of *B. hamiltonii* Balak (original magnification ×3500).

2. Rectangular pleurotreme type — P/E = 1.5 to 2.0; sexine thicker than or nearly equal to nexine; pores mostly pleurotreme; the exine ornamentation reticulate, coarsely reticulate and rarely striato-reticulate under LM; mostly foveolate along the colpi; verrucose, aggregate, verrucose, reticulate, striato-reticulate, and rarely rugulose on the mesocolpium under SEM. Examples are *B. smithii, B. commelynoideum* var. *flaviflorum, B. candolle, B. rockii, B. longicaule* var. *franchetii, B. malconense, B. chaishoui, B. hamiltonii, B. chinense.*

3. Subellipsoidal, nearly rhomboidal or subrectangular and goniotreme or pleurotreme type — P/E = 1.4 to 1.75; sexine thicker than or nearly equal to nexine; pores goniotreme or pleurotreme, rarely circular, ellipsoidal or rectangular; the exine ornamentation reticulate or striato-reticulate under LM; foveolate or subspilate along the colpi; aggregate verrucose or striato-reticulate, rarely verrucose, rugulose or reticulate on the mesocolpium under SEM. Examples are two varieties: *B. longicaule* var. *strictum, B. marginatum* var. *stenophyllum.*

Pollen morphology is presented in Table 3.2.

TABLE 3.2
Pollen Morphology of Sino-Himalaya

Species	P/E	Size (μm)		Ornamentation	
		Long	Wide	Polar Area	Mesocolpium
B. euphorbioides	1.4	20.1–25.7	14.3–18.6	Subspilate	Rugulose
B. triradiatum	1.35	31.6–37.8	23.1–29.1	Foveolate	Rugulose
B. exaltatum	1.4	23.1–27.3	16.8–18.9	Subspilate	Striato-reticulate
B. hoffmeisteri	1.8	23.7–38.6	14.7–21	Subspilate	Rugulose
B. commelynoideum var. *flaviflorum*	1.5	21.5–28.6	15.1–17.2	Subspilate	Rugulose
B. angustissimum	1.4	23.1–25.2	16.8–18.9	Subspilate	Foveolate
B. chinense var. *octoradiatum*	1.1	20.1–31.5	20.1–28.5	Foveolate	Verrucose
B. dalhousieanum	1.4	21.5–28.6	15.7–20.1	Subspilate	Rugulose
B. scorzonerifolium	1.5	25.7–29.1	16.8–20.9	Subspilate	Foveolate
B. longiradiatum	1.6	17.2–22.9	11.5–12.4	Foveolate	Verrucose
B. longicaule var. *strictum*	1.7	26.7–31.5	14.3–20.1	Foveolate	Striato-reticulate
B. marginatum var. *stenophyllum*	1.4	20.1–24.3	14.3–17.1	Foveolate	Striato-reticulate
B. gracillimum	1.5	23.1–27.3	16.8–18.9	Foveolate	Verrucose
B. malconense	1.5	21.5–25.7	14.3–17.2	Foveolate	Verrucose
B. candolle	2.0	22.9–28.6	11.4–14.3	Foveolate	Finely reticulate
B. hamiltonii var. *humile*	1.6	23.1–27.8	14.7–16.8	Subspilate	Reticulate
B. longicaule var. *giraldii*	1.6	24.3–28.6	15.7–17.2	Foveolate, striate	Aggregate, verrucose
B. longicaule	1.7	22.5–27.3	14.7–16.8	Foveolate	Striato-reticulate
B. smithii	1.56	23.1–31.5	16.8–19.3	Subspilate	Aggregate, verrucose
B. petiolulatum	1.64	21.0–25.7	11.5–17.2	Foveolate	Striato-reticulate
B. rockii	1.63	22.9–27.1	13.1–17.3	Foveolate	Striato-reticulate
B. yunnanense	1.6	19.1–25.8	12.9–17.2	Foveolate	Striato-reticulate
B. commelynoideum	1.3	21.5–24.5	15.7–20.1	Subspilate	Reticulate
B. longiradiatum var. *porphyranthum*	1.8	31.5–33.6	17.2–18.9		
B. marginatum	1.5	20.1–28.6	12.9–18.6	Foveolate	Striato-reticulate
B. microcephalum	1.75	22.9–29.3	12.9–17.2	Reticulate	Verrucose
B. wenchuanense	1.7	20.1–25.8	16.8–20.1	Foveolate	Striato-reticulate
B. chinense	1.3	23.1–25.2	16.8–21.0		
B. chinense f. *vanheurckii*	1.5	25.2–29.3	16.8–18.9	Foveolate	Rugulose verrucose
B. chaishoui	1.6	21.5–25.7	12.9–17.1	Foveolate	Striato-reticulate
B. hamiltonii	1.6	20.1–22.9	11.5–14.5	Reticulate	Perforations
B. himalayaense	1.6	23.1–33.6	16.8–21.0		
B. longicaule var. *franchetii*	1.5	23.1–28.6	15.7–17.2	Foveolate	Verrucose

3.3 CONCLUSIONS

A total of 44 species, 17 varieties, and 7 forms of *Bupleurum* occur in China. Nearly all of their roots have been used as crude drugs. The root appearance of most species is similar, but differences occur in their microscopical characters. According to Pan et al. (1996, 2002), the number of cork cell layers, oil cavities, starch grains, xylem fibers, and pitted vessels can be used for species classification and identification. In the aerial parts, ribs and pith cavity of stems, fibers of leaves, and the numbers of oil ducts at vallecula in the cremocarps can be used for classification and identification purposes. Furthermore, the size and ornamentation of pollen grains are important for the identification on some species.

REFERENCES

Nagoshi, K. and Odani, T. (1976) Pharmacognostical studies on *Bupleurum* Radix "Saiko" on the so-called collenchyma-like tissue and the resin ducts distributed in the same tissue, *Syoyakugaku Zasshi*, 30, 83–86.

Pan, S.L., Cheng, D.H., Huang, J.M., and Ohashi, H. (1996) Pharmacognostical studies on medicinal bupleurums of China, *J. Jpn. Med. Bot.*, 19, 6–19.

Pan, S.L., Shun, Q.S., Bo, Q.M., and Bao, X.S. (2002) *The Coloured Atlas of Medicinal Plants from Genus Bupleurum in China.* Shanghai Sci. Tech. Doc. Publishing House, Shanghai, China.

Wang, P.L. and Fu, F.D. (1995) Pollen morphology of *Bupleurum* L. from Sino-Himalaya and its systematic significance, *Chin. J. Appl. Environ. Biol.*, 1, 34–43.

4 Chromosomes of *Bupleurum* L. Especially for the Classification and Cross-Breeding of *B. falcatum* L. *sensu lato*

Shigeki Ohta, Eiji Miki, You-Chang Zhu, and Chang-Qi Yuan

CONTENTS

4.1 INTRODUCTION

The genus *Bupleurum* L. has been described to include 150 and more species (Engler, 1964; Linchevskii, 1973) and some of them (*B. fructicosum* L., *B. rotundifolium* L., etc.) are available for gardening, flower arrangement, or medical use (Wolff, 1910, Linchevskii, 1973, Guinea et al., 1994). In the Far East, dried roots of some species in *Bupleurum* (Bupleuri radix; "saiko" in Japanese) have been used in the therapy of disease. In Japan, saiko has recently become very important for treating chronic diseases such as hepatitis, neurosis, and asthma that could not be remedied by Western medicines alone. Saiko is mainly used in decoctions after mixing with other crude drugs according to the traditional prescriptions of "Kampo." These formulations/prescriptions are now manufactured in a convenient form for patients. In 2002, the gross proceeds of manufactured "saiko-zai," which is a prescription group including saiko as a constituent, amounted to about 27 billion yen for clinical use, accounting for approximately 26% of the total sales of Kampo clinical medicines.

However, despite such demand for saiko-zai in modern medical treatment, the source plants of saiko have been broadly defined in the *Japanese Pharmacopoeia* (14th rev. ed., 2001) since the first description at the 7th revision in 1966, as from *B. falcatum* L. *sensu lato*. This plant is widely distributed from Europe through the Caucasus and Central Asia to China, Korea, and Japan, and is well known to exhibit great variation in the external morphology (Wolff, 1910; Hiroe, 1952; Ohwi, 1965; Tutin, 1968). It is preferable to exclude crude drugs with no historical and clinical application from the provision. In addition, as noticed by Kampo medical doctors, wholesalers, manufactures, and investigators of the crude drug, major Bupleuri radixes from Japanese, Korean, and Chinese markets are mutually different in their morphology as well as quality, and hence their sources may also differ. So, it is desirable to identify at least source plants of the major Bupleuri radixes from these countries and to produce evidence for the later Japanese provision.

During several decades, chromosome studies have been carried out in many plant species and have contributed much information for understanding of the speciation, which is related to the classification (John and Lewis, 1965; Stebbins, 1971; Tanaka, 1982; Kayano, 1982). For *Bupleurum* L., about 100 species have been described based on their chromosome numbers (Darlington and Wylie, 1955; Cave, 1958–1959, 1959–1964; Federov, 1969; Ornduff, 1967–1969; Moore, 1970–1974, 1977; Goldblatt, 1981, 1984, 1985, 1988; Goldblatt and Johnson, 1990, 1991, 1994, 1996, 1998, 2000). Moreover, for some of the European species the basic number has been discussed in relation to their speciation and classification (Cauwet-Marc, 1979).

The present author has previously reported chromosome study in *B. falcatum* L. *s. l.* from Japan and abroad, with reference to the chromosome differentiation at metaphase and the speciation within the taxonomic group (Ohta et al., 1986; Ohta, 1991). Tanaka (1971, 1980, 1987) demonstrated that chromosome information at resting stage was useful to trace the speciation in Orchidaceae with a relationship to the cross-ability (affinity of crossing). In this chapter, we report the results of chromosome study at mitotic prophase and metaphase, and at resting stage in *B. falcatum* L. *s. l.* from Japan, Korea, China, Russia, and European countries including some of the other species, and based on them and their morphological study, propose the scientific names for Japanese and Korean plants of this species. Additionally, we describe for the first time artificial hybridization between the Japanese and the Korean source plants of Bupleuri radix.

4.2 THE CHROMOSOMES OF *BUPLEURUM* L.

4.2.1 Characteristics of Somatic Chromosomes in the Species of *Bupleurum* Investigated

For the purpose of this study, several species of *Bupleurum* were cytologically investigated. In Figure 4.1, somatic chromosomes of *B. fruticosum* L. (in A, C, E) and *B. ranuncuroides* L. (in B, D, F) at metaphase, prophase, and resting stage are shown. At the metaphase, $2n = 14$ and $2n = 42 + 5B$ (a new report) were counted in *B. fruticosum* (Figure 4.1A) and *B. ranuncuroides* (Figure 4.1B), respectively. Chromosomes at metaphase of the former were medium to large sized (ca. 3 to 6 µm in length) among the species of this genus observed, while those of the latter were small (ca. 1 to 2 µm). Sizes of chromosomes at metaphase in all the species of *Bupleurum* investigated were within those of the above two species. According to Tanaka (1971, 1980, 1987), *B. fruticosum* was found to be an interstitial type (Figure 4.1C) at prophase, and *B. ranunculoides* was a proximal type (Figure 4.1D). At resting stage, both species were categorized as a complex chromocenter type (Figure 4.1E, F). Besides, an intermediate between interstitial type and proximal type was observed at prophase of *B. scorzonerifolium* Willd. (Figure 4.1F), and an intermediate between complex chromocenter type and simple chromocenter type was at the resting stage of *B. falcatum* L. *s. str.* (Figure 4.1G).

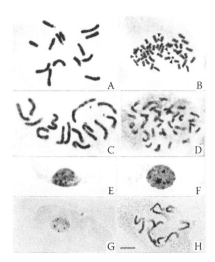

FIGURE 4.1 Somatic chromosomes in root tip cells of the species in *Bupleurum* L. at metaphase (A, B), prophase (C, D, H), and resting stage (E–G). (A, C, E) *B. fruticosum* L. (2*n* = 14); (B, D, F) *B. ranunculoides* L. (B, F: 2*n* = 42 + 5B; D: 2*n* = 42); (G) *B. falcatum* L. *s. str.* (2*n* = 16); (H) *B. scorzonerifolium* Willd. (2*n* = 12). C: interstitial type; D: proximal type; H: intermediate between interstitial type and proximal type. E, F: complex chromocenter type; G: intermediate between complex chromocenter type and simple chromocenter type. Arrowheads in B indicate B-chromosomes. Bar: 5 μm.

4.2.2 SOMATIC CHROMOSOMES AT METAPHASE OF THE PLANTS BELONGING TO *BUPLEURUM FALCATUM* L. *S. L.*

Somatic chromosomes at metaphase of the plants belonging to *B. falcatum* L. *s. l.* investigated are shown in Figure 4.2 and Figure 4.3, and the locality is presented in Figure 4.4 and Figure 4.5. *Bupleurum falcatum* L. *s. str.* from Europe had small chromosomes of 2*n* = 16 (Figure 4.2A), while the other plants of *B. falcatum* L. *s. l.* including *B. scorzonerifolium, B. chinense* DC., *B. komarovianum* Lincz., *B. microcephalum* Diels., and four *Bupleurum* sp. from Japan, Korea, China, and Russia, had medium to large chromosomes of 2*n* = 8, 12, 20, 20(+ 4B), 24, 26, and 32 (Figure 4.2B to H, Figure 4.3B to H). *Bupleurum falcatum* L. *s. l.* from Japan was found to comprise three cytotypes with 2*n* = 20, 26, and 32 (Ohta et al., 1986, Ohta, 1991), and each cytotype was distributed in the different regions (Figure 4.4).

The Korean plants that were morphologically identical to those of the cytotype with 2*n* = 20 from Japan were cytogenetically the same, as well. The plants of cytotype with 2*n* = 20 (Figure 4.2E, Figure 4.5) were found in Heilongjiang Province, China, and those with 2*n* = 26 were in Heilongjiang and Nei Mongol Province (Figure 4.2G, Figure 4.5). Figure 4.2F shows 2*n* = 20 chromosomes in the plant that has the same external morphology and karyotype except for chromosomes with a satellite. In the plants of cytotypes with 2*n* = 20 and 2*n* = 26 from China, aneuploidy, or a heterogeneous chromosome (Figure 4.2E, and as a pair of chromosomes with a satellite in Figure 4.2F), and a chromosome fragment (Figure 4.6H) were often observed as in the Japanese plants (Ohta, 1991).

Bupleurum scorzonerifolium and *B. chinense* had a common karyotype; that is, the same in number and morphology of their chromosomes, except for the number of chromosomes with a satellite (Figure 4.2B, C, Figure 4.3H). In addition, aneuploidy, or a heterogeneous chromosome, and a chromosome fragment were not observed in both species. In addition, presumable tetraploids were found in *B. chinense* (Figure 4.2D). In the tetraploids, heterogeneous chromosomes were detected at a considerable rate (Figure 4.6G), suggesting their autoploid origin (Ohta et al., 1995).

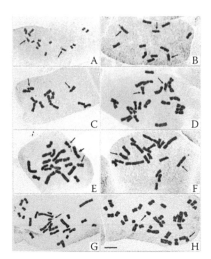

FIGURE 4.2 Somatic chromosomes at metaphase in root tip cells of the species belonging to *B. falcatum* L. *s. l.* (A) *B. falcatum* L. *s. str.* (2*n* = 16) from France; (B) *B. scorzonerifolium* (2*n* = 12) from Heilongjiang Prov., China; (C) *B. chinense* DC. (2*n* = 12) from Hubei; (D) *B. chinense* (2*n* = 24) from Liaoning; (E, F) *B. falcatum* L. *s. l.* (2*n* = 20) from Heilongjiang; (G) *B. falcatum* L. *s. l.* (2*n* = 26) from Heilongjiang; (H) *B. falcatum* L. *s. l.* (2*n* = 32) from Japan. Long arrows in A–H indicate chromosomes with a satellite, and short arrow in E shows a heterogeneous chromosome. Bar: 5 μm.

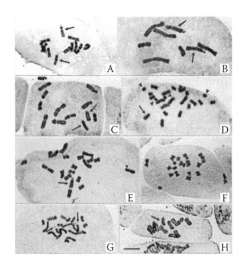

FIGURE 4.3 Somatic chromosomes at metaphase in root tip cells of the species belonging to *B. falcatum* L. *s. l.*, and the related species, *B. longiradiatum* Turcz. (A) *B. longiradiatum* (2*n* = 12) from Heilongjiang Prov., China; (B) *B. komarovianum* Lincz. (2*n* = 8) from Heilongjiang; (C) *B. microcephalum* Diels. (2*n* = 12) from Sichuan; (D) *Bupleurum* sp. (2*n* = 20 + 4B) from Shanxi; (E) *Bupleurum* sp. (2*n* = 20) from Sichuan; (F) *Bupleurum* sp. (2*n* = 20) from Hunan; (G) *Bupleurum* sp. (2*n* = 20) from Shaanxi; (H) *B. scorzonerifolium* (2*n* = 12) from Russia. Arrows in A–E, G, H indicate chromosomes with a satellite, and arrowheads in D indicate B chromosomes. Bar: 5 μm.

For *B. komarovianum*, 2*n* = 8 was counted and its chromosomes were the larger among the plants of *B. falcatum* L. *s. l.* investigated (Figure 4.3B). *Bupleurum microcephalum* had 2*n* = 12 chromosomes (Figure 4.3C); the same number as *B. scorzonerifolium* and *B. chinense*. However, its karyotype was much different from both species, since terminal and subterminal chromosomes

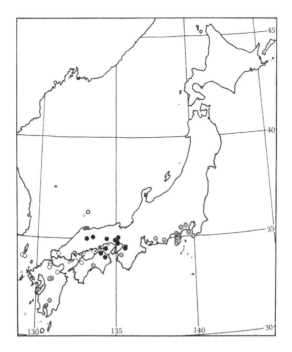

FIGURE 4.4 Map showing locality of *B. falcatum* L. *s. l.* investigated from Japan. One new site for $2n = 20$ (○), two for $2n = 26$ (◎), and seven for $2n = 32$ (●) were added to those in Figure 38 of a previous paper (Ohta, 1991).

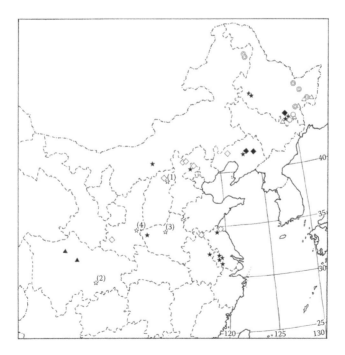

FIGURE 4.5 Map showing locality of the Chinese plants investigated, belonging to *B. falcatum* L. *s. l.* (△) *B. komarovianum* ($2n = 8$), (★) *B. scorzonerifolium* ($2n = 12$), (◇) *B. chinense* ($2n = 12$), (♦) *B. chinense* ($2n = 24$), (▲) *B. microcephalum* ($2n = 12$), (○) *B. falcatum* L. *s. l.* ($2n = 20$), (◎) *B. falcatum* L. *s. l.* ($2n = 26$), (☆) [1]*Bupleurum* sp. ($2n = 20 + 4B$), [2]*Bupleurum* sp. ($2n = 20$), [3]*Bupleurum* sp. ($2n = 20$), [4]*Bupleurum* sp. ($2n = 20$).

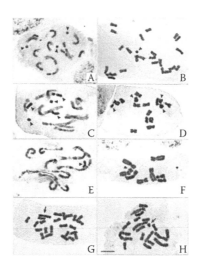

FIGURE 4.6 Somatic chromosomes in root tip cells of the species belonging to *B. falcatum* L. *s. l.* at prophase (A, C, E) and metaphase (B, D, F–H). (A) *B. sceorzonerifolium* ($2n = 12 + 3B$) from Jiangsu Prov., China; (B) *B. chinense* ($2n = 24 + 1B$) from Liaoning; (C, D) *B. chinense* (C) $2n = 12 + 3B_L + 2B_S$; (D) $2n = 12 + 3B_L + 1B_S$) from Shanxi; (E, F) *B. komarovianum* ($2n = 8 + 1B$) from Heilongjiang; (G) *B. chinense* ($2n = 24$) from Heilongjiang; (H) *B. falcatum* L. *s. l.* ($2n = 19 + 1f$) from Heilongjiang. Arrowheads in A–F indicate B chromosomes. Arrow in G shows a heterogeneous chromosome, and that in H a chromosome fragment. Bar: 5 μm.

were contained. Moreover, the plants included in *B. falcatum* L. *s. l.* from inner China having a peculiar external morphology each, but being not identified according to Shan and Li (1974) and Li and Sheh (1979), were observed. In those plants, $2n = 20$ or $20 + 4B$ was counted (Figure 4.3D through G). They were divided into two groups by their karyotypes; that is, "bimodal type" (Figure 4.3D, E, and G) and "gradual type" (Figure 4.3F). In both groups, the plant from Sichuan Province (Figure 4.3E) differed markedly from the others in external morphology. It was suggested that the plants cytologically and morphologically differentiated, belonging to *B. falcatum* L. *s. l.*, are growing in these areas (Figure 4.5).

Bupleurum longiradiatum Turcz., which was one of the four species of *Bupleurum* growing in Japan (Ohwi 1965), was also studied. The chromosome number was $2n = 12$ (observed as in the Chinese plants in Figure 4.3A), and the chromosome complement and morphological features of the chromosomes at prophase and at resting stage were the same as those in *B. scorzonerifolium* and *B. chinense*.

4.2.3 OTHER CHARACTERISTICS ON MITOTIC CHROMOSOMES OF THE SPECIES IN *BUPLEURUM* INVESTIGATED

Several species in *Bupleurum* have been reported to have so-called B chromosomes. We observed them in most of the taxa investigated (Figure 4.6). They varied in number among the different plants or the different root tip cells of one plant (Ohta, 1991) and indicated early condensed regions at mitotic prophase (Figure 4.6A, C, E). Moreover, they were not pairing with any A chromosomes at meiotic metaphase I (Ohta, 1991). The sizes of them were ca. 0.3 to 1.4 μm in length in the smaller (Figure 4.6A through D) and ca. 1.5 to 1.8 μm in the larger (Figure 4.6C through F). In the larger B chromosome, the centromere was found at the median (Figure 4.6D through F) or submedian position (Figure 4.6C). It was noticed that the plants containing B chromosomes often indicated a low stainability of their pollen (for example; 20.1%), with an aqueous solution of aniline blue.

4.3 SCIENTIFIC NAMES FOR THE JAPANESE AND THE KOREAN SOURCE PLANTS OF BUPLEURI RADIX

The chromosomal data mentioned above and gained previously are summarized in Table 4.1. Results cytologically and morphologically obtained in the present study are as follows:

1. Three plant groups that were cytologically differentiated (cytotypes with $2n = 20$, 26, and 32) were distributed in different regions of Japan (additionally, in northeastern China) (Figure 4.4 and Figure 4.5).
2. They each had their own characteristics in external morphology, such as phyllotaxis and adventitious root (Ohta, 1991).
3. The Japanese and the Korean source plants of Bupleuri radix belonged to the cytotypes with $2n = 26$, and with $2n = 20$, respectively (Ohta, 1991).
4. The Chinese source plants, *B. scorzonerifolium* and *B. chinense* (*Pharmacopoeia of the People's Republic of China*, 1992) had an identical chromosome number ($2n = 12$) and karyotype, while they could be morphologically distinguished from each other and from the Japanese and Korean cytotypes (Ohta et al., 1995).
5. Tetraploids ($2n = 24$) of *B. chinense*, showing a morphological similarity and a cytogenetical distinction to the Japanese and Korean cytotype with $2n = 20$, were found in Heilongjiang and Liaoning Province, China (Ohta et al., 1995).
6. The European plants had the different chromosome number ($2n = 16$) and karyotype from those of the Japanese, Korean, and Chinese plants, and had distinct morphological characteristics from those plants (Ohta, 1991).

Regarding the scientific name (species level) for the Japanese source plants of Bupleuri radix, three candidates are proposed from their taxonomic treatments. That is, (1) *B. falcatum* L., as included within the European species (Wolff, 1910; Hiroe, 1952, 1958; Hara, 1954; Ohwi, 1965; Kitamura, 1985); (2) *B. scorzonerifolium* Willd., as within the East Asian species (Nakai, 1937; Kitagawa, 1960; Linchevskii, 1973; Ohba, 1999; Yamazaki, 2001); and (3) *B. stenophyllum* (Nakai) Kitagawa (Kitagawa, 1947). In Japanese *Bupleurum* L., Ohwi (1965) recognized four species, and thought that the same species, *B. falcatum* L., as in Europe were distributed in Japan, as well. The present Japanese provision (*Pharmacopoeia*, 14th rev. ed.) for source plants of Bupleuri radix is derived from his opinion.

As summarized above, results from studies on the source plants indicate that the Japanese source plants, cytotype with $2n = 26$, are clearly distinguished from the Korean and the Chinese plants, as well as the European. In addition, data from RFLP analysis of chloroplast DNA in those plants strongly supported their distinction (Matsumoto et al., 2004). Moreover, at least in Japan, the distribution area of the cytotype with $2n = 26$ does not overlap with those of the others, and is limited to certain regions (Figure 4.4). Namely, it is suggested that the Japanese source plants of Bupleuri radix are recognized as a distinct species.

Nakai (1937) had previously recognized five species in the Japanese, Korean, and Chinese plants that had been treated as *B. falcatum* L. by Ohwi (1965). In that paper, he classified the plants growing in the Kanto, Tokai, Kinki, and Shikoku regions, and in a part of Khushu region, of Japan, as *B. scorzonerifolium* var. *stenophyllum* Nakai, including the allied plants in Korea and China. Thereafter, Kitagawa (1947) recognized that variety as a species, *B. stenophyllum* (Nakai) Kitag., excluding the plants occurring in China. Except for Korea, the distribution of *B. stenophyllum* almost coincides with that of the cytotype with $2n = 26$, and type locality (Hakone, Ashinoyu) of the species is in those distribution areas, as well (Figure 4.4). Therefore, at present, we suppose that the Japanese source plants of Bupleuri radix are identified as *B. stenophyllum*, and we could propose to use that name for their scientific treatment (Ohta, 1998).

On the other hand, the Korean source plants (cultivated) are of the cytotype with $2n = 20$ and are distributed in the northern Khushu and the western Chugoku of Japan, although their origin in the wild is unknown. According to the results of cytological and morphological studies described above, they would be also recognized as a certain taxon. Kitagawa (1947) regarded the plants growing in the northern Khushu and the western Chugoku as a variety of *B. stenophyllum*, i.e., var. *kiusianum* Kitag. The plants from type locality (Mt. Kawaradake) of that variety were of the cytotype with $2n = 20$ (Ohta, 1991). Accordingly, at this time, we consider that the Korean source plants are identified as *B. stenophyllum* var. *kiusianum*. It might be suggested to use that name for their scientific treatment, although they exhibit considerable difference in external morphology compared with the cytotype of $2n = 26$ (Ohta, 1998). As mentioned below, they are also cytogenetically distinct from that cytotype.

Recently, plants with $2n = 20$ and $2n = 26$ belonging to *B. falcatum* L. s. l. have been found to grow in northeastern China (Figure 4.2 and Figure 4.5; Ohta et al., 1993; Jiang et al., 1994; Li et al., 1994; Pan et al., 1995). Zhu (1977) classified the Chinese plants very similar to those of the cytotype with $2n = 26$ as *B. sibiricum* De Vest. He also considered the Chinese plants very similar to those of the cytotype with $2n = 20$, as *B. chinense* DC. var. *octoradiatum* (Bunge) Kitag. (Zhu, 1989). Therefore, further field and herbarium works on those plants from the cyto-geographical aspect will be needed to determine more precisely the scientific names for Japanese and Korean source plants of Bupleuri radix.

Through the present studies, we were able to indicate that the cyto-geographical aspect, including morphological features of mitotic chromosomes at prophase and resting stage, as well as at metaphase, was very useful for classifying the plants within the genus *Bupleurum*, especially the East Asian species. In addition, we found that a new taxon, the cytotype with $2n = 32$, was distributed in the regions surrounding the eastern part of the Setonaikai Inland Sea (Figure 4.4). Here, we name it "Setouchi-saiko" in Japanese. Moreover, the cytological studies on *Bupleurum* revealed that *B. falcatum* L. s. l. in Japan and northeastern China was related to *B. longiradiatum* rather than European *B. falcatum* L. s. str. (Table 4.1), together with the result of their DNA analyses (Matsumoto et al., 2004).

4.4 CROSS-BREEDING BETWEEN *BUPLEURUM STENOPHYLLUM* AND *BUPLEURUM STENOPHYLLUM* VAR. *KIUSIANUM*

Bupleurum radixes from Japanese and Korean markets are mutually different in quality as well as in morphology. That is, the Japanese products are known to have good quality in clinical use (Ohtsuka et al., 1954), while the Korean have been reported to be higher in the total content of pharmacologically effective saikosaponins (Kimata et al., 1979). Therefore, we tried to create new plants that have good clinical quality together with a high saponin content by crossing between the Japanese source plants, *B. stenophyllum*, and the Korean, *B. stenopyllum* var. *kiusianum*.

Figure 4.7 shows the somatic chromosomes ($2n = 46$) at metaphase of the amphidiploid that was obtained in 1988 for the first time in breeding of *Bupleurum* by colchicine treatment of the hybrid seeds — Korean ($♀$) × Japanese ($♂$). At meiotic metaphase I of the amphidiploid, 23 pairs of diad were found and the following stages progressed ordinarily, resulting in fully matured seeds. (This suggests that the Japanese and the Korean source plants are cytogenetically much different from each other, that is, different species.)

Then, after seed reproduction, the new plants were evaluated on quality and yield of their roots, as well as tolerance to plant diseases such as anthrax. Regarding the results, the final goal has not yet been accomplished, because of the lower yield of roots, although they had high saponin content and consistency in their external morphology and constituents (data not shown). Further trials to acquire the other strains of amphidiploid are in progress.

TABLE 4.1
Cytological Characteristics of *Bupleurum falcatum* L. *sensu lato* and Related Species from the Far East and Europe

Taxon	Chromosome Number (2n)	Chromosome Length (μm)	Karyotype			Aneuploidy	No. of B Chromosome	Length of B Chromosome(μm)	Source
			Res	Pro	Met				
B. falcatum L. *sensu lato*									
B. falcatum L. *sensu stricto*	16	1.9–0.7	S-C	P	G	ND	3–6	0.3	Germany,France, Hungary,Russia
B. scorzonerifolium Willd.	12	3.5–2.3	C	P-I	G	ND	1–3[a]	0.6, 0.8–1.1	China,Russia
B. chinense DC.	12	3.5–2.3	C	P-I	G	ND	1–5[a]	1.1–1.3, 1.6–1.8	China
	24	3.3–2.1	C	P-I	G	D	1–3	1.0–1.2	China
B. stenophyllum (Nakai) Kitag.	26	5.6–1.2	C	P-I	B	D	1–5	1.1–1.6	Japan, China
B. stenophyllum var. *kiusianum* Kitag.	20	5.6–2.4	C	P-I	B	D	1–6	1.1–1.3	Japan,Korea,China
Bupleurum sp. (a new taxon)	32	5.7–1.2	C	P-I	B	D	1–5	1.2–1.4	Japan
B. komarovianun Lincz.	8	5.7–3.0	C	P-I	B	ND	1–2[a]	1.0–1.2, 1.7	China
B. microcephalum Diels.	12	4.5–2.4	C	P-I	G	—	—	—	China
Bupleurum sp.[1] from Shanxi	20	3.3–1.1	C	P	B	—	4	0.8–0.9	China
Bupleurum sp.[2] from Sichuan	20	3.2–1.2	C	P	B	—	—	—	China
Bupleurum sp.[3] from Hunan	20	3.6–1.0	—	—	G	—	—	—	China
Bupleurum sp.[4] from Shaanxi	20	3.5–1.4	—	P-I	B	—	—	—	China
B. longiradiatum Turcz.	12	3.3–2.4	C	P-I	G	ND	1	1.0	Japan, China

Abbreviations: Res: resting stage, Pro: prophase, Met: metaphase; C: complex chromocenter type, S-C: intermediate between simple chromocenter type and complex chromocenter type; P:proximal type, I: interstitial type, P-I: intermediate between proximal type and interstitial type; G: gradual type, B: bimodal type; D: detected, ND: not detected.

[a] Two types of B chromosomes were observed.

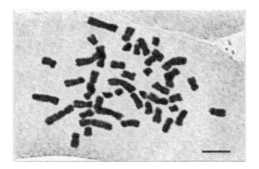

FIGURE 4.7 Somatic chromosomes at metaphase of an amphidiploid between the cytotype with $2n = 20(\female)$ and that with $2n = 26(\male)$ in *B. falcatum* L. s. l. Bar: 5 μm.

ACKNOWLEDGMENTS

For giving the materials and for guidance to the habitats, we express our thanks to the following persons: Mr. Tomiki Kobayashi, Hyogo Pref., Mr. Shiro Yamamoto and Mr. Watanabe, Ehime Pref., Dr. Toshiro Shibata and Mr. Osamu Iida, Tsukuba Med. Plant Res. Station, Natl. Inst. of Health Science, and Ms. Ze-Hui Pan, Assoc. Prof., and Mr. Shan-An He, Director, and the other members of Bot. Inst. of Jiangsu, Prov. & Chinese Acad. of Sci., Nanjing, China. Our cordial thanks are extended to Mr. Yoshihiro Shinotuka, Ms. Miyako Kurihara, and Ms. Kiyomi Suzuki for their technical assistance during the course of this study.

REFERENCES

Cauwet-Marc, A.-M. (1979) Contribution de la caryologie a la connaissance de la systematique et de la phylogenie du genre *Bupleurum* L., *Coden Cndlar,* 34(1), 49–86.

Cave, M.S., Ed. (1958–1959) *Index to Plant Chromosome Numbers 1956–1957 and Supplement prior to 1956.* California Botanical Society, Berkeley.

Cave, M.S., Ed. (1959–1964) *Index to Plant Chromosome Numbers 1958–1964.* University of North Carolina Press, Chapel Hill.

Compilation Committee of Explanation for Pharmacopoeia of Japan. (2001) *Explanation for Pharmacopoeia of Japan,* 14th rev. ed., Hirokawa, Tokyo, D407–412 [in Japanese].

Darlington, C.D. and Wylie, A.P., Eds. (1955) *Chromosome Atlas of Flowering Plants.* George Allen & Unwin, London.

Engler, A. (1964) *A. Engler's Syllabus der Pflanzenfamilien.* Gebruder Borntraeger, Berlin, 376.

Federov, A.A., Ed. (1969) *Chromosome Numbers of Flowering Plants.* Izdatel'stva Nauka, Leningrad.

Goldblatt, P., Ed. (1981, 1984, 1985, 1988) *Index to Plant Chromosome Numbers 1975–1978, 1979–1981, 1982–1983, 1984–1985.* Monogr. Syst. Bot. from the Missouri Botanical Garden, 5, 8, 13, 23.

Goldblatt, P. and Johnson, D.E. (1990, 1991, 1994, 1996, 1998, 2000) *Index to Plant Chromosome Numbers 1986–1987, 1988–1989, 1990–1991, 1992–1993, 1994–1995, 1996–1997.* Monogr. Syst. Bot. from the Missouri Botanical Garden, 30, 40, 51, 58, 69, 81.

Guinea, M.C., Parellada, J., Lacaille-Dubois, M.A., and Wagner, H. (1994) Biologically active triperpene saponins from *Bupleurum fruticosum, Planta Med.,* 60, 163–167.

Hara, H. (1954) *Bupleurum* L. In *Enumeratio supermatophytarum japonicarum* (III), Iwanami-Shoten, Tokyo, 300–303 [in Japanese].

Hiroe, M. (1952) *Bupleurum* of Japan, *Acta Phytotaxon. Geobot.,* 16, 142–146.

Hiroe, M. (1958) *Bupleurum* L. In *Umbelliferae of Asia (excluding Japan),* No. 1. Eikodo, Tokyo, 75–91.

Jiang, C., Xu, N., Wang, H., Li, R., and Liu, M. (1994) Cytotaxonomical studies on *Bupleurum* L. in northeast China. I. Karyology analyses of six taxa and their significance of taxonomy, *Bull. Bot. Res.,* 14, 267–272 [in Chinese].

John, B. and Lewis, K.R. (1965) *Protoplasmatologia, Handbuch der Protoplasmaforshung* IV-F1, *The Meiotic System*. Springer-Verlag, New York.

Kayano, H. (1982) Chromosome variation and speciation. In Sakai, K., Ed., *Seitai-iden to shinka*. Shoukabo, Tokyo, 324–349 [in Japanese].

Kimata, H., Hiyama, C., Yahara, S., Tanaka, O., Ishikawa, O., and Aiura, M. (1979) Application of high performance liquid chromatography to the analysis of crude drugs: separatory determination of saponins of Bupleuri radix, *Chem. Pharm. Bull.*, 27, 1836–1841.

Kitagawa, M. (1947) Miscellaneous notes on Apiaceae (Umbelliferae) of Japan (V), *J. Jpn. Bot.*, 21, 95–100 [in Japanese].

Kitagawa, M. (1960) Synoptical review of Umbelliferae from Japan, Korea Manchuria, *Bull. Natl. Sci. Mus.* (Tokyo), 5, 1–35.

Kitamura, S. (1985) Plants of "Honzo-Komoku"; Saiko. In *Plants of "Honzo."* Hoikusha, Osaka, 158–159 [in Japanese].

Li, R., Jiang, C., Wang, H., and Liu, M. (1994) Chromosomes of so-called *Bupleurum falcatum* in northeast China, *Cytologia*, 59, 365–368.

Li, Y. and Sheh, M. (1979) *Bupleurum* L. In *Flora Reipublicae Popularis Sinicae*, Vol. 55(1). Science Press, Beijing, 215–295 [in Chinese].

Linchevskii, I.A. (1973) *Bupleurum* L. In Shishkin, B.K., Ed., *Flora of the U.S.S.R*., Vol. 16, Israel Program for Scientific Translation, Jerusalem, 196–251.

Matsumoto, H., Ohta, S., Yuan, C., Zhu, Y., Okada, M., and Miyamoto, K. (2004) Phylogenetic relationships among subgroups in *Bupleurum falcatum* L. *sensu lato* (Umbelliferae) based on restriction site variation of chloroplast DNA, *J. Jpn. Bot.*, 79, 79–90.

Moore, R.J., Ed. (1970–1974, 1977) Index to plant chromosome numbers for 1968, 1969, 1970, 1967–1971, 1972, 1973–1974. *Regnum Veg.*, 68, 77, 84, 90, 91, 96.

Nakai, H. (1937) Notulae ad plantas asiae orientalis (II), *J. Jpn. Bot.*, 13, 471–491.

Ohba, H. (1999) *Bupleurum* L. In Iwatsuki, K., Boufford, D.E., and Ohba, H., Eds., *Flora of Japan*, IIc. Kodansha, Tokyo, 275–277.

Ohta, S. (1991) Cytogenetical study on the speciation of *Bupleurum falcatum* L. (Umbelliferae), *J. Sci. Hiroshima Univ., Ser. B, Div. 2*, 23, 273–348.

Ohta, S. (1998) Cytogenetical and morphological studies on the Japanese, Chinese and Korean source plants of Bupleuri radix, *Proceedings of the 7th International Symposium on Traditional Medicine in Toyama*, 187–190.

Ohta, S., Liu, M., Zhu, Y., and Okada, M. (1993) Common distribution of *Bupleurum falcatum* L. with 2n=26 in Japan and China. *Abst. of the 15th Int. Bot. Cong. in Yokohama*, 231.

Ohta, S., Mitsuhashi, H., and Tanaka, R. (1986) Aneuploidal variation in *Bupleurum falcatum* L. from Japan, *J. Jpn. Bot.*, 61, 212–216 [in Japanese].

Ohta, S., Yuan, C., Zhu, Y., Okada, M., and He, S (1995) Cytogenetical and taxonomical studies on the source plants of Chinese Bupleurum radixes; characteristics in *B. scorzonerifolium* Willd. and *B. chinense* DC., *Abst. of the 42nd Annual Meeting of the Jpn. Soc. Pharm. in Fukuyama*, 198 [in Japanese].

Ohtsuka, K., Yakazu, D., and Shimizu, T. (1954) Saiko. In *Kanposhinryou no zissai*. Nanzando, Tokyo, 355 [in Japanese].

Ohwi, J. (1965) *Bupleurum* L. In *Flora of Japan*, rev. ed. Shibundo, Tokyo, 973–974 [in Japanese].

Ornduff, R., Ed. (1967–1969) Index to plant chromosome numbers for 1965/66/67. *Regnum Veg.*, 50, 55, 59.

Pan, Z., Zhuang, T., Xhou, X., Yao, X., and Lin, X. (1995) Karyotype analysis of four taxa of *Bupleurum* used in Chinese drugs, *J. Plant. Resourc. & Environ.*, 4, 41–45 [in Chinese].

Pan, S.L., Shun, Q.S., Bo, Q.M., and Bao, X.S. (2002) *The Coloured Atlas of the Medicinal Plants from Genus Bupleurum in China*, Shanghai Science & Technol. Doc. Publishing House, Shanghai.

Pharmacopoeia Committee of PRC. (1992) *Pharmacopoeia of the People's Republic of China*, English ed., Guantong Sci. & Tech. Press, Guangzhou, 154–155.

Shan, R. and Li, Y. (1974) On the Chinese species of *Bupleurum* L., *Acta Phytotaxon. Sin*., 12, 261–294.

Stebbins, G.L. (1971) *Chromosomal Evolution in Higher Plants*. Edward Arnold, London.

Tanaka, R. (1971) Types of resting nuclei in Orchidaceae, *Bot. Mag.* (Tokyo), 84, 118–122.

Tamaka, R. (1980) Karyotype. In Yamashita, K., Ed., *Saibo-bunretsu to saibo-iden*, Shoukabo, Tokyo, pp. 335–358.

Tanaka, R. (1982) Karyotype evolution. In: Sakai, K., Ed., *Seitai-iden to shinka*. Shoukabo, Tokyo, 462–493 [in Japanese].

Tanaka, R. (1987) The karyotype theory and wide crossing as an example in Orchidaceae, *Proc. Sino-Jpn. Symposium Pl. Chromos. Pl. Chromos Res.*, 1–10.

Tutin, T.G. (1968) *Bupleurum* L. In Tutin, T.G. et al., Eds., *Flora Europaea,* Vol. 2. Cambridge University Press, London, 345–350.

Wolff, H. (1910) *Bupleurum* L. In Engler, A. and Prantl, K., Eds., *Pflanzenreich,* Vol. 43 (IV 228), Academie Verlag, Berlin, 36–173.

Yamazaki, T. (2001) *Bupleurum* L. Umbelliferae in Japan I, *J. Jpn. Bot.*, 76, 145–149.

Zhu, Y. (1977) *Bupleurum* L. In *Flora Plantarum Herbacearum Chinae Boreali-Orientalis*, Vol. 6. Science Press, Beijing, 188–200 [in Chinese].

Zhu, Y. (1989) Chaihu. In *Plantae Medicinales Chinae Boreali-Orientalis Redactoribus Principalibus*. Heilongjiang Sci. & Technol. Publishing House, Harbin, 811–814 [in Chinese].

Section II

Cultivation

5 Cultivation of *Bupleurum falcatum* in Japan

Osamu Iida

CONTENTS

5.1   INTRODUCTION

In Japan, *Bupleurum falcatum* L. is cultivated for its roots. The crude drug preparation obtained from the roots is called "Saiko" in Japanese, and only that from this species is official in Japan for use in Chinese medicines.

Bupleurum falcatum L. grows naturally in areas to the west of the Kanto region (central Japan on the Pacific Ocean side, Figure 5.1). Its wild roots have been used as medicine since ancient times, and those produced in the Izu and Kyushu areas are considered to be of good quality (Nanba and Tani, 1973). The production of Saiko in Japan from wild roots was 0.4 to 0.5 tons in 1943–1944 (Nagai, 1968), and reached a peak of 3.7 tons in 1963 (Mat. Drug Data, 1964), but decreased markedly thereafter due to excessive collection and changes in the natural environment. In the early 1980s, wild root-derived Saiko in Japan completely disappeared. In addition to the decreased domestic collection, the cost of producing Saiko in Japan was higher than overseas. Therefore, imports increased while cultivation in Japan was advanced. Most of the Saiko has been imported from China (but not from *B. falcatum*), and on occasion from Korea *B. falcatum*, with as much as 100 tons brought in 1973 (Mat. Drug Data, 1974).

The cultivation of *B. falcatum* L. in Japan was started in the latter half of the 1940s (Hatta, 1947), and spread to various areas from about 1955. In 1976, cultivation sharply increased. In September 1976, Chinese medicines began to be increasingly used in health care in Japan, and demand rapidly increased. In particular, the demand for "Sho-saiko-to" increased markedly, and

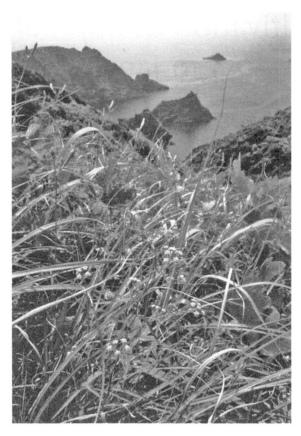

FIGURE 5.1 Wild plants of *B. falcatum* L. that grow at Irozaki in Shizuoka Prefecture. They grow in grassland that faces the Pacific Ocean, and have a salt tolerance.

as a result, the demand for its major component, Saiko, also increased. The cultivation of *B. falcatum* L. in Japan reached a peak in about 1990 (Figure 5.2), when the cultivation area was 722 ha, and production was 251 tons (Mat. Drug Data, 1992). In the early 1990s, drug poisoning due to the inappropriate use of Sho-saiko-to became a problem. In addition, a recession in Japan occurred, and the demand for Chinese medicines and Sho-saiko-to rapidly decreased, resulting in a rapid decline in the cultivation of *B. falcatum* L. The latest data (Mat. Drug Data, 2002) show that the cultivation area and production of Saiko in 2000 were 2.9 ha and 11.4 tons, respectively, and the cultivation area/farmer and the mean yield (dry roots) per 10 are were 10.4 are (are = 100 m^2) and 34 kg, respectively. The major cultivation areas were Kochi, Ibaragi, Gunma, Oita, Kumamoto, and Nara Prefectures.

In Japan, *B. falcatum* L. is cultivated mostly under prior contract with pharmaceutical manufacturers or dealers. This contract is important because of the limitations in the demand for and uses of Saiko, the necessity for a stable supply, and the guarantee of producers' price.

5.2 GROWTH CHARACTERISTICS

Bupleurum falcatum L. is a perennial herbaceous plant, and its growth is very slow in the wild. Bolting does not occur in the first year. However, during cultivation, many individual plants show bolting/flowering in the first year under good conditions, and are larger than the wild types.

There have been several studies on the growth of *B. falcatum* L. and seasonal changes in the constituents of its roots (Figure 5.3) (Tanaka et al., 1988; Minami et al., 1995). In this chapter, root

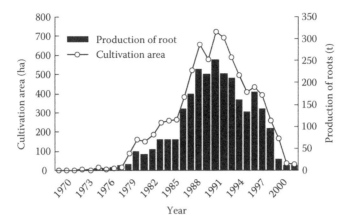

FIGURE 5.2 Cultivation area and production of roots (as crude drug) of *B. falcatum* L. in Japan, 1970–2000. (Sources: Shoyaku Shiryo, from 1970 through 1978; Yakuyo Sakumotsu (Shoyaku) Kankeishiryo, from 1979 through 2000.)

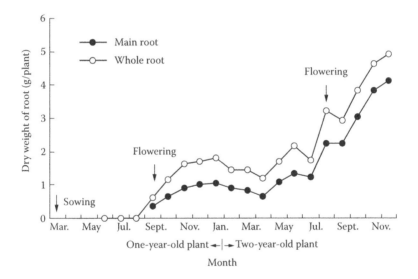

FIGURE 5.3 Seasonal variations of dry weight of whole and main root per *Bupleurum* plant cultivated at Tsukuba Medicinal Plant Research Station (Iida and Satake, 1986).

growth in the northern part of the Kanto region (Tsukuba, Ibaraki Prefecture) is described (Iida and Satake, 1986). In general, sowing is performed in spring, and germination occurs after 1 month. Bolting starts in July, budding occurs in August, and flowering in September. In November, frost causes the aerial part to wither and die. *Bupleurum* roots grow very slowly in the initial phase but rapidly develop from autumn to winter. The next year, sprouts occur in early March, and bolting/flowering occurs 1 to 2 months earlier than in the first year. Survival for about 3 years is possible in field cultivation.

5.3 METHOD OF CULTIVATION

In terms of quality, Saiko should be prepared from perennial plant roots that correspond to wild roots. However, due to disease, *B. falcatum* L. is mostly harvested after 1 year in Japan excluding some snowfall areas where the plant is harvested after 2 years. Seeds are obtained from biennial or older plants.

Cultivation may be performed by direct sowing or transplantation. At present, only the former method is used. The main points in cultivation are to select suitable land, to raise an adequate number of plants per unit area, to control weeds, and to supply fertilizers effectively.

There are many studies (Kawanishi et al., 1983) and books (Fujita, 1972; Ministry of Health and Welfare, 1992) on the cultivation of *B. falcatum* L. The basic cultivation method used in the Kanto region is introduced below.

5.3.1 SUITABLE CULTIVATION AREAS

For the economical cultivation of *B. falcatum* L., warm areas similar to its natural climate are suitable. Cultivation is possible in cold and snowfall areas, but growth is poor (Horikoshi et al., 1976a, 1976b). The other requirements are fertile loam and clay loam, much sunshine, and good water retention and drainage.

5.3.2 SPECIES

All *B. falcatum* L. cultivated at present in Japan has the chromosome number $2n = 26$ obtained by adaptation of wild plants (Ohta, 1991). There are no special cultivarieties obtained by breeding. Seeds for reproduction are renewed by means of home seed-raising in each cultivation group or by individual cultivators. Even using the seeds in the same lot, the plants in a population show variations in the time of bolting and flowering, plant height, and size of leaves and roots. These variations may be genetic, and selection breeding is necessary.

5.3.3 SOWING

The optimum temperature of germination for *B. falcatum* L. is 15 to 20°C, and seeding is generally performed from the middle of March to the middle of April. The other method is sowing immediately after seed collection in autumn. The advantages of sowing in autumn are an early germination the next spring and early growth compared with sowing in spring. However, this method is rarely utilized because much time is required for the prevention of seed scattering due to wind during the winter and for weed control.

Shallow sowing furrows (15 to 20 cm) are made with a ridge width of 60 to 70 cm. The amount of seeds sown is 600 to 800 g/10 are. Germination is slow, and it takes about 1 month before the cotyledons appear above the ground. Germination is promoted by exposing seeds to flowing water for 2 days before sowing (Liu et al., 1995). This may be because germination inhibitors (Momonoki et al., 1978, 1979, 1981) contained in seeds are removed by flowing water (Ohashi and Aikawa, 1965). Seeds are covered with about 5 mm of soil, which is softly pressed with the sole of the foot or an instrument. For good germination, chaff or straw is placed on the soil to prevent drying.

To prevent weeds, a herbicide is sometimes sprayed after sowing. Pendimethalin (commercial name: Go-Go-San in Japanese) is the only weed-killer approved for *B. falcatum* L. in Japan.

5.3.4 FERTILIZER APPLICATION

Before plowing, 2 tons of compost, 50 to 100 kg of exhausted rapeseed oilcake, 100 kg of magnesia lime, and 20 kg of chemical fertilizer per 10 are are applied as basal fertilizer, and the soil is plowed to a depth of about 20 cm. Due to slow early growth, slow-releasing chemical fertilizer is used. Later, 40 to 50 kg of chemical fertilizer is applied in June and September, the bolting and flowering periods, respectively. As additional fertilizer in the second year, 100 to 150 kg of organic fertilizers such as chicken droppings and rapeseed oilcake and 20 kg of chemical fertilizer are applied in

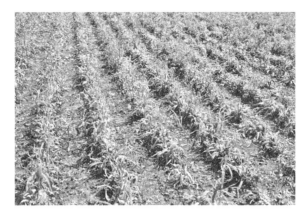

FIGURE 5.4 One-year-old *Bupleurum* plants at bolting stage (July).

March, the sprouting period, and 40 to 50 kg each of chemical fertilizer in May and September. When necessary, trace elements are applied.

5.3.5 PLANT CARE

When germination occurs, thinning is performed two to three times so that the plants form a zigzag with an intrarow spacing of 5 to 10 cm (Figure 5.4). After application of additional fertilizer, soil is brought to the base of plants partly for weed control (Figure 5.5 and Figure 5.6).

When growth is good, even annual plants bolt and flower, and therefore, the aerial parts are cut at a height of 70 cm in the early phase of budding. Subsequently, elongated floral branches are cut again. Top pinching is not always necessary for annual plants, but is necessary for dense planting or biennial cultivation (except for seed-producing plants). Top pinching is performed while leaves remain on the main stem, and has a marked effect in promoting root growth (Hatta, 1947) and allowing flexible root growth by inhibiting lignification (Hosoda and Noguchi, 1993).

5.3.6 PLANT PROTECTION

5.3.6.1 Disease

Dry root-rot disease is the most serious disease in the cultivation of *B. falcatum* L., preventing the production of good-quality Saiko (Kurata and Fujita, 1963a). This disease was the primary cause

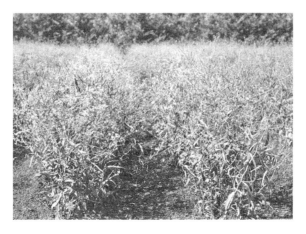

FIGURE 5.5 One-year-old *Bupleurum* plants at flowering time (October) in the standard row cultivation.

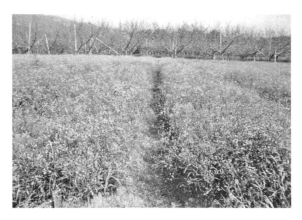

FIGURE 5.6 Dense planting in the bed cultivation. Although high root yield is produced, much labor is required in various activities.

of the establishment of an annual cultivation regime of this plant. Slightly depressed brown to dark brown pathological patches develop on the root head near the verge of the ground and gradually extend to the entire root, resulting in drying and decay. This disease is due to a complex infection of pathogenic fungi such as *Phoma terrestris* , *Fusarium oxysporum* , and *Phomopsis* sp. (Kurata and Fujita, 1963b).

Anthracnose (*Colletotrichum* sp.) is a major disease in the aerial parts of the plant and characterized by blackening and death from withering at the tip, stem, and branches of the plant (Sato et al., 1992). It occurs in June and September during rainy periods in Japan. The root is only slightly affected. However, when the disease is severe, root growth is inhibited, and no seeds are collected from seed-producing plants. There was a large outbreak of this disease throughout the country in 1985 (Iida et al., 1987), but no great damage has been observed since.

Other diseases include leaf spot (*Phoma* sp.) (Suyama and Nishi, 1981), sickle hare's ear yellows (*Mycoplasma* -like organisms) (Shiomi et al., 1983), southern blight, and damping-off.

Measures to combat these diseases include the disinfection of soil and seeds, avoidance of repeated cultivation on the same plots, selection of land with good drainage, and use of organic fertilizer as primary fertilizer, avoiding the frequent use of chemical fertilizers, especially nitrogenous ones.

5.3.6.2 Insect Damage

Common cutworms develop in the early stages of growth, armyworms after the middle stages, aphids and mites before and after the flowering stage, bugs in the fructification stage, and root-knot-nematodes (*Meloidogyne* sp.) (Sato et al., 1992) in the root.

5.3.7 HARVESTING

Roots are harvested after several frosts, which is from the middle of November to the middle of January in the Kanto region. The aerial parts are cropped from the verge of the ground, and the roots are dug out using hoes or harvest machines (Figure 5.7 and Figure 5.8). The remaining stem is then cut, and the roots are washed in the water by hand while being rubbed to remove soil and sand, dried in the sun for 1 to 2 days, and rubbed with the hands while the main root is still flexible to remove fibrous and thin roots (Figure 5.9). Subsequently, the roots are dried until they snap (water content, about 10%), further dried, and stored in paper bags at low humidity.

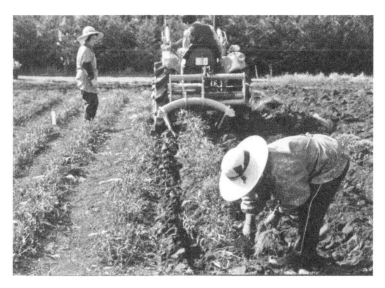

FIGURE 5.7 Harvesting of *Bupleurum* roots by the root digger attached to a tractor at Tsukuba Medicinal Plant Research Station.

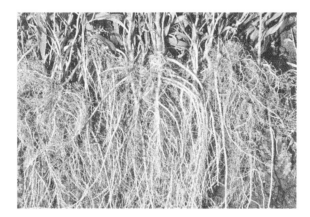

FIGURE 5.8 Harvested one-year-old *Bupleurum* roots. The remaining stems are cut, and the roots are washed in the water, and then are sun-dried.

The yield of roots markedly changes according to weather and cultivation conditions. The dry weight per 10 are varies from several kilograms to more than 100 kg. The mean dry yield of roots per 10 are prepared as Saiko in annual cultivation is 30 to 40 kg. In biennial cultivation, a mean yield of 70 to 90 kg/10 are can be expected.

5.3.8 REPRODUCTION OF SEEDS

Seeds are collected from biennial or older plants. Fructification is also observed in some annual plants, but the roots of these early flowering plants are generally small. Seeds collected from early flowering plants form a population showing even earlier flowering, with the risk of subsequent reduced root yield (Ohashi and Kuribayashi, 1972). Therefore, seed collection from annual plants should be avoided. Seeds yield of 2-year-old plants per 10 are is 40 to 50 kg (Fujita, 1972). After seed collection the roots are also used for medicine.

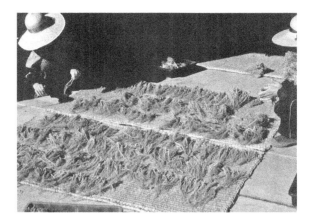

FIGURE 5.9 Sun-drying and preparation of the roots for crude drug. The roots are rubbed with hands to remove fibrous and thin roots.

5.4 QUALITY ASSESSMENT

The quality assessment method for Saiko is very important not only for cultivators but also for users. There is no single parameter for the quality assessment of crude drugs including Saiko, and multiple parameters are used.

The Japanese Pharmacopoeia (JP) gives the most basic criteria for quality assessment, providing the origin of the plant, description, identification, purity, and standard values. The JP 14th edition (2001) shows only *B. falcatum* L. as the original species for Saiko and provides the following purity and various standard values:

> Purity:
> 1. Stem and leaf — The amount of stems and leaves contained in *Bupleurum* root does not exceed 10.0%.
> 2. Foreign matter — The amount of foreign matter other than stems and leaves contained in *Bupleurum* root does not exceed 1.0%.
>
> Total ash: Not more than 6.5%
> Acid-insoluble ash: Not more than 2.0%
> Extract content: Dilute ethanol-soluble extract — not less than 11.0%

The dilute ethanol-soluble extract content (extract content) in Saiko produced in Japan is 15% or more, readily clearing the JP standard. The extract content shows seasonal variation (Figure 5.10) (Iida and Satake, 1986) and changes according to drying conditions after harvest. Air-drying for about 1 week after root harvest increases the extract content compared with warm wind drying at 50°C immediately after harvest (Aoyagi et al., 2001).

Saikosaponin (SS) is a major active component, and its content is also a parameter for the quality assessment of Saiko (Yamamoto, 1980). However, the JP has not yet provided the content of SS. The SS-a, -c, and -d content of roots cultivated in Japan is generally 1 to 2%. The SS content in roots also shows seasonal changes, increasing in spring and from autumn to winter (Iida and Satake, 1986). In addition, the SS content of roots differs according to the plant species (Shimokawa et al., 1980), conditions of cultivation (Kawanishi et al., 1983), size (Shimokawa and Ohashi, 1980), and position of the root (Tani et al., 1986). In the assessment of Saiko as a crude drug, an extremely high SS content does not always indicate quality, and Saiko with a stable SS content and stable drug efficacy is more desirable. Cultivation should aim at Saiko of uniform quality.

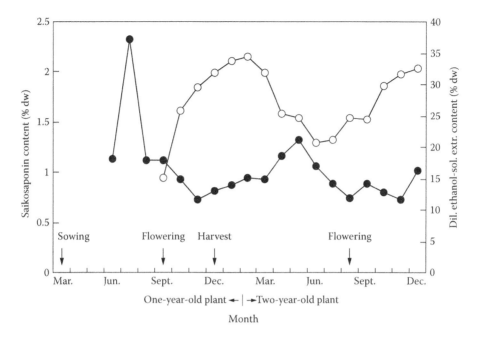

FIGURE 5.10 Seasonal variations of Saikosaponin (a–c–d) content and dilute ethanol-soluble extract content of *Bupleurum* roots cultivated at Tsukuba Medicinal Plant Research Station: (●), Saikosaponin (a–c–d); (○), dilute ethanol-soluble extract (Iida and Satake, 1986).

Compared with wild products, cultivated Saiko is hard, breaks easily, is poor in specific fat-like aroma, and has little oily moisture (Nanba and Tani, 1973). In other words, Saiko of good quality has a rich surface color, aroma, and few fibrous roots, and is less fibrous, which is close to the characteristics of the wild products (Nishimoto, 1981). The traditional method of assessment using the five senses is also important in the quality assessment of crude drugs, but requires long experience and is difficult to use. A new scientific quality assessment method that directly and readily evaluates the quality of Saiko is necessary.

REFERENCES

Aoyagi, M., Iida, O., and Anetai, M. (2001) Preparation and chemical evaluation of *Bupleurum* root. Preparation condition and variation of sugar and dilute ethanol-soluble extract contents, *Rep. Hokkaido Inst. Public Health*, 51, 100–102.

Fujita, S. (1972) Mishimasaiko. In *Yakuyo Shokubutu Saibai Zenka*. Nousan Gyoson Bunka Kyokai, Tokyo, 306–313.

Hatta, R. (1947) Study on the cultivation of *Bupleurum falcatum* L., *Shoyaku*, 1, 16–19.

Horikoshi, T., Homma, N., and Ishizaki, S. (1976a) Studies on the cultivation of medicinal plants — on the germination and growth of *Bupleurum falcatum* L., *Eisei Shikenjo Hokoku*, 94, 163–166.

Horikoshi, T., Homma, N., and Ishizaki, S. (1976b) Studies on the cultivation of medicinal plants on the growth and yield of *Bupleurum falcatum* L., *Eisei Shikenjo Hokoku*, 94, 166–169.

Hosoda, K. and Noguchi, M. (1993) Studies on the cultivation of *Bupleurum falcatum* L. — effects of disbudding and picking flower on the root growth and root morphology, *Shoyakugaku Zasshi*, 47, 39–42.

Iida, O. and Satake, M. (1986) Study on breeding of *Bupleurum falcatum* L. — on growth and component of the root. Proceedings of the 33rd Annual Meeting of the Japanese Society of Pharmacognosy, 54.

Iida, O., Satake, M., Ichinohe, M., Minoura, S., Okada, M., and Mitsuhashi, H. (1987) Study on anthracnose of *Bupleurum falcatum* L. — occurrence of the disease. *Proceedings of the 34th Annual Meeting of the Japanese Society of Pharmacognosy*, 58.

Kawanishi, F., Nagaoka, Y., Watanabe, H., Oshio, H., and Nakamoto, K. (1983) On the cultivation of *Bupleurum falcatum* L. (Mishima-saiko), *J. Takada Res. Lab.*, 42, 57–63.

Kurata, H. and Fujita, S. (1963a) Notes on the dry root-rot disease of *Bupleurum falcatum* L. — isolation of pathogenic fungi from the leaf, stem and root, *Eisei Shikenjo Hokoku*, 81, 182–183.

Kurata, H. and Fujita, S. (1963b) Notes on the dry root-rot disease of *Bupleurum falcatum* L. — inoculation experiment by use of isolates, *Eisei Shikenjo Hokoku*, 81, 184–186.

Liu, S., Wu, W., Wang, J., Son, L., Yen, M., and Lin, C. (1995) Studies on the agronomic characteristics, yield, and saikosaponin content of two *Bupleurum* species in Taiwan, *Am. J. Chin. Med.*, 23, 181–194.

Minami, M., Sugino, M., Sadaoka, M., Ashida, K., and Ogaki, K. (1995) Seasonal variation of growth and saikosaponin content of *Bupleurum falcatum* L., *Yakugaku Zasshi*, 115, 145–155.

Ministry of Health and Welfare (1960–1984) Mat. Drug Data 1959–1983. Ministry of Health and Welfare, Tokyo.

Ministry of Health and Welfare (1992) Mishimasaiko. In *Medicinal Plants, Cultivation and Quality Assessment*, Part 1. Yakuji Nippousha, Tokyo, 53–62.

Ministry of Health, Labour and Welfare (2001) *The Japanese Pharmacopoeia*, 14th ed. Ministry of Health, Labour and Welfare, Tokyo, 862.

Momonoki, Y., Hasegawa, T., Ota, Y., Kaneki, R., and Suzuki, T. (1978) Studies on the germination of seeds of *Bupleurum falcatum* L. — germination inhibitors of *B. falcatum* seeds, *Jpn. J. Crop Sci.*, 47, 197–205.

Momonoki, Y., Hasegawa, T., Ota, Y., Tanabe, T., Suzuki, T., and Kaneki, R. (1979) Studies on the germination of seeds of *Bupleurum falcatum* L. — germination inhibitors of *B. falcatum* seeds (2), *Jpn. J. Crop Sci.*, 48, 311–316.

Momonoki, Y., Ota, Y., and Hasegawa, T. (1981) Studies on the germination of seeds of *Bupleurum falcatum* L. — germination inhibitors of *B. falcatum* seeds (3), *Jpn. J. Crop Sci.*, 50, 143–147.

Nagai, Y. (1968) Present status of Saiko market. *Proceedings of the 3rd Medicinal Plants Cultivation Workshop*, 34th Annual Meeting of the Japanese Society of Pharmacognosy, 5.

Nanba, T. and Tani, T. (1973) Introduction of Bupleuri radix, *Taisha*, 10 (Extra ed. no.), 667–675.

Nishimoto, K. (1981) The quality of *Bupleurum* root (chaihu), *J. Trad. Sino-Jpn. Med.*, 1, 51–56.

Ohashi, H. and Aikawa, S. (1965) On some problems in the cultivation of Mishimasaiko, *Bupleurum falcatum* L., *Shoyakugaku Zasshi*, 19, 32–35.

Ohashi, H. and Kuribayashi, T. (1972) On the trial selection of annual crop in *Bupleurum falcatum* (preliminary report), *Shoyakugaku Zasshi*, 27, 41–43.

Ohta, S. (1991) Cytological study on the speciation of *Bupleurum falcatum* L. (Umbelliferae). *J. Sci. Hiroshima Univ. Ser. B, Div. 2* (Botany), 23, 273–348.

Sato, T., Matsuhashi, M., and Iida, O. (1992) Fungi isolated from diseased medicinal plants. *Eisei Shikenjo Hokoku*, 110, 60–66.

Shimokawa, Y. and Ohashi, H. (1980) Cultivation and breeding of *Bupleurum falcatum* L. — relation among cultivation years, root growth and saikosaponin content, *Shoyakugaku Zasshi*, 34, 235–238.

Shimokawa, Y., Okuda, I., Kuwano, M., and Ohashi, H. (1980) Cultivation and breeding of *Bupleurum falcatum* L. — geographical variation of *B. falcatum*, *Shoyakugaku Zasshi*, 34, 239–244.

Shiomi, T., Choi, Y.M., and Sugiura, M. (1983) Occurrence and host range of sickle hare's ear (*Bupleurum falcatum* L.) yellows in Japan. *Ann. Phytopathol. Soc. Jpn.*, 49, 228–238.

Suyama, K. and Nishi, K. (1981) Diseases of medicinal plants. *Shokubutu Boueki*, 35, 34–38.

Tanaka, T., Ito, T., Sakai, E., Mizuno, M., Kawamura, T., Hisata, Y., Okuda et al. (1988) Cultivation and saponin contents of Guangxi *Bupleurum, Shoyakugaku Zasshi*, 42, 236–239.

Tani, T., Katsuki, T., Kubo, M., and Arichi, S. (1986) Histochemistry — distribution of saikosaponins in *Bupleurum falcatum* root, *J. Chromatogr.*, 360, 407–416.

Yakuyo Sakumotsu (Shoyaku) Kankeishiryo 1979–2000 (1980–2002) Zaidanhojin Nihon Tokusan-nosanbutsu Kyokai, Tokyo.

Yamamoto, M. (1980) Biochemistry of *Bupleurum falcatum* L., *J. Trad. Sino-Jpn. Med.*, 1, 41–44.

6 Distribution of Saikosaponins of *Bupleurum falcatum* and Variation of Its Contents in Plant Organs by Environmental Factors

Nak-Sul Seong, Hae-Gon Chung, and Kwan-Su Kim

CONTENTS

6.1 INTRODUCTION

The useful components of *Bupleurum falcatum* are mainly saponin derivatives and polysaccharides, which are present in underground parts. Recently, flavonoids, lignans, essential oil, and steroids are reported in aboveground plant organs. Saikosaponin and sub-saponin are mainly distributed in the root and also found in the other plant organs such as the stem and leaf (Kim et al., 1997). Saikosaponin was detected among the plant organs in the order of the pericycle, periderm, phloem, and xylem (Tani et al., 1986). According to Zhang (1985), thick root contains a small amount of saikosaponins but these are higher in the side roots. The variation of saponin synthesis and accumulation of the compound mainly depended on the species, weather, soil condition, and environmental factors. However, the temperature of the cultivation area, soil condition, altitude, and precipitation are identified as the major factors influencing compound variations (Shimokawa et al., 1980b; Tanaka et al., 1988; Mizukami et al., 1991; Park et al., 1995; Watanabe et al., 1998). The variation of components was affected by plant condition, characteristics of individual plant, fertilization, and cultivation methods (Ohashi and Kuribayashi, 1967, 1972; Ostuka et al., 1977; Hosoda and Noguchi, 1990). A variation in saikosaponins and a decrease in growth rate and other compounds were detected during the plant developmental stages (Minami et al., 1995). Shimokawa (1980c) pointed out that the chemical content and growth characters did not show significant difference to the bolting rate at low temperature. Meanwhile the flowering and fertilization rate was high at moderate temperature, but a high capacity of root yield was observed at low temperature. However, saikosaponin content showed no difference (Shimokawa et al., 1980c). On the contrary, with cultivation of densely populated plants, dry root weight was reduced and the saikosaponin content was increased.

6.2 VARIATION OF SAIKOSAPONIN CONTENT BETWEEN THE CULTIVAR AND COLLECTED WILD POPULATIONS

Two cultivars (Korean local cultivar "Jeongsun" and Japanese cultivar "Mishima," hereafter called Jeongsun and Mishima) of *B. falcatum* in Korea were compared under different environmental factors to obtain useful information and selection for a high-yielding breeding line with a high content of saikosaponins.

Bupleurum euphorbiodes and *B. longiradiatum* were investigated to compare the saponin content and the ratio of outer phloem layer. We collected the species (*B. euphorbiodes, B. longiradiatum*) at Seorak mountain in Kangwon province and also *B. scorzonaefolium* at Hanla mountain on Jeju Island. Jeongsun was collected from Jeongsun, Kangwon province in Korea and Mishima was collected in Suwon and imported from Japan to compare the saikosaponin contents under the different ecological conditions in Korea. The saikosaponin content of plants from different collection areas is shown in Table 6.1. The content of saikosaponin-d was high in *B. scorzonaefolium,* and in cultivars Jeongsun and Mishima. Saikosaponin was detected only in the leaf of *B. scorzonaefolium* and Mishima. In comparing the saikosaponin content of the cultivars and collected lines, Jeongsun (1.01%) was higher than in other investigated populations (0.24 to 0.92%). Meanwhile the Mishima was high at root weight (1.0 g) and the ratio of outer phloem layer (74.0%). With these results, a high-yield productivity breeding line can be expected with the combination of good root growth character of Mishima with the high saikosaponin content of Jeongsun.

6.3 VARIATION OF SAIKOSAPONIN AND COMPARISON OF ITS CONTENT BETWEEN THE JEONGSUN AND MISHIMA CULTIVARS

The saikosaponin content of roots from 100 plants of the Jeongsun and Mishima cultivars was analyzed (Table 6.2). The saikosaponin content of Jeongsun was high: the maximum value was 2.15%, average 1.26%, and minimum 0.42%. The values were 1.94, 0.91, and 0.43% in the Mishima

TABLE 6.1
Comparison of Saikosaponins Content in Root and Leaf of Some *Bupleurum* Species Collected from Different Areas

Species	Saikosaponin (%) in Root				Saikosaponin (%) in Leaf			
	c	d	a	Total	c	d	a	Total
B. falcatum (Jeongsun)	0.14	0.35	0.52	1.01	0.00	0.00	0.00	0.00
B. falcatum (Mishima)	0.13	0.27	0.27	0.67	0.08	0.10	0.02	0.20
B. scorzonaefolium	0.08	0.44	0.39	0.92	0.02	0.19	0.02	0.24
B. longiradiatum	0.07	0.13	0.04	0.24	nd[a]	nd	nd	—
B. euphorbiodes	nd	nd	nd	—	nd	nd	nd	—

[a] nd: not detected in HPLC (0.05 AUFS).

TABLE 6.2
Mean, Range, Standard Deviation, and Coefficient of Variation of Saikosaponin Content (%) in Jeongsun and Mishima Cultivars

Cultivars	Components[a]	Min	Max	Range	Mean	SD	CV
Jeongsun	Sc	0.00	0.32	0.31	0.12	0.08	53.2
	Sd	0.17	0.95	0.78	0.50	0.18	33.0
	Sa	0.22	1.18	1.01	0.63	0.23	33.1
	Total	0.42	2.15	1.72	1.26	0.36	31.5
Mishima	Sc	0.06	0.35	0.29	0.17	0.06	32.6
	Sd	0.18	0.85	0.67	0.39	0.13	31.7
	Sa	0.17	0.77	0.60	0.35	0.11	31.2
	Total	0.43	1.94	1.50	0.91	0.26	28.6

[a] Sc: saikosaponin-c, Sd: saikosaponin-d, Sa: saikosaponin-a.

TABLE 6.3
Mean, Range, Standard Deviation, and Coefficient of Variation for Saikosaponin Content (%) in Leaf of Mishima Cultivar

Components[a]	Min	Max	Range	Mean	SD	CV
Sc	0.05	0.40	0.36	0.18	0.08	41.6
Sd	0.00	0.79	0.79	0.32	0.19	59.5
Sa	0.00	0.17	0.17	0.06	0.04	76.4
Total	0.05	1.27	1.22	0.55	0.29	53.6

[a] Sc: saikosaponin-c, Sd: saikosaponin-d, Sa: saikosaponin-a.

cultivar. The maximum content of saikosaponin was in leaf (1.27%), average (0.55%), and minimum (0.05%) at the time of flowering on apex, but in Jeongsun it was not detected (Table 6.3).

The negative correlation coefficient showed on the saikosaponin content mainly depended on the plant height, number of branches, number of peduncle, the length and width of leaf in Jeongsun population, but there was no significant difference among the characters of Mishima cultivar (Table 6.4).

Among the saikosaponin content and characters of the root and rhizome and flowering periods, there was negative correlation coefficient with root characters in the Jeongsun; however, there was no significant difference of the roots in both populations (Table 6.5).

Generally, between each growth character and saikosaponin content there was no difference in both populations due to high variation values among the individual plants in the two populations, which were assumed to be influenced by environmental factors. However, it was highly expected that the saikosaponin content was mainly dependent on the characters at the flowering time in both populations.

TABLE 6.4
Correlation Coefficients between Saikosaponin Content and Shoot Characters in Jeongsun and Mishima Cultivars

Cultivar	Saikosaponin	Plant Height	No. of Branches	No. of Peduncles	Leaf Area	Leaf W/L	No. of Nodes	Stem Thickness	Top Weight
Jeongsun	c	−0.07	−0.03	0.37*	−0.29*	−0.29*	0.11	−0.16	−0.03
	d	−0.16	−0.27*	0.08	−0.03	−0.17	−0.04	−0.18	−0.26*
	a	0.02	−0.19	0.32*	−0.04	−0.21*	−0.07	−0.15	−0.10
	Total	−0.04	−0.22	0.26*	−0.08	−0.23*	−0.04	−0.18	−0.17
Mishima	c	−0.03	−0.20	0.00	0.00	0.01	−0.08	−0.15	−0.19
	d	−0.04	−0.17	0.05	0.03	0.04	−0.11	−0.03	0.06
	a	−0.06	−0.10	0.07	−0.00	−0.00	−0.05	−0.00	0.09
	Total	−0.05	−0.16	0.06	0.02	0.02	−0.09	−0.05	0.02

Note: * Significant at the 0.05 probability level.

TABLE 6.5
Correlation Coefficients between Saikosaponin Content and Root Characters and Flowering Date in Jeongsun and Mishima Cultivars

Cultivar	Saikosaponin	Root Weight	Root Length	No. of Lateral Roots	Root Diameter	Flowering Date
Jeongsun	c	−0.18	−0.08	−0.07	−0.16	−0.32*
	d	−0.20	0.06	−0.13	−0.31*	−0.25*
	a	−0.13	0.06	−0.11	−0.20	−0.23*
	Total	−0.18	0.04	−0.13	−0.26*	−0.28*
Mishima	c	−0.26*	−0.12	−0.05	−0.17	−0.06
	d	0.01	−0.04	−0.05	0.02	−0.25*
	a	0.06	−0.08	0.03	0.02	−0.21*
	Total	−0.03	−0.07	−0.02	−0.02	−0.22*

Note: * Significant at the 0.05 probability level.

6.4 VARIATION OF SAIKOSAPONIN CONTENT BY DIFFERENT PLANT ORGANS AND DEVELOPMENTAL STAGES

To determine the distribution of saikosaponin content in different plant organs such as root, leaf, and stem, these were specially analyzed at the time of flowering on apex. The total saikosaponin content was 0.92% in root, 0.55% in leaf, 0.04% in stem, and saikosaponin-d was detected in the root and leaf but saikosaponin-c was relatively high in the stem (Table 6.6). Distribution of saikosaponin content in the root was high in the xylem and in the outer phloem layer of both cultivars. The main components were different: high saikosaponin-a in Jeongsun, high saikosaponin-d in Mishima cultivar (Table 6.7). The components were identified as the same in xylem and outer phloem layer of both cultivars. Comparison of saikosaponin content by planting years was high in both investigated populations as a high ratio of outer phloem layer in one-year-old root (Table 6.8). Since the chemical components were decreased during developmental stages, it was assumed that

TABLE 6.6
Comparison of Saikosaponin Content (%) and Its Composition in Root, Leaf, and Stem of Mishima Cultivar

Components[a]	Root	Leaf	Stem
Sc	0.17	0.18	0.03
Sd	0.40	0.31	0.01
Sa	0.35	0.06	0.01
Total	0.92	0.55	0.04
Composition	Sd > Sa > Sc	Sd > Sc > Sa	Sc > Sa > Sd

[a] Sc: saikosaponin-c, Sd: saikosaponin-d, Sa: saikosaponin-a.

TABLE 6.7
Comparison of Saikosaponin Content (%) in Xylem and Outer Phloem Layer (OPL) of Root in Jeongsun and Mishima Cultivars

Components[a]	Jeongsun		Mishima	
	Xylem	OPL	Xylem	OPL
Sc	0.05	0.19	0.03	0.17
Sd	0.14	0.45	0.05	0.35
Sa	0.20	0.67	0.04	0.34
Total	0.39	1.31	0.13	0.86
Composition	Sa > Sd > Sc		Sd > Sa > Sc	

[a] Sc: saikosaponin-c, Sd: saikosaponin-d, Sa: saikosaponin-a.

TABLE 6.8
Yearly Changes in Saikosaponin Content (%) of Jeongsun and Mishima Cultivars

Growing Years	Jeongsun[a]				Mishima			
	Sc	Sd	Sa	Total	Sc	Sd	Sa	Total
1	0.11	0.53	0.67	1.30	0.08	0.41	0.36	0.85
2	0.13	0.36	0.39	0.88	0.12	0.29	0.24	0.64
3	0.10	0.35	0.35	0.74	0.08	0.27	0.20	0.55

[a] Sc: saikosaponin-c, Sd: saikosaponin-d, Sa: saikosaponin-a.

the greater the increased root weights, the less the content that could be detected with low outer phloem ratio (Figure 6.1). The saikosaponin content during the developmental stages was not different in composition, and saikosaponin-a, -c, -d were always high in Jeongsun cultivar at the three successive stages.

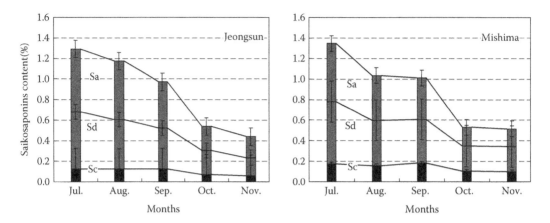

FIGURE 6.1 Seasonal changes in saikosaponin content of root in two cultivars of *B. falcatum* L.

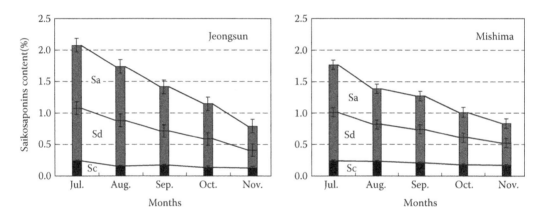

FIGURE 6.2 Seasonal changes in saikosaponin content in the outer phloem layer of root in two cultivars of *B. falcatum* L.

The variation of chemical components in the root during successive months in both populations decreased in the outer phloem layer of root (Figure 6.2). The variation of saikosaponin content in different plant organs and the decreased ratio of content in Jeongsun were not detected in the components in the leaves and stems during the plant developmental stages. Meanwhile, a higher saikosaponin content was detected in the leaf of Mishima and the highest content was detected in July at the time of bolting stage. The content decreased in August and September (0.36 to 0.37%) at the time of full flowering, in October (0.22%) at the time of end flowering, and in November (0.14%) at the time of ripening fruit stage in Mishima population.

At different growing stages the saikosaponin content increased. From July to October the highest content was in Jeongsun, decreasing a little in November. However, Mishima cultivar showed the content gradually increased until October and then re-increased in November. It is assumed that the result was due to flowering being 1 month late and the effect of this on the content.

6.5 VARIATION AND CORRELATION COEFFICIENT OF MAJOR GROWTH CHARACTERS

The morphological and growth character differences of both populations were investigated. Jeongsun cultivar did not show the variation of growth characters and started flowering 1 month earlier

TABLE 6.9
Mean, Range, Standard Deviation, and Coefficient of Variation for Plant Growth Characters in Jeongsun Cultivar

Characters	Min	Max	Range	Mean	SD	CV (%)
Plant height (cm)	42.0	81.0	39.0	61.0	8.10	13.3
Stem thickness (mm)	1.9	22.0	20.1	4.0	2.04	51.7
Branch number	3	17	14	8.8	2.88	32.6
Node number	12	26	14	18.0	3.03	16.8
Internode length (cm)	2.0	6.0	4.0	3.5	0.66	19.0
Peduncle number	5	14	9	9.0	1.94	21.6
Flowering date	Jul. 31	Sep. 6	38	Aug. 17	4.65	23.7
Dry top weight (g)	0.74	17.92	17.18	5.27	2.78	52.7
Leaf width (cm)	0.56	1.58	1.02	1.03	0.21	20.6
Leaf length (cm)	4.33	9.58	5.25	7.10	1.13	16.0
Leaf area[a]	2.60	13.90	11.30	7.44	2.34	31.6
Width/length (%)[b]	8.12	23.43	15.31	14.72	2.94	20.0
Root length (cm)	4.0	12.0	8.0	7.1	1.62	22.9
Root diameter (mm)	2.3	7.4	5.1	4.6	1.04	22.7
No. of lateral roots	0	12.0	12.0	5.1	2.63	51.1
Dry root weight (g)	0.15	1.69	1.54	0.57	0.27	53.5

[a] Leaf area = leaf length × leaf width.
[b] Width/Length (W/L) = (leaf width/leaf length) × 100.

than Mishima and fruit ripening was in mid-October in Suwon region. The main growth characters of a plant were plant height (61 cm), number of branches (8), number of nodes (18), number of flowers (9 to 10), width and length of leaf (14.7 cm), and flowering period was in mid-October in the Jeongsun population (Table 6.9). The average variation of coefficient for plant growth characters was 29% in Jeongsun cultivar. Stem thickness, leaf weight, and root weight characters showed high variation rate, but plant height, number of node, internode length, and leaf length showed low variation ratio. With these characters, it is assumed that the plant height, number of nodes, and leaf characters were even less affected by environmental conditions. The population of Mishima showed much more variable growth characters and the duration of the flowering period was 1 month, from mid-September to mid-October. To sustain a plant, the population was used to harvest seed from 2- and 3-year-old plants. Because Mishima has a late flowering habit, it could not produce fully ripened seeds compared with 1 month earlier flowering habit of the Jeongsun cultivar. The main growth characters in the Mishima population were plant height (53 cm), number of branches (12), number of nodes (20), number of flowers (6 to 7), width and length of leaf (10.8 cm), and the flowering period was in mid-September (Table 6.10). The averages of coefficient of variation for plant growth characters were high, over 50% in the Mishima cultivar. Among the characters of the Mishima, stem thickness, leaf weight, and root weight showed higher variation of characters than the Jeongsun population, but plant height, number of nodes, internode length, and leaf length showed a low variation rate, which was influenced by environmental factors.

Comparing the growth characters of the two populations, Jeongsun has a style of much earlier maturing habit, is taller, and exhibits less branching than the Mishima cultivar. Mishima has specific characters by the habits of 1 month later flowering and large leaf width and length, which showed vigorous developmental phases in an early stage (Table 6.11). The Mishima population showed a slightly higher outer phloem layer ratio in root and was stronger against some diseases than Jeongsun (Table 6.12). A highly significant correlation coefficient occurred for root weight, number of side roots, and root length in Jeongsun, while root weight, root length, root diameter, and number of

TABLE 6.10
Mean, Range, Standard Deviation, and Coefficient of Variation for Growth Characters in Mishima Cultivar

Characters	Min	Max	Range	Mean	SD	CV (%)
Plant height (cm)	26.0	97.0	71.0	53.1	12.18	22.9
Stem thickness (mm)	1.5	6.0	4.5	3.30	0.96	291
Branch number	4	24	20	12.4	4.40	35.4
Node number	12	30	18	20.1	4.01	20.0
Internode length (cm)	1.6	4.6	3.0	2.7	0.59	22.0
Peduncle number	3.5	10.5	7.0	6.2	1.31	21.1
Flowering date	Sep. 6	Sep. 27	21	Sep. 13	5.22	31.6
Dry top weight (g)	0.54	27.68	27.14	6.15	5.43	68.2
Leaf width (cm)	0.47	1.40	0.93	0.79	0.20	25.1
Leaf length (cm)	4.58	11.55	6.97	7.51	1056	20.8
Leaf area[a]	2.14	13.33	11.19	6.10	2.40	39.3
Width/Length (%)[b]	6.79	18.55	11.75	10.77	2060	24.1
Root length (cm)	5.0	20.0	15.0	9.85	3.02	30.6
Root diameter (mm)	1.9	7.2	5.3	4.15	1012	26.9
No. of lateral roots	0	13.0	13.0	3.78	2.78	73.6
Dry root weight (g)	0.10	1.65	1.58	0.53	0.36	57.7

[a] Leaf area = leaf length × leaf width.
[b] Width/Length(W/L) = (leaf width/leaf length) × 100.

TABLE 6.11
Comparison of Shoots Characters between Jeongsun and Mishima Cultivars

Cultivar	Plant Height (cm)	No. of Branches	No. of Nodes	Leaf Area[a]	Leaf W/L[b]	No. of Peduncles	Flowering Date	Stem Thickness (mm)
Jeongsun	61.0	8.8	18.0	7.44	14.72	9.0	Aug. 17	3.9
Mishima	53.1	12.4	20.1	6.10	10.77	6.2	Sep. 16	3.3

[a] Leaf area = leaf length × leaf width.
[b] Width/Length (W/L) = (leaf width/leaf length) × 100.

TABLE 6.12
Comparison of Root and Other Characters between the Jeongsun and Mishima Cultivars

Cultivar	Root Weight (g)	No. of Lateral Roots	Root Diameter (mm)	Root Length (cm)	Disease[a] Tolerance	Root Yield (kg/10 a)	OPL[b]/ Whole Root (%)
Jeongsun	0.57	5.1	4.6	7.1	Medium	45.5	67.1
Mishima	0.53	3.8	4.1	9.9	High	43.0	74.0

[a] Mainly anthracnose.
[b] OPL: the ratio of outer phloem layer to whole root.

TABLE 6.13

Correlation Coefficients among Root Characters in Jeongsun and Mishima Cultivars (above diagonal: Mishima; below diagonal: Jeongsun)

Characters	1 Root Weight	2 Root Length	3 No. of Lateral Roots	4 Root Diameter
1		0.375*	0.598*	0.777*
2	0.090		−0.033	0.245*
3	0.642*	−0.017		0.529*
4	0.776*	0.070	0.642*	

Note: * Significant at the 0.05 probability level.

side roots did not show a significant correlation coefficient in the Mishima population. However, there was no significant correlation coefficient in the root length and number of side roots in the case of both populations (Table 6.13). The correlation coefficients of underground and aboveground characters such as plant height, leaf area, and leaf weight were highly significant with root weight in Jeongsun. The Mishima cultivar also had a highly significant correlation in the number of branches, leaf area, and leaf weight with root weight, respectively (Table 6.14). The growth characters of aboveground organs have a highly significant correlation with root characters in both populations. With these results, an excellent breeding material could be selected with broad leaf, thick stem, multiple branches, and the required root characters.

TABLE 6.14

Correlation and Coefficients between the Growth Characters of Root and Shoot Parts in Jeongsun and Mishima Cultivars

Cultivar	Characters[a]	Plant Height	No. of Branches	Leaf Area	Stem Thickness	Top Weight
Jeongsun	1	0.345*	0.465*	0.532*	0.215*	0.719*
	2	−0.047	−0.090	0.028	0.028	−0.042
	3	0.294*	0.467*	0.455*	0.130	0.552*
	4	0.503*	0.610*	0.521*	0.300*	0.797
Mishima	1	−0.014	0.523*	0.290*	0.677*	0.758*
	2	0.126	0.045	0.317*	0.252*	0.144
	3	0.087	0.371*	0.018	0.472*	0.523*
	4	0.047	0.541*	0.286*	0.734*	0.686**

Note: *, ** Significant at the 0.05 and 0.01 probability levels, respectively.

[a] 1: root weight, 2: root length, 3: no. of roots, 4: root diameter.

REFERENCES

Chen, X.K., Zhan, R.Y., Zhang, Z.L., Jiang, T.Y., and Wang. B. (1993) Isolation and identification of two new saponins from *Bupleurum smithii, Acta Pharm. Sin.,* 28(5), 352–357.

Hosoda, K. and Noguchi, M. (1990) Studies on the cultivation of *Bupleurum falcatum* L. I. Effects of cultivation condition on the root growth and saponin contents, *Chem. Pharm. Bull.,* 38(2), 436–438.

Kim, K.S., Ryu, S.N., Seong, N.S., Lee, S.T., and Chae, Y.A. (1997) Distribution of saikosaponins and their variation due to plant growth characters in *Bupleurum falcatum* (SHIHO), *Proc. Int. Symp. Breeding Research on Medicinal and Aromatic Plants,* 177–180.

Minami, M., Sugino, M., Sadaoka, M., Ashida, K., and Ogaki, K. (1995) Seasonal variation on growth and saikosaponins content of *Bupleurum falcatum* L., *Jpn. J. Pharm. Soc.,* 115(2), 145–155.

Mizukami, H., Matsunaga, K., Ohashi, H., Amano, A., Maekawa, T., and Fujimoto, K. (1991) Variation of saikosaponin content of *Bupleurum falcatum* L. of different geographical origins, *Jpn. J. Pharmacogn.,* 45(4), 342–344.

Ohashi, H. and Kuribayashi, T. (1967) On the comparative cultivation of *Bupleurum falcatum* L. from Miyazaki, *Jpn. J. Pharmacogn.,* 21(1), 41–43.

Ohashi, H. and Kuribayashi, T. (1972) On the trial selection of annual crop in *Bupleurum falcatum* (preliminary report), *Shoyakugaku Zasshi,* 27, 41–43.

Ostuka, H., Kobayashi, S., and Shibata, S. (1977) Studies on the cultivation of *Bupleurum falcatum* L., *Jpn. J. Pharmacogn.,* 31(2), 195–197.

Park, C.H., Seong, N.S., Lee, S.T., Jeong, H.G., and Park, E.S. (1995) Callus formation and plantlet regeneration for anther culture in *Bupleurum falcatum* L., *Kor. J. Breeding,* 27(4), 387–393.

Shimokawa, Y., Okuda, I., Kuwano, M., and Ohashi, H. (1980a) Cultivation and breeding of *Bupleurum falcatum* L, Geographical variation of *B. falcatum, Jpn. J. Pharmacogn.,* 34(3), 239–244.

Shimokawa, Y., Okuda, I., Kuwano, M., Ushio, N., Uno, N., and Ohashi, H. (1980b) Cultivation and breeding of *Bupleurum falcatum* L. Effect of planting density on the growth, *Jpn. J. Pharmacogn.,* 34(3), 215–220.

Shimokawa, Y., Ushio, N., Uno, N., and Ohashi, H. (1980c) Cultivation and breeding of *Bupleurum falcatum* L. Effect of temperature on growth, development and saikosaponin content of one-year-old plants, *Jpn. J. Pharmacogn.,* 34(3), 209–214.

Tanaka, T., Sakai, E., Mizuno, M., Kawamura, T., Hista, Y., Okuda, K., Noro, Y., Zheng, Z.X.Z., and Fang, D. (1988) Cultivation and saponin contents of Guangxi *Bupleurum, Jpn. J. Pharmacogn.,* 42(3), 236–239.

Tani, W. and Eisenbrand, G. (1992) *Bupleurum* spp. In *Chinese Drugs of Plant Origin.* Springer-Verlag, New York, chap. 30, 223–232.

Tani, T., Katsuki, T., Kubo, M., and Arichi, S. (1986) Histochemistry. IX. Distribution of saikosaponins in *Bupleurum falcatum* root, *J. Chromatogr.,* 360, 407–416.

Watanabe, T., Yoshikawa, T., Isoda, S., Takada, A., Ishiguro, G., Namera, A., Kohda, H., Malla, K.J., and Takano, A. (1998) Studies on the medicinal plant resources of the Himalayas (2). Qualitative and quantitative evaluation of saikosaponins of some *Bupleurum* root collected in Nepal, *Nat. Med.,* 52(5), 421–425.

Zhang, J. (1985) Comparison on saikosaponin content in the root of *Bupleurum* chinense of different sizes, *Bull. Chin. Mat. Med.,* 10, 157–158.

Section III

Chemistry

7 Main Chemical Constituents of *Bupleurum* Genus

Sheng-Li Pan

CONTENTS

7.1   INTRODUCTION

There are more than 150 species in the genus *Bupleurum,* nearly a quarter of which have been subjected to phytochemical investigation. The main constituents from the genus are triterpene glycosides of the oleanane series. Furthermore, the occurrence of essential oils, lignans, flavonoids, coumarins, polysaccharides, polyacetylenes, phytosterols, and phenylpropanoids are also reported.

7.2   MAIN CHEMICAL CONSTITUENTS IN *BUPLEURUM* GENUS

7.2.1   TRITERPENOID SAPONINS

Triterpine glycosides of the oleanane series occurring in the genus are named saikosaponins, derived from the Japanese name "Saiko," the common name of *Bupleurum* spp. used in Kampo medicine. They proved to possess much pharmacological activity, e.g., anti-inflammatory (Takagi and Shibata, 1969b; Benito et al., 1998; Navarro et al., 2001), hepatoprotective (Abe et al., 1980, 1982, 1985; Guinea et al., 1994), anodynic and sedative (Takagi and Shibata, 1969a), antibacterial and antiviral (Kumazawa et al., 1990; Bermejo et al., 2002), immunomodulatory (Kumazawa et al., 1989; Ushio and Abe, 1992; Kato et al., 1995; Hsu et al., 2000), and antiallergic effect (Park et al., 2002).

Research on saikosides of *Bupleurum* started with Ezawa, who reported the presence of saponins in 1916. Subsequently, Robate (1931) isolated a glycoside from *B. rotundifolium* L. and named it rutoside. Since the 1960s, saponins from *Bupleurum* have been studied extensively. Shibata and co-workers (Shibata et al., 1965; Aimi and Shibata, 1966) and Kubota and co-workers (Kubota and Hinoh, 1966, 1968b; Kubota and Tonami, 1967; Kubota et al., 1967) independently clarified the structures of its triterpenoid sapogenins, named saikogenins A.-G. Kubota (Kubota and Hinoh, 1968b) suggested that saikogen E, F, and G were genuine sapogenins, which have the ether linkage between C-13 and C-28. Saikogenin A, B, C, and D, having conjugated dienes, were artifacts formed during the acid hydrolysis. Kubota and Hinoh (1968a) reported the structure elucidation of the major saponin constituents as well, i.e., the structures of saikosaponin-a through -d. Several years later, Shimaoka et al. (1975) reinvestigated the components of the saikosaponin-a and -b, and pointed out that Kubota's "saponin-a" contained saikosaponin-b_1 and b_3, while Kubota's "saponin-b" consisted of saikosaponin-b_2 and -b_4. From a recent investigation using nuclear magnetic resonance (NMR), many minor saikosaponins have been isolated and identified from *Bupleurum*. To date, more than 100 saikosaponins have been reported from it, which can be divided into six types. The structures of these and their references are as in Figure 7.1 and Table 7.1, respectively.

Saikosaponins from type I are genuine saponins enclosing saikosaponin-a, -d and -c, the major saponins existing in *Bupleurum*. Their aglycones are 13β, 28-epoxyolean-11-ene-16-ol. The pharmacological experiments demonstrated activity of saikosaponin-d > saikosaponin-a > saikosaponin-c, so it is suggested that the –OH of C-23 is necessary for their pharmacological effects, and α-OH of C-16 has more pharmacological activity than β-OH.

Saikosaponins from type II have aheteroannular diene. Nearly all of them were derived from genuine saikosaponins. While the 13,28-oxide bridge opened, saikosaponin-a would transform to saikosaponin-b_1 and -b_3, saikosaponin-d would transform saikosaponin-b_2 and -b_4, and then partly lose their pharmacological activity.

Saikosaponins from type III, IV, and V are also mainly derived from genuine saikosaponins.

Nose et al. (1989) reported, that saikosaponin-a, -c and -d could form 27 metabolites in the alimentary tract (Figure 7.2, Figure 7.3, and Figure 7.4).

The content of saikosaponins in *Bupleurum* genus is approximately ca 1 to 2%. Pan et al. (2000a, 2000b) determined the content of saikosaponins by high-performance liquid chromatography (HPLC) on 23 species and some of the same species growing in different districts of China. It was discovered that the content of saikosaponins in *B. polyclonum* was up to 7.44%, and it is the species with the highest content in this genus. In contrast, some species, e.g., *B. hamiltonii, B. candollei, B longicaule* var. *franchetii, B. bicaule,* contain very little saikosaponin. The content of saikosaponins of 23 species and of the same species from different districts are presented in Table 7.2 and Table 7.3.

7.2.2 ESSENTIAL OIL

As a main constituent of *Bupleurum*, research on essential oil composition began early. In 1913, Francesconi et al. reported the presence of a terpenic alcohol in *Bupleurum*, and named it bupleurol. Later, Peyron and Roubaud (1970), Pu (Pu et al., 1983), Gil (Gil et al., 1989), Manunta (Manunta et al., 1992), Yang (Yang et al., 1993), Barrero (Barrero et al., 1998), and Dugo (Dugo et al., 2002) identified many constituents of essential oil from several species in the genus. Notably Guo et al. (1990) studied the essential oils of 19 species from China, and identified more than 150 constituents. To date, more than 20 species have been studied and more than 200 constituents have been identified (Table 7.4). Based on such identification, Guo et al. (1990) suggested that the aliphatic compounds could be regarded as the characteristic chemical constituents of the essential oils of the Chinese species.

7.2.3 LIGNANS

Studies on lignans from *B. fruticescens* were started in 1975 (Gonzalez et al., 1975). Subsequently, a number of lignans have been isolated from *B. salicifolium* by A.G. Gonzalez and co-workers (Gonzalez et al., 1989, 1990a, 1990b, 1990c; Estevez-Reyes et al., 1992, 1993; Estevez-Braun

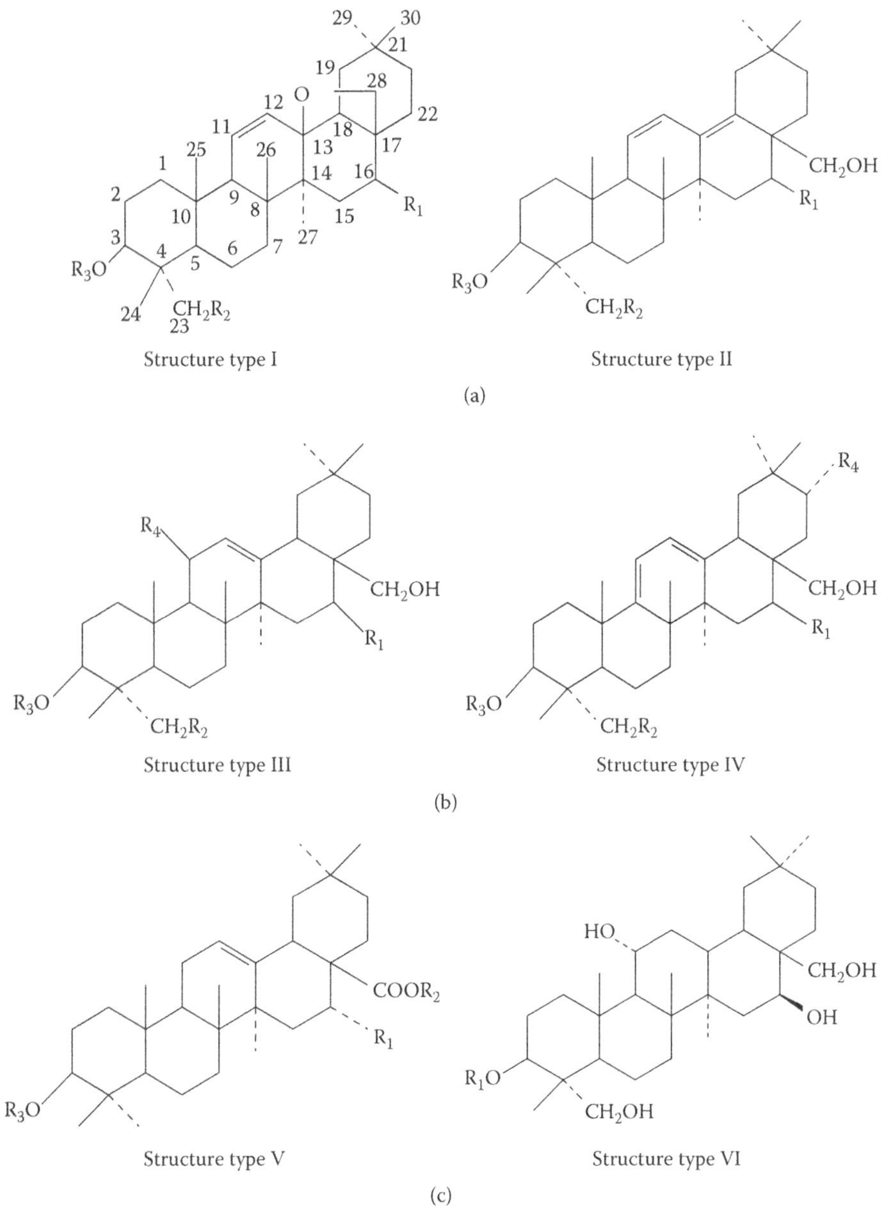

FIGURE 7.1 Structures of saikosaponins.

et al., 1994, 1995). Three new lignans were isolated from *B. handiense* by Lopez and Valera (1996), and some by Barrero et al. (1999) from *B. acutifolium*. The names and structures of lignans from *B. salicifolium* and *B. handiense* and *B. acutifolium* are described in Chapter 8.

Luo et al. (1993) of China reported two new lignan glucosides from *B. wenchuanense*, a Chinese endemic species of *Bupleurum*, and named them phillyrin and wenchuanensin (Figure 7.5).

7.2.4 FLAVONOIDS

Many flavonoids occur in the aerial parts of *Bupleurum*. In 1964, Minaeva et al. isolated rutin and narcissin from *B. multinerve*. Subsequently, quercetin, isoquercetin, isorhamnetrin, narcissin, and

TABLE 7.1
Saikosaponins and Their Structures

	Name of Saponin	Structure Type	Structure	Ref.
1.	Saikosaponin-a	I	R_1=β-OH R_2=-OH R_3=β-D-glu-(1~3)-β-D-fuc-	Kubota T and Hinoh H, 1968a
2.	23-*O*-Acetylsaikosaponin a	I	R_1=β-OH R_2=-OAc R_3=β-D-glu-(1~3)-β-D-fuc-	Ishii H et al., 1980
3.	2″-*O*-Acetylsaikosaponin a	I	R_1=β-OH R_2=-OH R_3=2″-*O*-acetyl-β-glu-(1~3)-β-D-fuc-	Ding JK et al., 1986
4.	3PP-*O*-Acetylsaikosaponin a	I	R_1=β-OH R_2=-OH R_3=3″-*O*-acetyl-β-D-glu-(1~3)-β-D-fuc-	Ding JK et al., 1986
5.	4″-*O*-Acetylsaikosaponin a:	I	R_1=β-OH R_2=-OH R_3=4″-*O*-acetyl-β-D-glu-(1~3)-β-D-fuc-	Seto H et al., 1986a
6.	6″-*O*-Acetylsaikosaponin a	I	R_1=β-OH R_2=-OH R_3=6″-*O*-acetyl-β-D-glu-(1~3)-β-D-fuc-	Ishii H et al., 1980
7.	2″,3′-Diacetylsaikosaponin a	I	R_1=β-OH R_2=-OH R_3=2″,3′-diacetyl-β-D-glu-(1~3)-β-D-fuc-	Seto H et al., 1986c
8.	3″,4″-Diacetylsaikosaponin a	I	R_1=β-OH R_2=-OH R_3=3″,4″-diacetyl-β-D-glu-(1~3)-β-D-fuc-	Seto H et al., 1986c
9.	3″,6″-Diacetylsaikosaponin a	I	R_1=β-OH R_2=-OH R_3=3″,6″-diacetyl-β-D-glu-(1~3)-β-D-fuc-	Seto H et al., 1986c
10.	Malonylsaikosaponin a	I	R_1=β-OH R_2=-OH R_3=6″-O-malonyl-glu-(1~3)-β-D-glu-	Ebata N et al., 1990
11.	Saikosaponin d	I	R_1=α-OH R_2=-OH R_3=β-D-gluc-(1~3)-β-D-fuc-	Kubota T and Hinoh H, 1968a
12.	2″-*O*-Acetylsaikosaponin d	I	R_1=β-OH R_2=-OH R_3=2″-*O*-acetyl-β-D-glu-(1~3)-β-D-fuc-	Seto H et al., 1986a
13.	3″-*O*-Acetylsaikosaponin d	I	R_1=α-OH R_2=-OH R_3=3″-*O*-acetyl-β-D-glu-(1~3)-β-D-fuc-	Ishii H et al., 1980
14.	4″-*O*- Acetylsaikosaponin d	I	R_1=α-OH R_2=-OH R_3=4″-*O*-acetyl-β-D-glu-(1~3)-β-D-fuc-	Ebata N et al., 1996
15.	6″-*O*-Acetylsaikosaponin d	I	R_1=α-OH R_2=-OH R_3=6″-*O*-acetyl-β-D-glu-(1~3)-β-D-fuc	Ishii H et al., 1980
16.	2″,3″-Diacetylsaikosaponin d	I	R_1=α-OH R_2=-OH R_3=2″,3″-diacetyl-β-D-glu-(1~3)-β-D-fuc-	Seto H et al., 1986c
17.	3″,4″-Diacetylsaikosaponin d	I	R_1=α-OH R_2=-OH R_3=3″,4″-diacetyl-β-D-glu-(1~3)-β-D-fuc-	Seto H et al., 1986c
18.	3″,6″-Diacetylsaikosaponin d	I	R_1=α-OH R_2=-OH R_3=3″,6″-diacetyl-β-D-glu-(1~3)-β-D-fuc-	Seto H et al., 1986c
19.	4″,6″-Diacetylsaikosaponin d	I	R_1=α-OH R_2=-OH R_3=4″,6″-diacetyl-β-D-glu-(1~3)-β-D-fuc-	Seto H et al., 1986c
20.	Malonylsaikosaponin d	I	R_1=α-OH R_2=-OH R_3=6″-O-malonyl-glu-(1~3)-β-D-glu-	Ebata N et al., 1990
21.	Saikosaponin c	I	R_1=β-OH R_2=-H R_3=β-D-glu-(1~6)-[α-L-rha-(1~4)-]-β-D-glu-	Kubota T and Hinoh H, 1968a
22.	Saikosaponin e	I	R_1=β-OH R_2=-H R_3=β-D-glu-(1`3)-β-D-fuc-	Ishii H et al., 1977
23.	3″-*O*-Acetylsaikosaponin e	I	R_1=β-OH R_2=-H R_3=3″-*O*-acetyl-β-D-glu-(1~3)-β-D-fuc-	Seto H et al., 1986c
24.	Prosaikogenin F	I	R_1=β-OH R_2=-OH R_3=β-D-fuc-	Shimizu K et al., 1985

TABLE 7.1 (CONTINUED)
Saikosaponins and Their Structures

	Name of Saponin	Structure Type	Structure	Ref.
25.	Prosaikogenin G	I	$R_1=\alpha$-OH $\quad R_2=$-OH $R_3=\beta$-D-fuc-	Shimizu K et al., 1985
26.	Chikusaikoside I	I	$R_1=\beta$-OH $\quad R_2=$-OH $R_3=\beta$-D-xyl-(1~2)-β-D-glu-(1~3)-β-D-fuc-	Ding JK et al., 1986
27.	16-Epi-chikusaikoside I	I	$R_1=\alpha$-OH $\quad R_2=$-OH $R_3=\beta$-D-xyl-(1~2)-β-D-glu-(1~3)-β-D-fuc-	Seto H et al., 1986a
28.	Chikusaikoside II	I	$R_1=\beta$-OH $\quad R_2=$-OH $R_3=\beta$-D-glu-(1~6)[β-L-rha-(1~4)]-β-D-glu-	Ding JK et al., 1986
29.	Rotundioside F	I	$R_1=\alpha$-OH $\quad R_2=$-H $R_3=\beta$-L-rha-(1~2)-β-D-glu-(1~2)-β-D-fuc-	Akai E et al., 1985
30.	Rotundioside G	I	$R_1=\alpha$-OH $\quad R_2=$-H $R_3=\beta$-D-xyl-(1~2)-β-D-glu-(1~2)-β-D-fuc-	Akai E et al., 1985
31.	Buddlejasaponin IV	I	$R_1=\beta$-OH $\quad R_2=$-OH $R_3=\beta$-D-glu-(1~2)-[β-D-glu-(1~3)-]-β-D-fuc-	Guinea MC et al., 1993
32.	Malonylbuddlejasaponin IV	I	$R_1=\beta$-OH $\quad R_2=$-OH $R_3=6''$-O-malonyl-β-D-glu-(1~2)-[β-D-glu-(1~3)-]-β-D-fuc-	Guinea MC et al., 1993
33.	Sandrosaponin I	I	$R_1=\beta$-OH $\quad R_2=$-OH $R_3=\beta$-D-glu-(1~2)-[4-O-sulfo-β-D-glu-(1~3)-]-β-D-fuc-	Sanchez-Contreras S et al., 1998
34.	Sandrosaponin II	I	$R_1=\beta$-OH $\quad R_2=$-OH $\quad 29$-CH$_2$OH $R_3=\beta$-D-glu-(1~2)-[4-O-sulfo-β-D-glu-(1~3)-]-β-D-fuc-	Sanchez-Contreras S et al., 2000b
35.	Sandrosaponin III	I	$R_1=\beta$-OH $\quad R_2=$-OH $\quad 29$-CH$_3$ $\quad 30$-COOH $R_3=\beta$-D-glu-(1~2)-[4-O-sulfo-β-D-glu-(1~3)-]-β-D-fuc-	Sanchez-Contreras S et al., 2000b
36.	Sandrosaponin IV	I	$R_1=\beta$-OH $\quad R_2=$-OH $\quad 29$-CH$_2$OH 30-COOH $R_3=\beta$-D-glu-(1~2)-[4-O-sulfo-β-D-glu-(1~3)-]-β-D-fuc-	Sanchez-Contreras S et al., 2000b
37.	Sandrosaponin V	I	$R_1=\beta$-OH $\quad R_2=$-OH $\quad 29$-CH$_3$ $\quad 30$-CH$_2$OH $R_3=\beta$-D-glu-(1~2)-[4-O-sulfo-β-D-glu-(1~3)-]-β-D-fuc-	Sanchez-Contreras S et al., 2000b
38.	Sandrosaponin VII	I	$R_1=\beta$-OH $\quad R_2=$-OH $\quad 29$-CH$_2$OH $R_3=\beta$-D-glu-(1~2)-[4-O-sulfo-β-D-glu-(1~3)-]-β-D-fuc-	Sanchez-Contreras S et al., 2000a
39.	Bupleuroside I	I	$R_1=\beta$-OH $\quad R_2=$-OH $R_3=\beta$-D-glu-(1~2)-β-D-glu-(1~3)-β-D-fuc-	Yoshikawa M et al., 1997b
40.	23-Acetoxy. 16α-hydroxy-13,28-epoxyolean-11-en-3β-yl-[β-D-glucopyranosyl (1-2)]-[β-D-glucopyranosyl (1-3)]-β-D-fucopyranoside	I	$R_1=\beta$-OH $\quad R_2=$-OCOCH$_3$ $R_3=\beta$-D-glu-(1~2)-[β-D-glu-(1~3)-]-β-D-fuc-	Pistelli L et al., 1996

TABLE 7.1 (CONTINUED)
Saikosaponins and Their Structures

	Name of Saponin	Structure Type	Structure	Ref.
41.	3-Acetoxy. 16α-hydroxy-13,28-epoxyolean-11-en-3 β-yl-[β-D-glucopyranosyl (1-2)]-[β-D-glucopyranosyl (1-3)]-β-D-fucopyranoside	I	R_1=α-OH R_2=-OCOCH$_3$ R_3=β-D-glu-(1~2)-[β-D-glu-(1~3)-]-β-D-fuc-	Pistelli L et al., 1996
42.	3β,16β,23-Trihydroxy-13,28-epoxyolean-11-en-3β-yl-[β-D-glucopyranosyl(1-2)]-[β-D-glucopyranosyl(1-3)]-β-D-fucopyranoside	I	R_1=β-OH R_2=-OH R_3=β-D-glu-(1~2)-[β-D-glu-(1~3)-]-β-D-fuc-	Pistelli L et al., 1993a
43.	Saikosaponin b1	II	R_1=β-OH R_2=-OH R_3=β-D-glu-(1~3)-β-D-fuc-	Shimaoka et al., 1975
44.	Saikosaponin b2	II	R_1=α-OH R_2=-OH R_3=β-D-glu-(1~3)-β-D-fuc	Shimaoka et al., 1975
45.	2''-O-Acetylsaikosaponin b2	II	R_1=α-OH R_2=-OH R_3=2''-O-acetyl-β-D-glu-(1~3)-β-D-fuc-	Seto H et al., 1986b
46.	3''-O-Acetylsaikosaponin b2	II	R_1=α-OH R_2=-OH R_3=3''-O-acetyl-β-D-glu-(1~3)-β-D-fuc-	Seto H et al., 1986b
47.	6''-O-Acetylsaikosaponin b2	II	R_1=α-OH R_2=-OH R_3=6''-O-acetyl-β-D-glu-(1~3)-β-D-fuc-	Ishii H et al., 1980
48.	2''-O-Glucosylsaikosaponin b2	II	R_1=α-OH R_2=-OH R_3=β-D-glu-(1~2)-β-D-glu-(1~3)-β-D-fuc-	Ding JK et al., 1986
49.	2''-O-Xylosylsaikosaponin b2	II	R_1=α-OH R_2=-OH R_3=2''-β-D-xyl-(1~2)-β-D-glu-(1~3)-β-D-fuc-	Luo SQ et al., 1993
50.	3'',6''-Diacetylsaikosaponin b2	II	R_1=α-OH R_2=-OH R_3=3'',6''-diacetyl-β-D-glu-(1~3)-β-D-fuc	Seto H et al., 1986c
51.	30-O-Glucosylsaikosaponin b2	II	R_1=α-OH R_2=-OH R_3=β-D-glu-(1~3)-β-D-fuc- 30-O-β-D-glu-	Seto H et al., 1986b
52.	Prosaikogenin A	II	R_1=β-OH R_2=-OH R_3=β-D-fuc-	Shimizu K et al., 1985
53.	Prosaikogenin D	II	R_1=α-OH R_2=-OH R_3=β-D-fuc-	Shimizu K et al., 1985
54.	Saikosaponin h	II	R_1=β-OH R_2=-H R_3=β-D-glu-(1~6)-[-L-rha-(1~4)-]-β-D-glu-	Shimizu K et al., 1985
55.	Saikosaponin k	II	R_1=β-OH R_2=-OH 30-OH R_3=β-D-xyl-(1~2)-β-D-glu-(1~3)-β-D-fuc-	Chen XK et al., 1993
56.	Saikosaponin l	II	R_1=α-OH R_2=-OH 30-CH$_2$OH R_3=β-D-xyl-(1~2)-β-D-glu-(1~3)-β-D-fuc-	Chen XK et al., 1993
57.	Saikosaponin m	II	R_1=H R_2=-OH R_3=β-D-glu-(1~3)-β-D-fuc-	Zhang RY et al., 1994
58.	Saikosaponin n	II	R_1=β-OH R_2=-OH R_3=β-D-glu-(1~6)-[α-L-rha-(1~4)-]-β-D-glu-	Zhang RY et al., 1994
59.	Saikosaponin o	II	R_1=β-OH R_2=-OH R_3=β-D-glu-(1~2)-β-D-glu-(1~6)-[β-D-glu-(1~2)-]-β-D-glu-O-	Ma LB et al., 1996

TABLE 7.1 (CONTINUED)
Saikosaponins and Their Structures

	Name of Saponin	Structure Type	Structure	Ref.
60.	Saikosaponin p	II	R_1=β-OH R_2=-OH R_3=β-D-glu-(1~6)-[β-D-glu-(1~2)-]-β-D-glu-	Luo HS et al., 1996
61.	Saikosaponin q	II	R_1=β-OH R_2=-OH 30-CH$_2$OH R_3=β-D-glu-(1~6)-[α-L-rha-(1~4)-]β-D-glu-	Luo HS et al., 1995
62.	Saikosaponin q-2	II	R_1=α-OH R_2=-OH 30-CH$_2$OH R_3=β-D-glu-(1~6)-[α-L-rha-(1~4)-]β-D-glu-	Lian H et al., 2001
63.	Saikosaponin r	II	R_1=α-OH R_2=-OH 30-CH$_2$OH R_3=β-D-glu-(1~2)-β-D-glu-(1~3)-β-D-fuc-	Tan L et al., 1996
64.	Saikosaponin s	II	R_1=α-OH R_2=-OH R_3=β-D-glu-(1~6)-[β-L-rha-(1~4)-]-β-D-glu-	Tan L et al., 1998
65.	Rotundioside:E	II	R_1=α-OH R_2=-H R_3=α-L-rha-(1~2)-β-D-glu-(1~2)-β-D-fuc-	Akai E et al., 1985
66.	Saponin BK1	II	R_1=α-OH R_2=H R_3=β-D-glu-(1~6)-α-Lrha-(1~4)-β-D-glu-	Luo SQ et al., 1987
67.	Saponin BK2	II	R_1=α-OH R_2=-H 30-CH$_2$OH R_3=β-D-glu-(1~6)-α-L-rha-(1~4)-β-D-glu-	Luo SQ et al., 1987
68.	Saponin BK3	II	R_1=β-OH R_2=-H 28-O-β-D-glu- R_3=β-D-glu-(1~6)-α-L-rha-(1~4)-β-D-glu-	Luo SQ et al., 1987
69.	Sandrosaponin VI	II	R_1=α-OH R_2=-OH 30-CH$_2$OH R_3=β-D-glu-(1~2)-[4-O-sulfo-β-D-glu-(1~3)-]-β-D-fuc-	Sanchez-Contreras S et al., 2000b
70.	Sandrosaponin VIII	II	R_1=α-OH R_2=-OH 30-CH$_2$OH 28-COOH R_3=β-D-glu-(1~2)-[4-O-sulfo-β-D-glu-(1~3)-]-β-D-fuc-	Sanchez-Contreras S et al., 2000a
71.	Saikosaponin u	II	R_1=α-OH R_2=-OH R_3=β-D-glu-(1~2)-β-D-glu-(1~3)-β-D-fuc- 30-oic acid-30-0-[pentito(1~1)-β-D-glu-(6~)]ester	Tan L et al., 1999
72.	Saikosaponin v	II	R_1=α-OH R_2=-OH R_3=β-D-glu-(1~3)-β-D-fuc- 30-oic acid-30-0-[pentito(1~1)-β-D-glu-(6~)]ester	Lian H et al., 1998b
73.	Saikosaponin v-2	II	R_1=α-OH R_2=-OH R_3=β-D-glu-(1~2) -D-glu-(1~3)-β-D-fuc- 30-oic acid-30-0-[pentito(1-1)-β-D-glu-(6-)]ester	Hong L et al., 2000
74.	Scorzoneroside A	II	R_1=α-OH R_2=-OH R_3=β-D-glu-(1~3)-β-D-rha- 30-β-D-glu-(1~5)-pentito-(1~)	Yoshikawa M et al., 1997a
75.	Scorzoneroside B	II	R_1=α-OH R_2=-OH 30- pentito R_3=β-D-glu-(1~3)-β-D-rha-	Yoshikawa M et al., 1997a
76.	Scorzoneroside C	II	R_1=α-OH R_2=-OH R_3=β-D-rha- 30- pentito	Yoshikawa M et al., 1997a

TABLE 7.1 (CONTINUED)
Saikosaponins and Their Structures

Name of Saponin	Structure Type	Structure	Ref.
77. 16α,23,28,30-Tetrahydroxyolean-11,13(18)-dien-3β-yl-β-D-glucopyranol-(1-3)-β-D-fucopyranoside	II	R_1=α-OH R_2=-OH 30-CH$_2$OH R_3=β-D-glu-(1~3)-β-D-fuc-	Pistelli L et al., 1993b
78. 3β,16α,23,28-Tetrahydroxyolean-11,13(18)-dien-30-oic acid 3-*O*-β-D-glucopyranosyl-(1-2)-β-D-glucopyranosyl-(1-3)-β-D-fucopyranoside	II	R_1=α-OH R_2=-OH 30-COOH R_3=β-D-glu-(1~2)-β-D-glu-(1~3)-β-D-fuc-	Barrero AF et al., 2000
79. 3β,16α28-Trihydroxyolean-11,13(18)-dien-3β-yl-β-D-glucopyranosyl-(1-6)-[α-L-rhampyranosyl-(1-4)]-β-D-glucopyranoside	II	R_1=α-OH R_2=H R_3=β-D-glu-(1~6)-[α-L-rha-(1~4)]-β-D-glu-	Luo SQ and Jin HF, 1991
80. 3β,16α28, 30-Tetrahydroxyolean-11,13(18)-dien-3β-yl-β-D-glucopyranosyl-(1-6)-[α-L-rhampyranosyl-(1-4)]-β-D-glucopyranoside	II	R_1=α-OH R_2=H 30-CH$_2$OH R_3=β-D-glu-(1~6)-[α-L-rha-(1~4)]-β-D-glu-	Luo SQ and Jin HF, 1991
81. 3β,16α28-Trihydroxyolean-11,13(18)-dien-O-β-D-glucopyranosyl-3β-yl-β-D-glucopyranosyl-(1-6)-[α-L-rhampyranosyl-(1-4)]-β-D-glucopyranoside	II	R_1=α-OH R_2=H 28-O-β-D-glu- R_3=β-D-glu-(1~6)-[α-L-rha-(1~4)]-β-D-glu-	Luo SQ and Jin HF, 1991
82. Saikosaponin b3	III	R_1=β-OH R_2=-OH R_4=α-OMe R_3=β-D-glu-(1~3)-β-D-fuc-	Shimaoka et al., 1975
83. 2″-*O*-Acetylsaikosaponin b3	III	R_1=β-OH R_2=-OH R_4=α-OMe R_3=2″-O-acetyl-β-D-glu-(1~3)-β-D-fuc-	Ding JK et al., 1986
84. 3″-*O*-Acetylsaikosaponin b3	III	R_1=β-OH R_2=-OH R_4=α-OMe R_3=3″-O-acetyl-β-D-glu-(1~3)-β-D-fuc-	Ding JK et al., 1986
85. 6″-*O*-Acetylsaikosaponin b3	III	R_1=β-OH R_2=-OH R_4=α-OMe R_3=6″-O-acetyl-β-D-glu-(1~3)-β-D-fuc-	Ding JK et al., 1986
86. Saikosaponin b4	III	R_1=α-OH R_2=-OH R_4=α-OMe R_3=β-D-glu-(1~3)-β-D-fuc-	Shimaoka et al., 1975
87. 3″-*O*-Acetylsaikosaponin b4	III	R_1=α-OH R_2=-OH R_4=α-OMe R_3=3″-O-acetyl-β-D-glu-(1~3)-β-D--fuc-	Ding JK et al., 1986
88. 6″-*O*-acetylsaikosaponin b4	III	R_1=α-OH R_2=-OH R_4=α-OMe R_3=6″-O-acetyl-β-D-glu-(1~3)-β-D-fuc-	Ishii H et al., 1980
89. 3″,4″-Diacetylsaikosaponin b4	III	R_1=α-OH R_2=-OH R_4=α-OMe R_3=3″,4″-diacetyl-β-D-glu-(1~3)-β-D-fuc-	Seto H et al., 1986c
90. Saikosaponin f	III	R_1=β-OH R_2=-H R_4=-H R_3=β-D-glu-(1~6)-[α-L-rha-(1~4)-]-β-D-glu-	Ishii H et al., 1980

TABLE 7.1 (CONTINUED)
Saikosaponins and Their Structures

	Name of Saponin	Structure Type	Structure	Ref.
91.	11α-Methoxysaikosaponin f	III	R_1=β-OH R_2=-H R_4=α-OMe R_3=β-D-glu-(1~6)-[α-L-rha-(1~4)-]-β-D-glu-	Ding JK et al., 1986
92.	Saikosaponin t	III	R_1=β-OH R_2=-H R_4=α-OMe R_3=β-D-glu-(1~3)-β-D-fuc-	Liang H et al., 1998a
93.	Saikosaponin 15	III	R_1=β-OH R_2=-OH R_4=α-OMe R_3=β-D-xyl-(1~2)-β-D-glu-(1~3)-β-D-fuc-	Ding JK et al., 1986
94.	Saikosaponin 16	III	R_1=β-OH R_2=-OH R_4=α-OMe R_3=β-D-glu-(1~6)-[α-L-rha-(1~4)-]-β-D-glu-	Ding JK et al., 1986
95.	Rotundioside D	III	R_1=α-OH R_2=-H R_4=α-H R_3=α-L-rha-(1~2)-β-D-glu-(1~2)-β-D-glu-	Akai E et al., 1985
96.	Bupleuroside III	III	R_1=-OH R_2=-OH R_4=α-OMe R_3=β-D-glu-(1~3)-β-D-fuc-(1~)	Matsuda H et al., 1997
97.	Bupleuroside VI	III	R_1=-OH R_2=-OH R_4=α-OMe C_{11}=O R_3=β-D-glu-(1~3)-β-D-fuc-	Matsuda H et al., 1997
98.	Bupleuroside IX	III	R_1=-OH R_2=-H R_4=α-OMe R_3=β-D-glu-(1~3)-β-D-fuc-	Matsuda H et al., 1997
99.	Hydroxysaikosaponin a	III	R_1=β-OH R_2=-OH R_4=α-OH R_3=β-D-glu-(1~3)-β-D-fuc-	Ebata N et al., 1996
100.	Hydroxysaikosaponin d	III	R_1=α-OH R_2=-OH R_4=α-OH R_3=β-D-glu-(1~3)-β-D-fuc-	Ebata N et al., 1996
101.	Hydroxysaikosaponin c	III	R_1=β-OH R_2=-OH R_4=α-OH R_3=β-D-glu-(1~6)-[α-L-rha-(1~4)-]-β-D-glu-	Ebata N et al., 1996
102.	11α,16,23β,28-Tetrahydroxyolean-12-en-3β-yl-[β-D-glucopyranosyl-(1-2)]-[β-D-glucopyranosyl-(1-3)]-β-D-fucopyranoside	III	R_1=β-OH R_2=-OH R_4=α-OH R_3=β-D-glu-(1~2)-[β-D-glu-(1~3)-]-β-D-fuc-	Pistelli L et al., 1993a
103.	16α,23,28-Trihydroxyolean-12-en-3β-yl-[β-D-glucopyranosyl-(1-2)][β-D-glucopyranosyl-(1-3)]-β-D-fucopyranoside	III	R_1=β-OH R_2=-OH R_4=α-OMe R_3=β-D-glu-(1~2)-[β-D-glu-(1~3)-]-β-D-fuc-	Pistelli L et al., 1993a
104.	Saikosaponin g	IV	R_1=β-OH R_2=-OH R_4=-H R_3=β-D-glu-(1~3)-β-D-fuc-	Shimizu K et al., 1985
105.	Saikosaponin i	IV	R_1=β-OH R_2=-H R_4=-H R_3=α-D-glu-(1~6)-[α-L-rha-(1~4)-]-β-D-glu-	Shimizu K et al., 1985
106.	Prosaikogenin H	IV	R_1=β-OH R_2=-OH R_4=-H R_3=β-D-fuc-	Shimizu K et al., 1985
107.	saikosaponin $S_{1:}$	V	R_1=-H R_2=β-D-glu- R_3=α-L-arab-(1~3)-β-D-glu-	Seto et al., 1986d
108.	Rotundioside A	V	R_1=β-OH R_3=-SO_3H R_2=β-D-glu-(1~6)-β-D-glu-(1~2)-β-D-glu-(1~6)-β-D-glu-	Akai E et al., 1985

TABLE 7.1 (CONTINUED)
Saikosaponins and Their Structures

	Name of Saponin	Structure Type	Structure	Ref.
109.	Rotundioside B	V	R_1=-H R_3=-SO$_3$H R_2=β-D-glu-(1~6)-β-D-glu-(1~2)-β-D-glu-(1~6)-β-D-glu-	Akai E et al., 1985
110.	Rotundioside C	V	R_1=-H R_3=-SO$_3$H R_2=β-D-glu-(1~6)-β-D-glu-(1~2)-β-D-glu-(1~2)-β-D-glu-	Akai E et al., 1985
111.	Sandrosaponin IX	V	R_1=-H R_2=β-D-glu- R_3=β-D-glu-(1~2)-β-D-gal-(1~2)-β-D-glc-	Sanchez-Contreras S et al., 2000a
112.	Sandrosaponin X	V	R_1=-H R_2=-H R_3=β-D-glu-(1~2)-β-D-gal-(1~2)-β-D-glc-	Sanchez-Contreras S et al., 2000a
113.	Bupleuroside XII	VI	R_1=β-D-glu-(1~3)-β-D-fuc-	Matsuda H et al., 1997

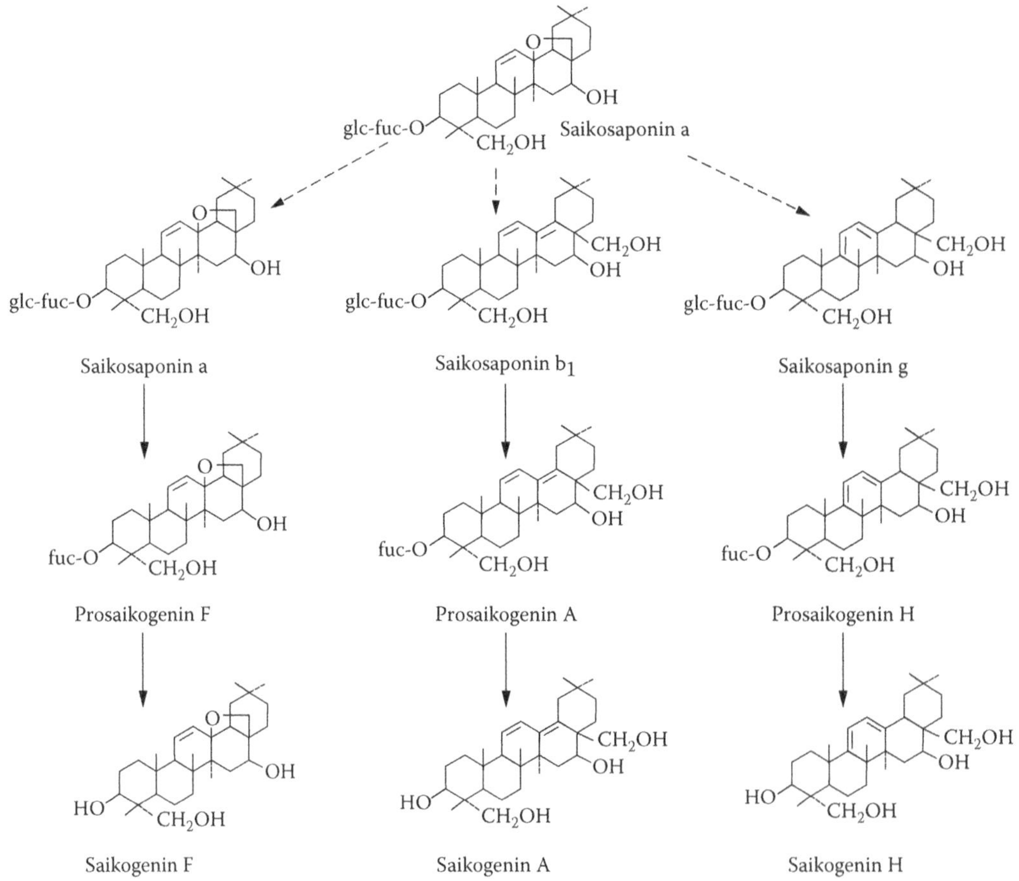

FIGURE 7.2 Metabolites of saikosaponin-a formed in the alimentary tract. ·······▶ Structural transformation in gastric juice. ——▶ Structural transformation in intestinal contents.

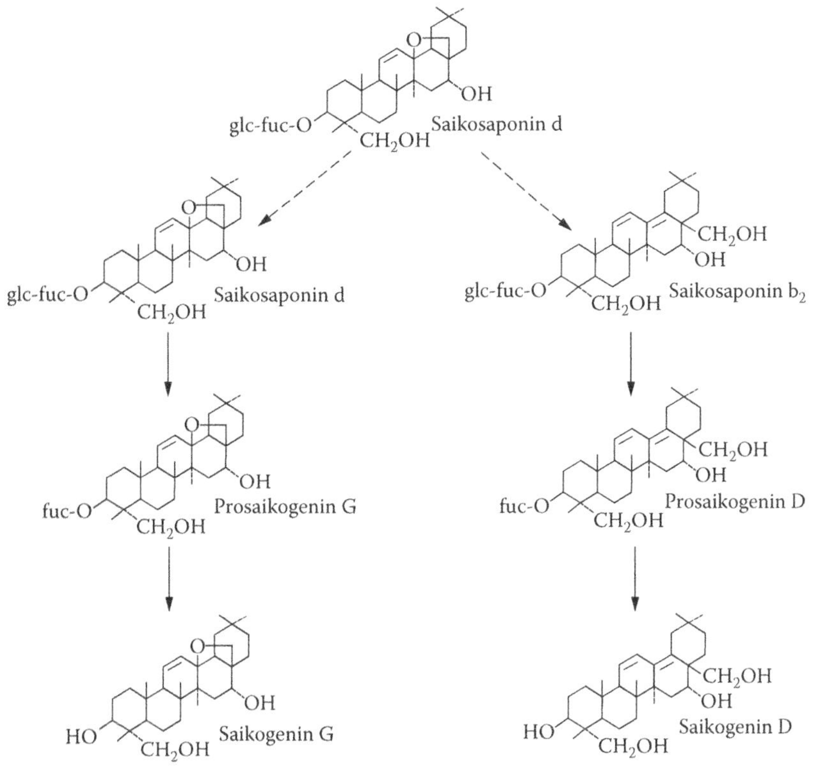

FIGURE 7.3 Metabolites of saikosaponin-d formed in the alimentary tract. ·······▶ Structural transformation in gastric juice. ——▶ Structural transformation in intestinal contents.

cacticin were isolated from *B. scorzonerifolium, B. aureum, B.triradiatum, B. bicaule, B. pusillum B. rotundifolium, B. ranunculoides,* and *B. martjanovii* (Minaeva et al., 1965, 1970; Sobolevskaya et al., 1967; Inoue and Ogihara, 1978). In 1980, Shi and Xu isolated kaempheritin and kaempferol-7-rhamnoside from *B. chinense.* Luo and Jing (1991) isolated quercetin-3-arabinofuranosids, quercetin-3-glucoside, isorhamnetin, and isorhamnetin-3-glucoside. Pistelli et al. (1993b) also isolated quercetin-3-arabinofuranoside and quercetin-3-arabinopyranoside from *B. falcatum* subsp. *cernuum* and isolated kaempferol, isokaempferide, gossipetin, luteolin, kaempferol-3-glucoside, kaempferol-3-rutinoside from *B. flavum* as well.

In 1998, Tan et al. isolated an isoflavonoside from *B. scorzonerifolium* and named it saikoisoflavonoside A (Figure 7.6).

In reference to aglycones, the flavonoids from *Bupleurum* can be divided into three series: quercetin series, kaempferol series and isorhamnetin series (Figure 7.6) Quercetin-3-glucoside, quercetin-3-rhamnoside, quercetin-3-arabipyranoside, quercetin-3-arabifuranoside, rutin, and isoquercetrin belong to the quecetin series. Kaempferol-7-rhamnoside, kaempferol-3-arabiferanol-7-rhamnopyranoside, kaempferol-3,7-dirhamnoside, and robinin belong to the kaempferol series. And isorhamnetin-3-rutinoside, isorhamnetin-3-glucoside, and narcissin belong to the isorhamnetin series (Pan et al., 2002).

7.2.5 COUMARINS

Coumarins are characteristic compounds in the plants of Umbelliferae, but are less common in the *Bupleurum* genus. They are mainly simple coumarins, e.g., scopoletin, scoparone, isoscoparone,

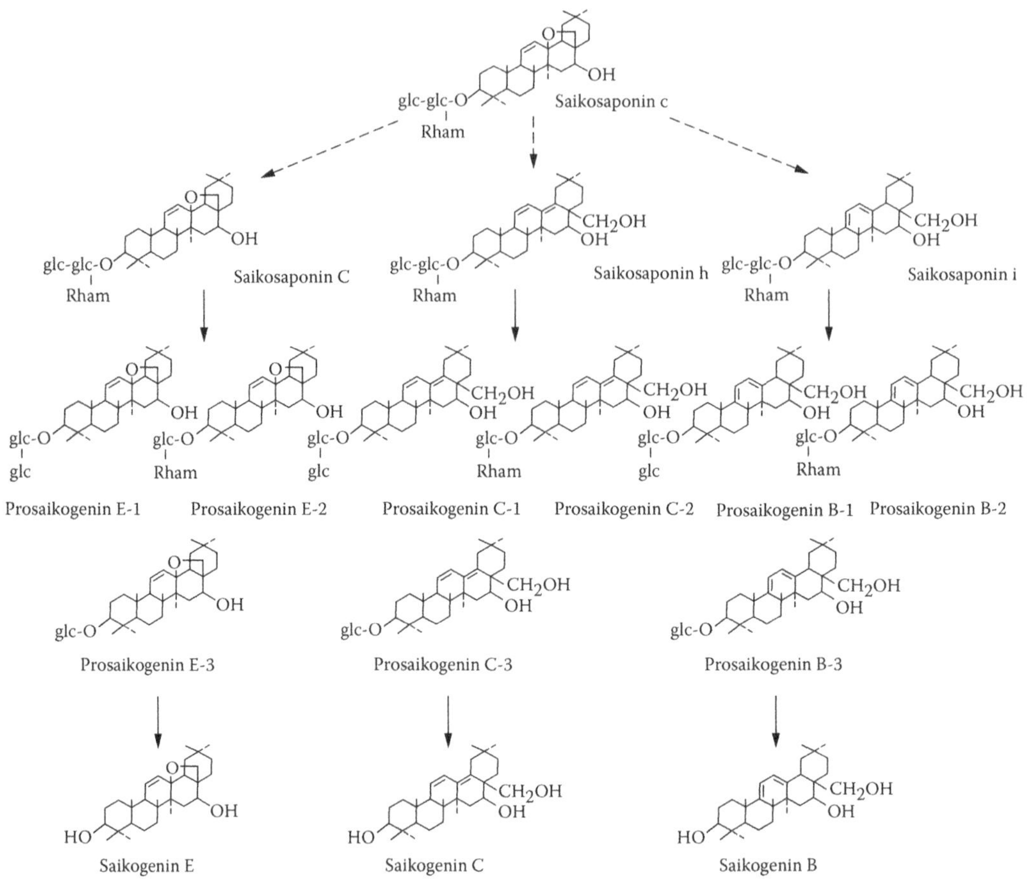

FIGURE 7.4 Metabolites of saikosaponin-c formed in the alimentary tract. ·······▶ Structural transformation in gastric juice. ──▶ Structural transformation in intestinal contents.

capensin, fraxetin, herniarin, limettin, prenyletin, aesculetin, angelicin, anomalin, etc. Their structures are shown in Chapters 8 and 9.

7.2.6 POLYACETYLENES

Zhao et al. (1987) isolated four new polyacetylenes from *B. longiradiatum* Turcz., and named them bupleurotoxin, bupleuronol, acetyl-bupleurotoxin, and bupleurynol. Bupleurotoxin and acetyl-bupleurotoxin are the toxic principles of the species. The LD_{50} for bupleurotoxin in mice (ip injection) is 3.03 mg/kg and for acetyl-bupleurotoxin 3.13 mg/kg. Physical, chemical, and spectroscopic evidence supports bupleurynol as heptadecatren-(2Z, 8E, 10E)-diyne-(4, 6)-ol-1, bupleurotoxin as 14-hydroxyl-bupleurynol, acetyl-bupleurotoxin as 14-acetoxy-bupleurynol and bupleuronol as 14-carbonyl-bupleurynol.

Morita et al. (1991) isolated three new polyacetylenes from the root of *B. falcatum*, and named them saikodiynes A, B, and C. Saikodiyne A was determined to be 2Z, 8E-pentadecadiene-4, 6-diyne-1, 10-diol. Sikodiyne B was identified as 10-hydroxy-2E, 8E-diene-4, 6-diyne-pentadecanal. Saikodiyne C was identified as 2Z, 9Z-pentadecadiene-4, 6-diyn-1-yl acetate.

Another 11 polyacetylenes have been isolated from the Spanish species *B. salicifolium, B. gibraltaricum,* and *B. acutifolium* (see Chapter 8).

TABLE 7.2
Content of Saikosaponin-a, -c, and -d in 23 Species from
***Bupleurum* Genus**

Species	Content of Saikosaponins (%)				
	ss-a	ss-c	ss-d	a + c + d	a + d
B. chinense	0.47	0.56	0.52	1.55	0.99
B. scorzonerifolium	0.41	0.15	0.35	0.91	0.76
B. smithii var. *parvifolium*	0.13	0.19	0.35	0.67	0.48
B. smithii	0.43	0.42	0.48	1.33	0.91
B. marginatum var. *stenophyllum*	3.55	0.19	0.11	3.85	3.66
B. yinchowense	0.68	0.15	0.37	1.20	1.05
B. polyclonum	3.66	0.82	2.96	7.44	6.62
B. longiradiatum	0.19	0.04	0.15	0.38	0.34
B. bicaule	0.15	0.07	0.15	0.37	0.30
B.angustissimum	0.27	0.17	0.28	0.72	0.55
B. krylovianum	0.59	0.04	0.16	0.79	0.75
B. kunmingense	1.71	0.68	2.01	4.40	3.72
B. luxiense	0.64	0.53	0.58	1.75	1.22
B. candollei	Trace	Trace	Trace	—	—
B. rockii	1.38	0.31	0.84	2.53	2.22
B. petiolulatum var. *tenerum*	1.09	0.38	0.88	2.35	1.97
B. hamiltonii	0.11	0.02	0.08	0.21	0.19
B. wenchuanense	1.47	0.73	2.25	4.45	3.72
B. sichuanense	1.08	0.19	1.06	2.33	2.14
B. candolle var. *franchetii*	0.05	Trace	0.03	0.08	0.08
B. malconense	0.52	0.18	0.51	1.21	1.03
B. chaishoui	0.88	0.30	0.71	1.89	1.59
B. commelynoideum var. *flaviflorum*	0.13	0.19	0.15	0.47	0.28

7.2.7 POLYSACCHARIDES

Polysaccharides from *Bupleurum* possess antiulcer, antitumor, and immunomodulatory activities. They are composed of galacturonic acid, arabinose, rhamnose, galactose, ribose, and xylose. Their molecular masses are from 3600 to 63000. Yamada et al. (1991) reported the pectic polysaccharide from *B. falcatum* has antiulcer activity. Zhang et al. (1986) demonstrated that the *B. kunmingense* polysaccharides (BKP) injected with ip 50 or 200 mg/kg qd for 4 days could increase the weight of mouse spleen. BKP with ip 50 mg/kg qd for 4 days could enhance the proliferative response of mouse splenocytes to lipopolysaccharides (LPS) but not to Con A as measured by [³H]TdR incorporation. On the other hand, the number of plaque-forming cells (PFC) in 2×10^7 splenocytes of mice treated with BKP was lower than that of the control group. These results suggested that BKP has selective activity on the immune system.

7.2.8 OTHER CONSTITUENTS

There also occur phenylpropanoids, sterols, organic acids, and chromones in some species of genus *Bupleurum.* Ten phenylpropanoids have been isolated from *B. frucicosum* and *B. actutifolium* (see Chapter 8).

The sterols from *Bupleurum* are stigmasterol, Δ^7-stigmastenol, Δ^{22}-stigmastenol, α-spinasterol, and β-sitosterol. Organic acids are petroselic acid, petrolidic acid, angelic acid, linolenic acid, lignoceric acid, palmitic acid, oleic acid, and stearic acid (Tomimatsu, 1969; Pan et al., 2002). One new chromone named saikochromone A has also been reported (Kobayashi et al., 1990; Figure 7.7).

TABLE 7.3
Content of Saikosaponins of *Bupleurum* Collected in Different Districts of China

Species	Collected District	Content of Saikosaponins (%)				
		ss-a	ss-c	ss-d	a + c + d	a + d
B. chinense	Shijiazhuang (Hebei)	0.48	0.26	0.63	1.37	1.11
B. chinense	Zhanhuang (Hebei)	0.59	0.20	0.49	1.28	1.08
B. chinense	Chengde (Hebei)	0.30	0.17	0.23	0.70	0.53
B. chinense	Luoyang (Henan)	0.50	0.24	0.48	1.22	0.98
B. chinense	Handan (Henan)	0.75	0.27	0.52	1.54	1.27
B. chinense	Tianjin	0.41	0.25	0.36	1.02	0.77
B. chinense	Shenyang (Liaoning)	0.58	0.13	0.28	0.99	0.86
B. chinense	Qing'an (Heilongjiang)	0.34	0.25	0.34	0.93	0.68
B. chinense	Wuhan (Hubei)	0.47	0.56	0.52	1.55	0.99
B. chinense	Taiyuan (Shanxi)	0.34	0.13	0.29	0.76	0.63
B. chinense	Xi'an (Shaanxi)	0.51	0.33	0.39	1.23	0.90
B. chinense	Luiyang (Shaanxi)	0.84	0.68	0.78	2.30	1.62
B. chinense	Gao'an (Jiangxi)	0.67	1.28	1.09	3.04	2.37
B. chinense	Pingxiang (Jiangxi)	0.36	0.18	0.30	0.84	0.66
B. chinense	Fuyang (Anhui)	0.24	0.23	0.28	0.75	0.51
B. chinense	Lin'an (Zhejiang)	0.87	0.39	0.64	1.84	1.51
B. chinense	Fuzhou (Fujian)	0.46	0.30	0.36	1.12	0.82
B. chinense	Quanzhou (Fujian)	0.27	0.21	0.32	0.80	0.59
B. chinense	Xiamen (Fujian)	0.22	0.16	0.27	0.65	0.49
B. chinense	Nanning (Guangxi)	0.24	0.13	0.25	0.62	0.49
B. smithii var. parvifolium	Tianzhu (Gansu)	0.51	0.47	0.36	1.34	0.87
B. smithii var. parvifolium	Yuzhong (Gansu)	0.15	0.01	0.30	0.46	0.45
B. smithii var. parvifolium	Yuzhong (Gansu)	0.38	0.09	0.22	0.69	0.60
B. smithii var. parvifolium	Yingchuan (Ningxia)	0.20	0.11	0.32	0.63	0.52
B. smithii var. parvifolium	Tongxin (Ningxia)	0.10	0.10	0.16	0.36	0.26
B. smithii var. parvifolium	Tongxin (Ningxia)	0.13	0.19	0.35	0.67	0.48
B. smithii var. parvifolium	Baotou (Nuimenggu)	0.12	0.07	0.14	0.33	0.26
B. smithii var. parvifolium	Yushan (Jiangxi)	0.25	0.10	0.25	0.60	0.50
B. scorzonerifolium	Tiangjin	0.37	0.18	0.31	0.86	0.68
B. scorzonerifolium	Chengde (Hebei)	0.41	0.15	0.35	0.91	0.76
B. scorzonerifolium	Chuxian (Anhui)	0.38	0.17	0.28	0.83	0.66
B. scorzonerifolium	Jinhua (Zhejiang)	0.13	0.18	0.09	0.40	0.22
B. marginatum var. stenophyllum	Kunming (Yunnan)	2.15	0.20	1.46	3.81	3.61
B. marginatum var. stenophyllum	Huize (Yunnan)	3.55	0.19	0.11	3.86	3.66
B. marginatum var. stenophyllum	Guangzhou (Guangdong)	0.66	0.15	0.51	1.32	1.17
B. marginatum var. stenophyllum	Dianbai (Guangdong)	0.45	0.13	0.31	0.89	0.76
B. marginatum var. stenophyllum	Nanning (Guangxi)	0.48	0.14	0.46	1.08	0.94
B. marginatum var. stenophyllum	Liuzhou (Guangxi)	0.75	0.13	0.64	1.52	1.39
B. yinchowense	Tiangshui (Gansu)	0.45	0.16	0.30	0.91	0.75
B. yinchowense	Heshui (Gansu)	0.28	0.10	0.22	0.60	0.50
B. yinchowense	Zhenning (Gansu)	0.55	0.18	0.42	1.15	0.97
B. yinchowense	Wuzhong (Ningxia)	0.68	0.15	0.37	1.20	1.05
B. bicaule	Xilinghaote (Neimenggu)	0.04	0.04	0.01	0.09	0.05
B. bicaule	Hulunbei'er (Neimenggu)	0.15	0.07	0.15	0.37	0.30
B. polyclonum	Kunming (Yunnan)	3.06	0.72	2.94	6.72	6.00
B. polyclonum	Huize (Yunnan)	3.66	0.82	2.96	7.44	6.62

TABLE 7.4
The Constituents of Oil and Their Original Plants

Constituents	Original Plants[a]																				
	A	B	C	D	E	F	G	H	I	J	K	L	M	N	O	P	Q	R	S	T	U
1. Acoradiene				+								+									
2. Aromadendrene		+			+			+									+	+			
3. Alloaromadendrene																			+		
4. (E)-Anethole																				+	
5. (Z)-Anethole																				+	
6. *p*-Anysaldehyde																				+	
7. Azulene				+				+	+												
8. Phenyl, ethyl-2-methylbenzoate																				+	
9. Benzyl benzoate																				+	
10. 1-Methyl-3-isopropylbenzene														+							
11. *p*-Isopropylbenzoic acid			+					+						+	+	+	+				
12. β-Bisabolene				+		+								+							
13. Borneol								+			+									+	
14. Isoborneol		+																			
15. Bornelene				+									+							+	
16. Isobornyl acetate																				+	
17. Phenyl, ethyl-3-methylbutanoate																				+	
18. β-Bourbonene																				+	+
19. Bupleurol																				+	
20. Hexyl-2-methylbutyrate																				+	
21. Cadinol																				+	
22. α-Cadinol																				+	
23. Cadinene								+													
24. γ-Cadinene			+	+				+			+						+				+
25. *cis*-γ-Cadinene																				+	
26. δ-Cadinene	+		+	+	+			+								+	+			+	+
27. *cis*-Calamenene																					+
28. *trans*-Calamenene																					+
29. Calarene																				+	
30. γ-Calcorene																					+
31. Camphene		+													+					+	
32. δ-3-Carene			+	+			+				+					+	+			+	+
33. Carvacrol											+					+				+	
34. Carvacrol methyl ether																				+	
35. [+]-Carvone	+												+			+				+	+
36. *cis*-Carveol																				+	
37. *trans*-Carveol	+					+	+									+				+	
38. Dihydro carveol																				+	
39. *cis*-Carvyl acetate																				+	
40. β-Caryophyllene																				+	+
41. *cis*-Caryophyllene		+	+		+						+					+	+				
42. *trans*-Caryophyllene	+	+									+										
43. Caryophyllene oxide																					+
44. β-Cedrene											+				+						
45. Cedrenol														+	+						
46. Methyl chavicol																				+	
47. *p*-Cimen-9-ol																				+	
48. 2,5-Dimethossy-*p*-cimene																				+	

TABLE 7.4 (CONTINUED)
The Constituents of Oil and Their Original Plants

	Constituents	A	B	C	D	E	F	G	H	I	J	K	L	M	N	O	P	Q	R	S	T	U
																					Original Plants[a]	
49.	p-Methoxy-cinnamal dehyde																				+	
50.	1,8-Cineole																				+	
51.	Dihydro-1,8-cineole												+								+	
52.	Citral	+																				
53.	Citronellol																			+		
54.	Citronellyl acetate																			+		
55.	Copaene							+												+		
56.	α-Copaene		+	+	+	+			+		+				+	+	+	+	+	+	+	+
57.	Cryptone																			+		
58.	α-Cubebene	+		+	+	+	+					+				+	+		+	+	+	+
59.	β-Cubebene																+					
60.	Cubebol																			+		
61.	Epi-cubebol																			+		
62.	Cubenol																			+		
63.	m-Cymene																					+
64.	p-Cymene	+																			+	+
65.	γ-Decalactone				+																	
66.	n-Decanal							+														
67.	Decanol																			+		
68.	n-Decane							+	+													
69.	5-Methyldecane															+						
70.	2,5-Dimethyldecane							+														
71.	5-Methyl-5-ethyldecane				+			+		+		+			+		+					
72.	n-Dodecanal							+														
73.	2,4-Dodecadienal							+														
74.	2-Methyldodecane									+		+										
75.	3-Methyldodecane															+						
76.	α-Elemene							+								+						
77.	β-Elemene		+	+	+	+							+			+				+	+	+
78.	γ-Elemene				+															+		
79.	δ-Elemene																			+		
80.	Elemicin																			+		
81.	β-Elemol																					+
82.	1,10-Epicubenol																			+		
83.	2,6-Dimethyl-5-epitanal																			+		
84.	Eudesmol													+								
85.	α-Eudesmol																					+
86.	Eugenol	+																				
87.	Methyl eugenol																			+		
88.	α-Farnesene		+	+	+			+	+		+					+				+		
89.	(E,E)-Farnesene																			+		
90.	trans-β-Farnesene				+										+					+		
91.	Farnesylacetone																			+	+	
92.	Hexahydrofarnesylacetone	+			+		+									+						
93.	α-Fenchene				+														+			
94.	β-Fenchene		+																			
95.	Fenchane							+														
96.	Fenchone															+						

TABLE 7.4 (CONTINUED)
The Constituents of Oil and Their Original Plants

	Constituents	A	B	C	D	E	F	G	H	I	J	K	L	M	N	O	P	Q	R	S	T	U
																		Original Plants[a]				
97.	2-Pentyl-furan	+						+									+	+				
98.	Geraniol	+		+	+								+									
99.	Geranyl acetate																				+	
100.	[*E*]-Geranylacetone	+				+		+														
101.	Germacrene D																				+	+
102.	Biciclogermacrene																				+	
103.	α-Guaiene																	+		+		
104.	β-Guaiene									+												
105.	Guaiol																					+
106.	β-Gurjunene					+		+	+							+	+	+				
107.	1-Heptadecene								+													
108.	Heptadecane				+																	
109.	8-Methylheptadecane								+													
110.	γ-Heptalactone				+																	
111.	*n*-Heptaldehyde									+					+							
112.	Heptanoic acid								+													
113.	1-Heptanol								+													
114.	3-Heptanone																	+				
115.	4-Methyl-3-heptanone														+							
116.	3,3,5-Trimethylheptane						+															
117.	Heptyl acetate																				+	
118.	Hexadecanal																	+				
119.	Hexadecanoic acid	+					+						+									
120.	2-Methylhexadecane								+						+							
121.	Cyclohexanone			+					+	+												
122.	1-Hexene																			+		
123.	*cis*-3-Hexene-1-ol																				+	
124.	(*Z*)-3-Hexenyl acetate																				+	
125.	α-Himachalene													+								
126.	Humulene	+	+	+	+		+		+					+		+		+				
127.	α-Humulene																				+	+
128.	α-Humulene oxide																					+
129.	Khusilol								+	+												
130.	Limonene	+	+	+	+	+	+	+	+			+		+			+	+	+	+	+	+
131.	Linalool	+	+			+						+									+	+
132.	Linalyl acetate																				+	
133.	Ledol		+															+	+	+	+	
134.	Longicyclene																					+
135.	Longifolene	+																			+	
136.	*cis-p*-Mentha-2,8-dien-1-ol																				+	
137.	*trans-p*-Mentha-2,8-dien-1-ol																				+	
138.	Menthone								+			+										
139.	Messoialactone	+																				
140.	T-Muurolol																				+	
141.	γ-Muurolene		+						+	+								+	+			+
142.	Myrcene			+	+						+			+						+	+	
143.	Myrcenone																				+	
144.	Myrcenol																			+		

TABLE 7.4 (CONTINUED)
The Constituents of Oil and Their Original Plants

Constituents	A	B	C	D	E	F	G	H	I	J	K	L	M	N	O	P	Q	R	S	T	U
145. Myrtenol	+		+	+	+									+						+	
146. Myrtenal			+							+										+	
147. Neral														+			+				
148. Nerol									+											+	
149. Nerolidol																				+	+
150. Nerolidol isomer			+							+						+					
151. Nonadecane											+										
152. Nonanal																				+	
153. 2-Nonenal																			+		
154. *cis*-6-Nonenal																			+		
155. Nootkatone	+	+				+	+										+				
156. (*E*)-β-Ocimene																				+	
157. (*Z*)-β-Ocimene																				+	
158. γ-Octalactone	+																				
159. Octanal	+						+		+	+											
160. 2,6-Dimethyloctane			+	+									+								
161. Octyl acetate																				+	
162. Patchoulane			+			+							+								
163. Patchouli alcochol								+													
164. γ-Patchoulene						+				+											
165. Pentanoic acid													+								
166. 2-Methylcyclopentanone	+		+	+	+	+				+				+	+	+	+	+			
167. Perillen								+										+			
168. *n*-Pentadecane	+										+						+				
169. α-Phellandrene																				+	
170. β-Phellandrene																				+	
171. Phytol																				+	
172. Phytol acetate																				+	
173. (*E*)-Phytol acetate																				+	
174. α-Pinene				+															+	+	
175. β-Pinene	+		+	+		+					+			+					+	+	+
176. Isopinocamphone											+										
177. Pinocarvone																				+	
178. *trans*-Pinocarvone																				+	
179. *trans*-Pipritol																				+	
180. 3-(Methoxyphenyl)-2-propen-1-ol																				+	
181. Pulegone	+	+		+							+		+			+	+				
182. Isopulegol											+								+		
183. Sabinene																				+	+
184. *trans*-Sabinene-hydrate																				+	
185. Salvial-4(14)-en -1-one																				+	
186. β-Selinene											+										
187. Spatulenol																				+	
188. 2.5-Dimethyl stirene																				+	
189. α-Terpineol	+		+	+	+	+		+			+		+	+			+				
190. β-Terpineol		+										+		+					+	+	
191. α-Terpinene																				+	
192. β-Terpinene														+					+	+	

TABLE 7.4 (CONTINUED)
The Constituents of Oil and Their Original Plants

Constituents	A	B	C	D	E	F	G	H	I	J	K	L	M	N	O	P	Q	R	S	T	U
193. γ-Terpinene			+							+				+				+		+	
194. Terpineol-4-ol			+	+				+												+	+
195. α-Terpineolene			+																		
196. 2,5-Dimethyltetradecane																	+				
197. n-Tetradecane			+				+							+		+	+				
198. Tetradecanoic acid				+	+																
199. α-Thujene				+										+						+	
200. β-Thujene				+																	
201. Thujone																				+	
202. Thymol	+									+	+									+	
203. Thymol methyl ether																				+	
204. Thymoquinone methyl ether																				+	
205. Torreyol																	+				
206. n-Tridecane	+		+	+			+							+		+					
207. 7-Methyltridecan																+					
208. 7-Tridecanone			+																		
209. 4,8-Dimethyltridecane			+		+		+	+	+	+						+	+				
210. n-Undecan	+		+	+	+	+	+	+	+	+						+	+				
211. Undecanal							+								+	+					
212. 5-Undecanone								+													
213. 3,8-Dimethylundecane									+												
214. Valensene																				+	+
215. (E)-Cinnamyl valerate																				+	
216. Amil isovalerate																				+	
217. Cinnamyl isovalerate																				+	
218. Hexyl isovalerate																				+	
219. Vanillin acetate	+																				
220. Veratryl alcohol													+								
221. trans-Verbenol																					
222. Verbenone																+					

[a] Original Plants — A: *Bupleurum chinense* DC.; B: *B. scorzonerifolium* Willd.; C: *B. smithii* Wolff; D: *B. smithii* Wolff var. *parvifolium* Shan et Y. Li; E: *B. marginatum* Wall. ex DC.; F: *B. marginatum* Wall. ex DC. var. *stenophyllum* (Wolff) Shan et Y. Li; G: *B. euphorbioides* Nakai; H: *B. polyclonum* Y. Li et S.L. Pan; I: *B. kunmingense* Y. Li et S.L. Pan; J: *B. luxiense* Y. Li et S.L. Pan; K: *B. longicaule* Wall. ex DC. var *franchetii* de Boiss.; L: *B. rockii* Wolff; M: *B. hamiltonii* Belak; N: *B. angustissimum* (Franch.) Kitagawa; O: *B. malconense* Shan et Y. Li; P: *B. wenchuanense* Shan et Y. Li; Q: *B. chaishoui* Shan et Sheh; R: *B. qinghaiense* Y. Li et Guo; S: *B. longiradiatum* Turcz.; T: *B. fruticosum* L.; U: *B. gibraltaricum* Lam.

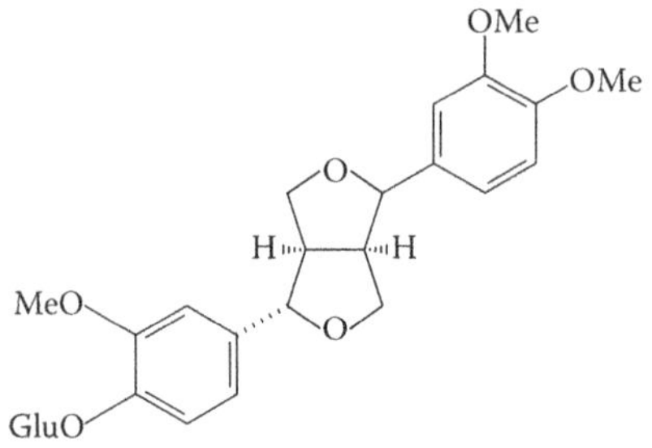

Phillyrin

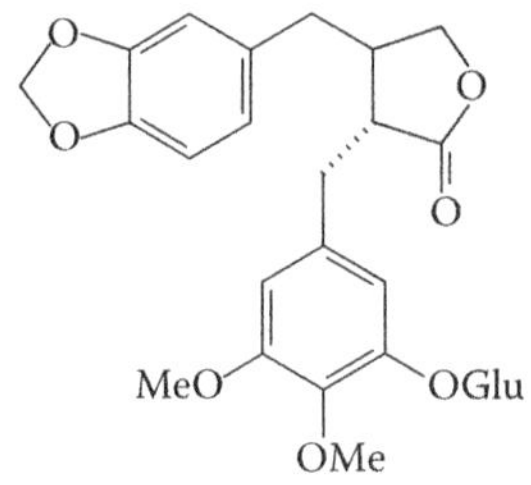

Wenchuanensin

FIGURE 7.5 Structures of phillyrin and wenchuanensin.

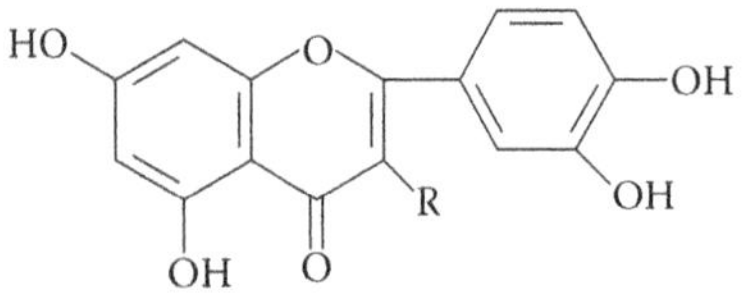

Quercetin: R=H

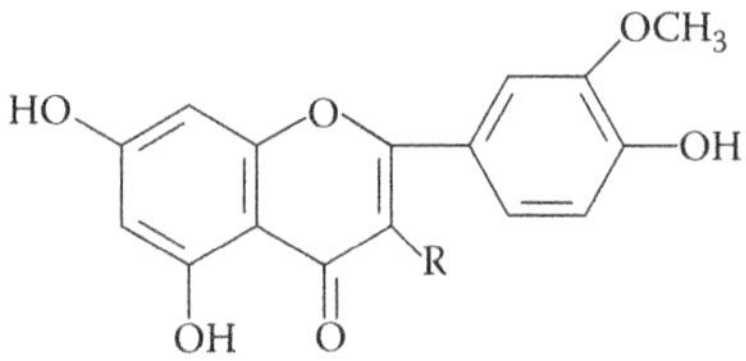

Isorhamnetin: R=OH

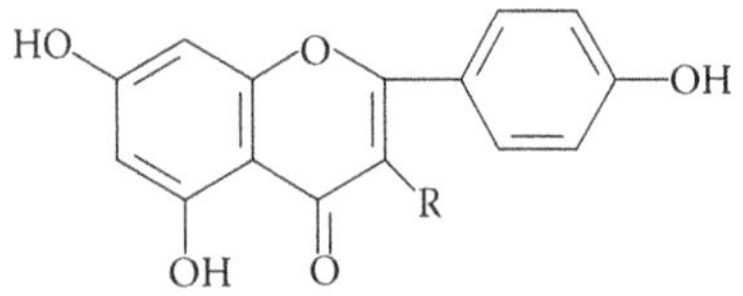

Kaempferol: R=OH

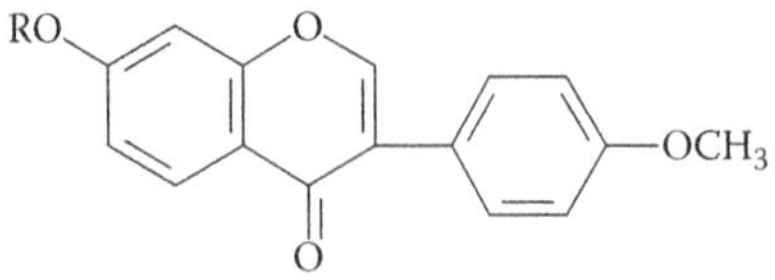

Saikoisoflavonoside A: R=glu (p)–(1~6)-glu (p)

FIGURE 7.6 The structure of flavonoids in *Bupleurum*.

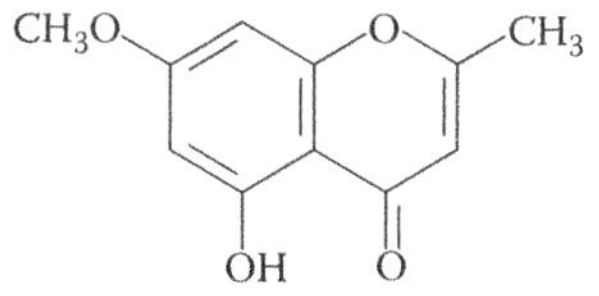

FIGURE 7.7 The structure of saikochromone a.

REFERENCES

Abe, H., Sakaguchi, M., Yamada, M., Arich, S., and Odashima, S. (1980) Pharmacological actions of saiko-saponins isolated from *Bupleurum falcatum*, *Planta Med.*, 40, 366–372.

Abe, H., Sakaguchi, M., Odashima, S., and Arich, S. (1982) Protective effect of saikosaponin-d isolated from *Bupleurum falcatum* L. on CCl_4-induced liver injury in the rat, *Nauyn-Schmiedeberg's Arch. Pharmacol.*, 320, 266–271.

Abe, H., Orita, M., Konishi, H., Arichi, S., and Odashima, S. (1985) Effects of saikosaponin-d on enhanced CCl_4-hepatotoxicity by phenobarbitone, *J. Pharm. Pharmacol.*, 37, 555–559.

Aimi, N. and Shibata, S. (1966) Saikosaponin E, a genuine saponin of *Bupleurum* roots. *Tetrahedron Lett.*, 39, 4721–4724.

Akai, E., Takeda, T., Kobayashi, Y., and Ogihara, Y. (1985) Sulfated triterpenoid saponins from the leaves of *Bupleurum rotundifolium* L., *Chem. Pharm. Bull.*, 33, 3715–3723.

Barrero, A.F., Haidour, A., and Reyes F. (1998) Monoterpene aldehydes from *Bupleurum gibraltaricum, J. Nat. Prod.*, 61, 506–507.

Barrero, A.F., Haidour, A., Sedqui, A., Mansour, A.I., Rodriguez-Garcia, I., Lopez, A., and Munoz-Dorado, M. (2000) Saikosaponins from roots of *Bupleurum gibraltaricum* and *Bupleurum spinosum, Phytochemistry,* 54, 741–745.

Barrero, A.F., Herrador, M.M., Akssira, M., Arteaga, P., and Romera J. L. (1999) Lignans and polyacetylenes from *Bupleurum acutifolium, J. Nat. Prod.*, 62, 946–948.

Benito, P.B., Abad-Marinez, M.J., Silvan-Sen, A.M., Sanz-Gomez, A., Femandez-Matellano, L., Sanchez-Contreras, S., and Diaz-Lanza, A.M. (1998) *In vivo in vitro* antiinflammatory activity of saikosaponins, *Life Sci.*, 63, 1147–1156.

Benito, P.B., Abad-Marinez, M.J., Diaz-Lanza, A.M., Femandez-Matellano, L.,.,Santos, J.D., Sanchez-Contreras, S., Villaescusa, L., Carrasco, L., and Iruzun, A. (2002) Antiviral activity of seven iridoids, three saikosaponins and one phenylpropanoid glycoside extracted from *Bupleurum rigidum* and *Scrophularia scorodonia, Planta Med.,* 68, 106–110.

Bermejo, P., Abad, M.J., Diaz, A.M., Fernandez, L., Santos, J.D., Sanchez, S., Villaescusa, L., Carrasco, L., and Irurzun, A. (2002) Antiviral activity of seven iridoids, three saikosaponins and one phenylpropanoid glycoside extracted from *Bupleurum rigidum* and *Scrophularia scorodonia, Planta Medica,* 68, 106–110.

Chen, X.K., Zhang, R.Y., Zhang, Z.L., and Wang, B. (1993) Isolation and identification of two new saponins from *Bupleurum smithii* Wolff, *Acta Pharm. Sin.*, 28, 352–357.

Ding, J.K., Fujino, H., Kasal, R., Fujimoto, N., Tanaka, O., Zhou, J., Matsuura, H., and Fuwa, T. (1986) Chemical evaluation of *Bupleurum* species collected in Yunnan, China, *Chem. Pharm. Bull.*, 34, 1158–1167.

Dugo, G., Trozzi, A., Verzera, A., and Rapisarda, A. (2002) Essential oils from leaves of typical Mediterranean plants, Note I, *Bupleurum fruticosum, Essenze. Derivati Agrumari.*, 70, 201–204.

Ebata, N., Nakajima, K., Taguchi, H., and Mitsuhashi, H. (1990) Isolation of new saponins from the root of *Bupleurum falcatum* L., *Chem. Pharm. Bull.*, 38, 1432–1434.

Ebata, N., Nakajima, K., Hayashi, K., Okada, M., and Maruno, M. (1996) Saponins from the root of *Bupleurum falcatum, Phytochemistry*, 41, 895–901.

Estevez-Braun, A., Estevez-Reyes, R., and Gonzalez, A.G. (1994) Structural elucidation and conformational analysis of new lignan butenolides from the leaves of *Bupleurum salicifolium, Tetrahedron,* 50, 5203–5210.

Estevez-Braun, A., Estevez-Reyes, R., Gonzalez-Perez, J.A., and Gonzalez, A.G. (1995) Busaliol and busalic-
    ifol, two new lignans from *Bupleurum salicifolium, J. Nat. Prod.*, 58, 887–892.
Estevez-Reyes, R., Estevez-Braun, A., and Gonzalez, A.G. (1992) Lignanolides from *Bupleurum salicifolium,
    Phytochemistry*, 31, 2841–2845.
Estevez-Reyes, R., Estevez-Braun, A., and Gonzalez, A.G. (1993) New lignan butenolides from *Bupleurum
    salicifolium, J. Nat. Prod.*, 56, 1177–1181.
Ezawa, T. (1916) *Rep. Taiwan Central Res. Lab.*, 5, 179.
Francesconi, L. and Sernagiotto, E. (1913) Bupleurol, the alcohol of the essence of *Bupleurum fruticosum,
    Gazz. Chim. Ital.*, 43, 153–161.
Gil, M.L., Jimenez, J., Ocete, M.A., Zarzuelo, A., and Cabo M.M. (1989) Comparative study of different
    essential oils of *Bupleurum gibraltaricum* Lamarck, *Pharmazie*, 44, 284–287.
Gonzalez, A.G., Trujillo, J.M., Estevez, R., and Perez, J.P. (1975) Componentes de Umbeliferas IV. Lignanos
    del *Bupleurum fruticescens* L., *An. Quim.*, 71, 109–110.
Gonzalez, A.G., Estevez-Reyes, R., and Mato, C. (1989) Salicifoliol, a new furolactone-type lignan from
    Bupleurum salicifolium, J. Nat. Prod., 52, 1139–1142.
Gonzalez, A.G., Estevez-Reyes, R., Mato, C., and Estevez-Braun, A. (1990a) Isokaerophyllin, a butyrolactone
    from *Bupleurum salicifolium, Phytochemistry*, 29, 675–678.
Gonzalez, A.G., Estevez-Reyes, R., Mato, C., and Estevez-Braun, A. (1990b) Three lignans from *Bupleurum
    salicifolium, Phytochemistry*, 29, 1981–1983.
Gonzalez, A.G., Estevez-Reyes, R., and Estevez-Braun, A.M. (1990c) Buplerol and guayarol, new lignans
    from *Bupleurum salicifolium, J. Chem. Res.*, 220–221.
Guinea, M.C., Parellada, J., Lacaille-Dubois, M.A., and Wagner, H. (1994) Biologically active triterpene
    saponins from *Bupleurum fruticosum, Planta Med.*, 60, 163–167.
Guo, J.X., Pan, S.L., Li, Y., Hong, X.K., and Wang, Z.H. (1990) A study on the chemical constituents of
    volatile oils from 19 species of the genus *Bupleurum* in China, *Acta Acad. Med. Shanghai*, 17,
    278–282.
Hong L, Cui Y.J. et al. (2000) Saikosaponin v-2 from *Bupleurum chinense, Chin. Chim. Lett.,*
Hsu, M.J., Cheng, J.S., and Huang, H.C. (2000) Effect of saikosaponin, a triterpene saponin, on apoptosis in
    lymphocytes: association with c-myc, p53, and bcl-2 mRNA. *Br. J. Pharmacol.*, 131, 1285–1293.
Inoue, O. and Ogihara, Y. (1978) Studies on the constituents of *Bupleurum rotundifolium* L. I, *Shoyakugaku
    Zasshi*, 32, 100–103.
Ishii, H., Seo, S., Tori, K., Tozyo, T., and Yoshimura, Y. (1977) The structures of saikosaponin-e and acetyl-
    saikosaponins, minor components isolated from *Bupleurum falcatum* L., determined by C-13 NMR
    spectroscopy. *Tetrahedron Lett.*, 14, 1227–1230.
Ishii, H., Nakamura, M., Seo, S., Tori, K., Tozyo, T., and Yoshimura, Y. (1980) Isolation, characterization, and
    nuclear magnetic resonanse spectra of new saponins from the roots of *Bupleurum falcatum* L., *Chem.
    Pharm. Bull.*, 28, 2367–2383.
Just, M.J., Recio, M.C., Giner, R.M., Cuellar, M.J., Manez, S., Bilia, A.R., and Rios, J.L. (1998) Anti-
    inflammatory activity of unusual lupane saponins from *Bupleurum fruticescens, Planta Med.*, 64,
    404–407.
Kato, M., Pu, M., Isobe, K.L., Hattori, T., Yamagita, N, and Nakashima, I. (1995) Cell type-oriented differential
    modulatory action of saikosaponin-d on growth responses and DNA fragmentation of lymphocytes
    triggered by receptor-mediated and receptor-bypassed pathways, *Immunopharmacology*, 29, 207–213.
Kobayashi, M., Takashi, T., Tsuchida, T., and Mitsuhashi, H. (1990) Studies on the constituents of Umbelliferae
    plants. XVIII. Minor constituents of *Bupleurum* radix: occurence of saikogenins, polyhydroxysterols,
    a trihydroxy C18 fatty acid, a lignan and a new chromone, *Chem. Pharm. Bull.*, 38, 3169–3171.
Kubota, T. and Hinoh, H. (1966) Isolation of saikosaponin e, a new triterpene from *Bupleurum falcatum,
    Tetrahedron Lett.*, 39, 4725–4728.
Kubota, T. and Hinoh, H. (1968a) The constitution of saponins isolated from *Bupleurum falcatum* L.,
    Tetrahedron Lett., 3, 303–306.
Kubota, T. and Hinoh, H. (1968b) Triterpenoids from *Bupleurum falcatum* L. III, Isolation of genuine
    sapogenins saikogenins E, F and G, *Tetrahedron*, 24, 675–686.
Kubota, T. and Tonami, F. (1967) Triterpenoids from *Bupleurum falcatum* L. II, Isolation of saikosaponin b
    and lengispinogenin, *Tetrahedron*, 23, 3353–3362.

Kubota, T., Tonami, F., and Hinoh, H.. (1967) Triterpenoids from *Bupleurum falcatum* L. I. The structure of saikosaponins a, c and d, *Tetrahedron*, 23, 3333–3351.

Kumazawa, Y., Takimoto, H., Nishimura, C., Kawakita, T., and Nomoto, K. (1989) Activation of murine peritoneal macrophages by saikosaponin-a, saikosaponin-d and saikogenin d, *Int. J. Immunopharmacol.*, 11, 21–28.

Kumazawa, Y., Kawakita, T., Takimoto, H., and Nomoto, K. (1990) Protective effect of saikosaponin-a, saikosaponin-d and saikogenin d against *Pseudomonas aeruginosa* infection in mice, *Int. J. Immunopharmacol.*, 12, 531–537.

Liang, H., Zhao, Y.Y., Qiu, H.Y., Huang, J., and Zhang, R.Y. (1998a) A new saikosaponin from *Bupleurum chinense* DC., *Acta Pharm. Sin.*, 33, 37–41.

Liang, H., Zhao, Y.Y., Bai, Y.J., Zhang, R.Y., and Tu, G.Z. (1998b) A new saikosaponin from *Bupleurum chinense* DC., *Acta Pharm. Sin.*, 33, 282–285.

Liang, H., Cui, Y.J., Zhao, Y.Y., Wang, B., Yang, W.X., and Yu, Y. (2001) Saikosaponin v-2 from *Bupleurum chinense, Chin. Chem. Lett.*, 12, 331–332.

Liang, H., Han Z.Y., Zhao, Y.Y. et al. (2001) The structure of new saikosaponin q-2, *Acta Pharm. Sin.*, 42, 198.

Lopez, H. and Valera A. (1996) Lignans from *Bupleurum handiense, J. Nat. Prod.*, 59, 493–494.

Luo, H.S., Zhao, Y.Y., Ma, Y.Z., Peng, J.R., and Zhang R.Y. (1995) Isolation and identification of saikogenin q and saikosaponin q from *Bupleurum smithii* Wolff var. *parvifolium* Shan et Y. Li, *Acta Pharm. Sin.*, 30, 435–439.

Luo, H.S., Zhao, Y.Y., Qia, L., Ma, L.B., and Zhang, R.Y. (1996) Structure identification of saikosaponin p. *Acta Bot. Sin.*, 38, 910–913.

Luo, S.Q. and Jing, H.F. (1991) Studies on chemical constituents from the aerial parts of 6 medicinal *Bupleurums* in the Southwest District of China, *Zhongguo Zhongyao Zazhi*, 16, 353–356.

Luo, S.Q., Jin, H.F., Kawai, H., Seto, H., and Otake, N. (1987) Isolation of new saponins from the aerial part of *Bupleurum kunmingense* Y. Li et S. L. Pan, *Agric. Biol. Chem.*, 51, 1515–1519.

Luo, S.Q., Lin, L.Z., and Cordell G.A. (1993) Lignan glucosides from *Bupleurum wenchuanense, Phytochemistry*, 33, 193–196.

Ma, L.B., Jin, Y.Z., Tu, G.Z., Luo, H.S., Zhao, Y.Y., Hu, C.F., Zhang, R.Y., Lai, L.H., Xu, X.J., and Tang, Y.Q. (1996) The structure study of a new saikosaponin, *Acta Chem. Sin.*, 54, 1200–1208.

Manunta, A., Tirillini, B., and Fraternale, D. (1992) Secretory tissue and essential oil composition of *Bupleurum fruticosum* L., *J. Essent. Oil Res.*, 4, 461–466.

Matsuda, H., Murakami, T., Ninomiya, K. et al. (1997) New hepatoprotective saponins, bupleuroside III, VI, IX, and XII from Chinese *Bupleuri* radix: structure-requirements for the cytoprotective activity in primary cultured rat hepatocytes. *Bioorg. Med. Chem. Lett.*, 7, 2193.

Minaeva, V.G. and Volkhonskaya, T.A. (1964) Flavonoids of *Bupleurum multinerve*. *Dokl. Akad. Nauk SSSR*, 154, 956–959.

Minaeva, V.G., Volkhonskaya, T.A., and Valutskaya, A.G. (1965) Comparative investigation of the flavonoid composition of some Siberian species of *Bupleurum, Rast. Resursy*, 1, 233–235.

Morita, M., Nakajima, K., Ikeya, Y., and Mitsuhashi, H. (1991) Polycetylenes from the root of *Bupleurum falcatum, Phytochemistry*, 30, 1543–1545.

Navarro, P., Giner, R.M., Carmen Recio, M., Manes, S., Cer-Nicolas, M., and Rios, J.L. (2001) *In vivo* anti-inflammatory activity of saponin from *Bupleurum rotundifolium, Life Sci.*, 68, 1199–1206.

Nose, M., Amagaya, S., and Ogihara, Y. (1989) Corticosterone secretion-inducing activity of saikosaponin metabolites formed in the alimentary tract, *Chem. Pharm. Bull.*, 37, 2736–2740.

Pan, S.L., Wang, Z.H., Hong, X.K., Lin, D.H., Mao, R.G., and Ohashi, H. (2000a) Determination on saikosaponin-a, -c and -d in 23 species of *Bupleurum* by HPLC, *J. Jpn. Med. Bot.*, 23, 35–39.

Pan, S.L., Wang, Z.H., Hong, X.K., Lin, D.H., Mao, R.G., and Ohashi, H. (2000b) Determination on saikosaponin-a, -c and -d by HPLC in *Bupleurums* from different districts of China, *J. Jpn. Med. Bot.*, 23, 40–44.

Pan, S.L., Shun, Q.S., Bo, Q.M., and Bao, X.S. (2002) *The Coloured Atlas of Medicinal Plants from Genus Bupleurum in China,* Shanghai Sci. Tech. Doc. Publishing House, Shanghai, China.

Park, K.H., Park, J., Koh, D., and Lim, Y. (2002) Effect of saikosaponin-a, atriterpenoid glycoside, isolated from *Bupleurum falcatum* on experimental allergic asthma, *Phytother. Res.*, 16, 359–363.

Peyron, L. and Roubaud, M. (1970) *Bupleurum fruticosum* essential oil, *Plant. Med. Phytother.*, 4, 172–175.

Pistelli, L., Bilia, A.R., Marsili, A., Tommasi, N., and Manunta, A. (1993a) Triterpenoid saponins from *Bupleurum fruticosum, J. Nat. Prod.*, 56, 240–244.

Pistelli, L., Cammilli, A., Manunta, A., Marsili, A., and Morelli, I. (1993b) Triterpenoid saponins and flavonoid glycosides from *Bupleurum falcatum* subsp. *cernuum, Phytochemistry*, 33, 1537–1539.

Pistelli, L., Bertoli, A., Bilia, A.R., and Morelli, I. (1996) Minor constituents from *Bupleurum fruticosum* roots, *Phytochemistry*, 41, 1579–1582.

Pu, Q.L., Ji, X.D., Xu, P., Huang, L., Guo, Q.Y., and Chen, X.X. (1983) Studies on constituent of essential oil of *Bupleurum chinense* DC., *Acta Chim. Sin.*, 41, 559–561.

Robate, J. (1931) *Chem. Zentralbl.*, 102, 1772.

Sanchez-Contreras, S., Diaz-Lanza, A.M., Matellano, L.F., Bernabe, M., Ollivier, E., Balansard, G., and Faure, R. (1998) A sulfated saponin from *Bupleurum rigidum, J. Nat. Prod.*, 61, 1383–1385.

Sanchez-Contreras, S., Diaz-Lanza, A.M., and Bernabe, M. (2000a) Four new triterpenoid saponins from the roots of *Bupleurum rigidum, J. Nat. Prod.*, 63, 1479–1482.

Sanchez-Contreras, S., Diaz-Lanza, A.M., Bartolome, C., and Bernabe, M. (2000b) Minor sulfated saikosaponins from the aerial parts of *Bupleurum rigidum* L., *Phytochemistry*, 54, 783–789.

Seto, H., Otake, N., Luo, S.Q., Qian, F.G., Xu, G.Y., and Pan, S.L. (1986a) Isolation of triterpenoid glycosides (saikosaponins) from *Bupleurum kunmingense* and their chemical structures, *Agric. Biol. Chem.*, 50, 943–948.

Seto, H., Otake, N., Kawai, H., Luo, S.Q., Qian, F.G., and Pan, S.L. (1986b) Isolation of triterpenoid glycosides (saikosaponins) from *Bupleurum polyclonum* Y. Li et S. L. Pan and their chemical structures, *Agric. Biol. Chem.*, 50, 1607–1611.

Seto, H., Kawai, H., Otake, N., Luo, S.Q., Qian, F.G., and Pan, S.L. (1986c) Structures of new saponins from *Bupleurum kunmingense* Y. Li et L. S. Pan, *Agric. Biol. Chem.*, 50, 1613–1620.

Seto, H. et al. (1986d) A new triterpenoid glycoside from *Bupleurum chinense* DC., *Agric. Biol. Chem. Soc.*, 50, 939–942.

Shi, Y.N. and Xu, L. (1980) Extraction, isolation and identification of kaempferitrin and kaempferol-7-rhamnoside from *Bupleurum, Zhong Cao Yao*, 11, 241–243.

Shibata, S., Kitagawa, I., and Fujimoto, H. (1965) The structure of saikogenin a, a sapogenin of *Bupleurum* species, *Tetrahedron Lett.*, 42, 3783–3788.

Shimaoka, A., Seo, S., and Minato, H. (1975) Saponins isolated from *Bupleurum falcatum* L., components of saikosaponin b, *J. Chem. Sci. Perkin Trans.*, 20, 2043–2048

Shimizu, K., Amagaya, S., and Ogihara, Y. (1985) New derivatives of saikosaponins, *Chem. Pharm. Bull.*, 33, 3349–3355.

Sobolevskaya, K.A., Volkhonskaya, T.A., and Minaeva, V.G. (1967) Hare's ear (*Bupleurum*) of Western Siberia as a source of bioflavonoids, *Polez. Rast. Prir. Flory Sib.*, 92–99.

Takagi, K. and Shibata, M. (1969a) Pharmacological studies on *Bupleurum falcatum* L. I. Acute toxicity and Central depressant actions of crude saikosides, *Yakugaku Zasshi*, 89, 712–720.

Takagi, K. and Shibata, M. (1969b) Pharmacological studies on *Bupleurum falcatum* L. II. Antiinflammatory and other pharmacological actions of crude saikosides, *Yakugaku Zasshi*, 89, 1367–1378.

Tan, L., Zhao, Y.Y., Zhang, R.Y., and Hong, S.L. (1996) A new saikosaponin from *Bupleurum scorzonerifolium, J. Chin. Pharm. Sci.*, 5, 128–131.

Tan, L., Zhao, Y.Y., Wang, B., and Zhang, R.Y. (1998) Identification of saikosaponins, *Acta Bot. Sin.*, 40, 176–179.

Tan, L., Zhao, Y.Y., Tu, G.Z., Wang, B., Cai, S.Q., and Zhang, R.Y. (1999) Saikosaponins from roots of *Bupleurum scorzonerifolium, Phytochemistry*, 50, 139–142.

Tomimatsu, T. (1969) Isolation of sucrose and α-spinasterol from the roots of *Bupleurum longiradiatum* Turcz., *Yakugaku Zasshi*, 89, 589–590.

Ushio, Y. and Abe, H. (1992) Inactivation of measles virus and herpes simplex virus by saikosaponin d, *Planta Med.*, 58, 171–173.

Yamada, H., Hirano, M., and Kiyohara, H. (1991) Partial structure of an anti-ulcer pectic polysaccharide from the roots of *Bupleurum falcatum* L., *Carbohydrate Res.*, 219, 173–192.

Yang, Y.J., Xiang, B.R., Liang, X., An, D.K., Yuan, C.Q., Cao, R., Pen, J.H., and Sheng, L.S. (1993) Analyses on components of essential oils in genus *Bupleurum, Zhong Cao Yao*, 24, 289–291.

Yoshikawa, M., Murakami, T., Hirano, K. et al. (1997a) Scorzoneroside A, B and C, novel triterpene, *Tetrahedron Lett.*, 38, 7395.

Yoshikawa, M., Murakami, T., Inadzuki, M., Hirano, K., Ninomiya, K., Yamahara, J., and Matsuda, H. (1997b) Hepatoprotective principles from chinese natural medicine "bupleuri radix" — structure–activity relationships and chemical modification of bupleurosides, *Tennen Yuki Kagobutsu Toronkai Koen Yoshishu*, 39, 205–210.

Zhang, L.X., Xu, W.M., Pan, S.L., Ding, L., and Lu, Y.F. (1986) Effect of *Bupleurum kunmingense* polysaccharides on the weight of spleen, thymus proliferation of lymphocyte and plaque forming cell in mice, *Acta Pharmacol. Sin.*, 7, 479–481.

Zhang, R.Y., Chen, X.K., Yang, X.B., He, W.Y., and Tan, L. (1994) The structures of saikosaponin m and n from *Bupleurum smithii* Wolff, *Acta Pharm. Sin.*, 29, 684–688.

Zhao, J.F., Guo, Y.Z., and Meng, X.S. (1987) The toxic principles of *Bupleurum longiradiatum, Acta Pharm. Sin.*, 22, 507–511.

8 The Chemistry and Biological Activity of the Genus *Bupleurum* in Spain

Alejandro F. Barrero, M. Mar Herrador, Pilar Arteaga, and José F. Quílez

CONTENTS

8.1 INTRODUCTION

The genus *Bupleurum* is represented in Spain by 23 species (Table 8.1), of which *B. salicifolium* subsp. *acciphyllum* and *B. hadiense* are endemic plants from the Canary Islands, and *B. barceloi* and *B. bourgaei* are endemic plants from the Baleares Islands and the Spanish Southeast (Sierra de Alcaraz), respectively. *Bupleurum acutifolium* is endemic from the Southwest of the Iberian Peninsula (Sierra Bermeja, Spain and near Odemira, Portugal). Seven of these have been studied phytochemically (Table 8.2).

TABLE 8.1
***Bupleurum* Species Located in Spain**

Species	Location
B. acutifolium Boiss.	Sierra Bermeja
B. angulosum L.	Mountains of the Northeast
B. baldense Turra	Calcareous soils
B. barceloi Cosson ex Willk.	Baleares Islands
B. bourgaei Boiis. & Ruter in Boiss.	Sierra de Alcaraz
B. falcatum L.	Pirineos and Centre
B. foliosum Salzm. ex DC.	Campo de Gibraltar
B. fruticescens L.	East and center
B. fruticosum L.	Calcareous and wetted places
B. gerardi All.	Calcareus soils
B. gibraltaricum Lam.	Center and south (fissure of limestone rocks)
B. hadiense (Bolle) G. Kunker	Canary Islands
B. lancifolium Hornem.	Temperate zones near the coasts
B. praealtum L.	Northeast
B. ranunculoides L.	Mountains of the Northeast
B. rigidum L.	Center and Mediterranean region (rocky places)
B. rigidum L. subsp. *Paniculatum* (Brot)	South and southwest
B. rotundifolium L.	Clay and marl soils
B. salicifolium R. Br. in Buch	Canary Islands
B. salicifolium R. Br. in Buch subsp. *aciphyllum* (Webb ex Parl) Sunding & G. Kunker	Canary Islands
B. semicompositum L.	Mediterranean region and Canary Islands (sandy soils)
B. spinosum Gouan	Mediterranean region
B. tenuissimum L.	Center, northeast, and Mediterranean region (saline habitats)

TABLE 8.2
Species of *Bupleurum* Studied in Spain

Species	Place of Collection
B. acutifolium	Sierra Bermeja (Málaga)
B. fruticescens	Sierra de Baza (Granada)
B. fruticosum	Serrania de Grazalema (Cádiz), Sierra de Cogollos (Granada), near Tarragona
B. gibraltaricum	Quéntar Reservoir, Sierra de Cázulas and Balcón de Canales (Granada)
B. hadiense	Centro de Productos Naturales Antonio González (Tenerife)
B. rigidum	San Andrés del Congosto (Guadalajara)
B. salicifolium	Río Badajoz Barranco (Tenerife), Guayadeque Barranco (Gran Canarias)

8.2 CHEMICAL COMPOSITION OF *BUPLEURUM* SPECIES

The secondary metabolites isolated from the different species studied of *Bupleurum* fall under the following groups:

Polyacetylenes
Lignans
Flavonoids and Coumarins
Terpenes
Phenylpropanoids

8.2.1 POLYACETYLENES

In all, 11 polyacetylenes have been identified in different species of *Bupleurum*. Polyacetylene 1 was isolated from *B. salicifolium* (Estévez-Braun et al., 1994b), 2 through 4 from *B. gibraltaricum* (Bohlmann et al., 1975), and 5 through 11 from *B. acutifolium* (Barrero et al., 1999). Of them, 5 through 8 were described for the first time and 6 through 8 are the first polyacetylenes possessing a skeleton of 18 carbon atoms isolated from the *Bupleurum* genus.

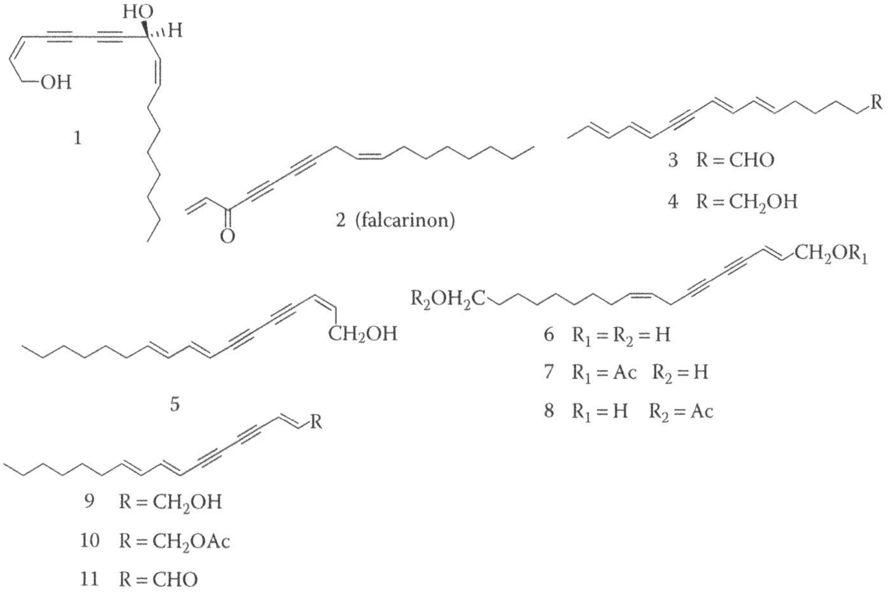

8.2.2 LIGNANS

In all, 20 new lignans have been obtained from *B. salicifolium* (González et al., 1989, 1990a, 1990b, 1990c; Estévez-Reyes et al., 1992, 1993; Estévez-Braun et al., 1994a, 1995), *B. acutifolium* (Barrero et al., 1999), and *B. fruticescens* (González et al., 1975). Their structures were shown to be 12 through 31. Other lignans isolated from these species were 32 through 49. Lignans 24 and 41 also have been identified in *B. hadiense* (López et al., 1996), together with 50. Salicifoliol 51, a furolactone-type lignan, has been isolated from the aerial parts of *B. salicifolium*, excluding leaves or flowers (González et al., 1989).

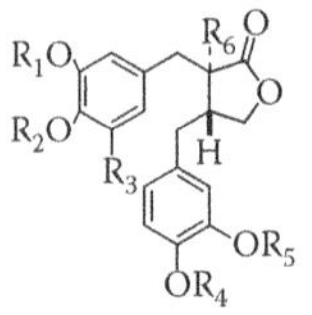

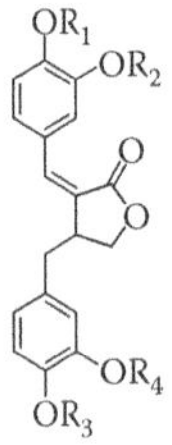

16 R$_1$ = R$_2$ = R$_5$ = Me R$_3$ = R$_4$ = R$_6$ = H (Buplerol)

17 R$_1$ = R$_2$ = Me R$_3$ = R$_4$ = R$_5$ = R$_6$ = H (Guayarol)

18 R$_1$ = R$_3$ = R$_6$ = H R$_2$ = Me R$_4$R$_5$ = -CH$_2$- (Guamarolin)

19 R$_1$ = R$_2$ = Me R$_3$ = H R$_4$R$_5$ = -CH$_2$- R$_6$ = OH (Benchequiol)

32 R$_1$ = R$_2$ = Me R$_3$ = R$_6$ = H R$_4$R$_5$ = -CH$_2$-(Bursehernin)

33 R$_1$ = Me R$_2$ = R$_3$ = R$_6$ = H R$_4$R$_5$ = -CH$_2$-(Pluviatolide)

34 R$_1$ = R$_5$ = Me R$_2$ = R$_3$ = R$_4$ = R$_6$ = H (Matairesinol)

35 R$_1$ = R$_2$ = R$_4$ = R$_5$ = Me R$_3$ = R$_6$ = H (Matairesinol dimethyl ether)

36 R$_1$ = R$_5$ = Me R$_2$ = R$_4$ = R$_6$ = H R$_3$ = OMe (Thujaplicatin methyl ether)

37 R$_1$ = R$_2$ = Me R$_3$ = R$_6$ = H R$_4$R$_5$ = -CH$_2$- (Methyl pluviatolide)

38 R$_1$ = R$_5$ = Me R$_2$ = R$_4$= H R$_3$ = OMe R$_6$ = OH (2-Hydroxythujaplicatin methyl ether)

12 R$_1$ = R$_2$ = R$_3$ = R$_4$ = Me

13 R$_1$ = R$_2$ = Me R$_3$R$_4$ = -CH$_2$-(Isokaerophyllin)

14 R$_1$= Me R$_2$ = H R$_3$R$_4$ = -CH$_2$-(Isoguamarol)

15 R$_1$ = R$_3$ = H R$_2$ = R$_4$ = Me (Salicifoline)

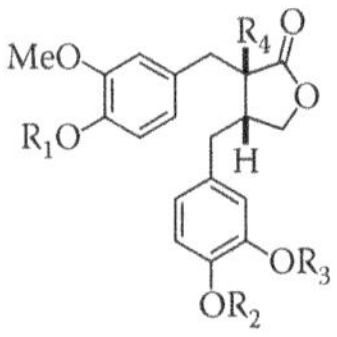

20 R$_1$ = R$_2$ = R$_3$ = Me R$_4$ = OAc

21 R$_1$ = Me R$_2$R$_3$ = -CH$_2$- R$_4$ = OH (Guayadequiol)

22 R$_1$ = Me R$_2$R$_3$ = -CH$_2$- R$_4$ = OAc (Guayadequiol acetate)

23 R$_1$ = R$_2$ = H R$_3$ = Me R$_4$ = OH ((-)-Epinortrachelogenin)

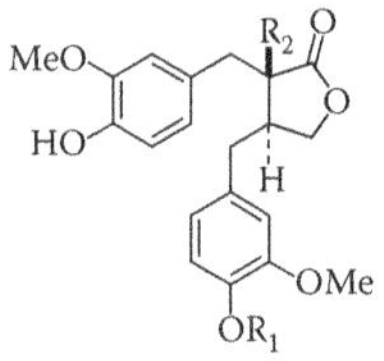

39 R$_1$ = H R$_2$ = OH ((-)-Nortrachelogenin)

40 R$_1$ = Me R$_2$ = H (Arctigenin)

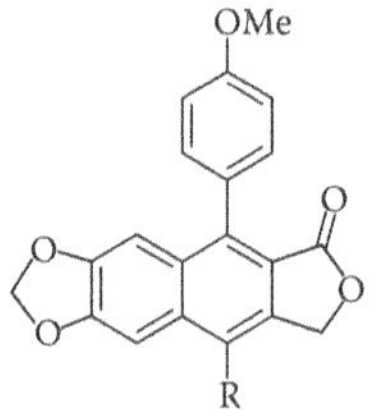

24 R = OH (Isodiphyllin)

41 R = H (Chinensin)

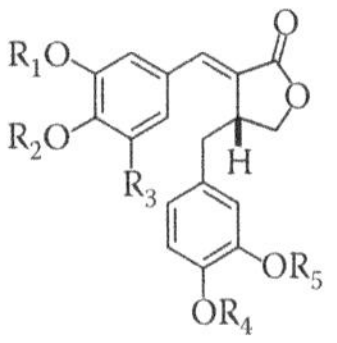

25 R$_1$ = R$_3$ = H R$_2$ = Me R$_4$R$_5$ = -CH$_2$- (Guamarol)

26 R$_1$ = R$_5$ = Me R$_2$ = R$_3$ = R$_4$ = H (Isosallcifoline)

42 R$_1$ = R$_2$ = Me R$_3$ = H R$_4$R$_5$ = -CH$_2$- (Kaerophyllin)

43 R$_1$ = R$_5$ = Me R$_2$ = R$_4$ = H R$_3$ = OMe (2, 5-Dehydrothujaplicalin methyl ether)

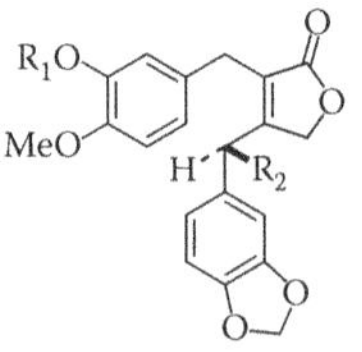

27 R$_1$ = Me R$_2$ = H (Guayadequiene)

28 R$_1$ = Me R$_2$ = OH (Methylchasnarolide)

29 R$_1$ = H R$_2$ = OH (Chasnarolide)

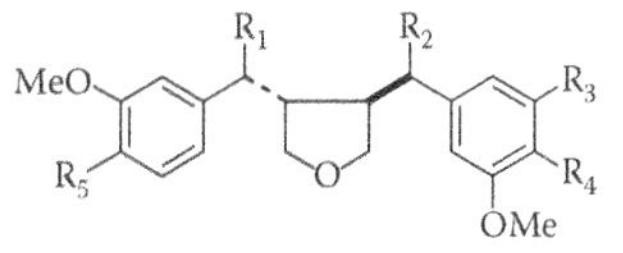

MeO   R$_1$ R$_2$ R$_3$ R$_4$ R$_5$ OMe

30 R$_1$ = H R$_2$ = R$_4$ = R$_5$ = OH R$_3$ = OMe (Busaliol)

31 R$_1$ = OEt R$_2$ = R$_4$ = R$_5$ = OH R$_3$ = H (Busalicifol)

44 R$_1$ = R$_3$ = H R$_2$ = R$_4$= R$_5$ = OH

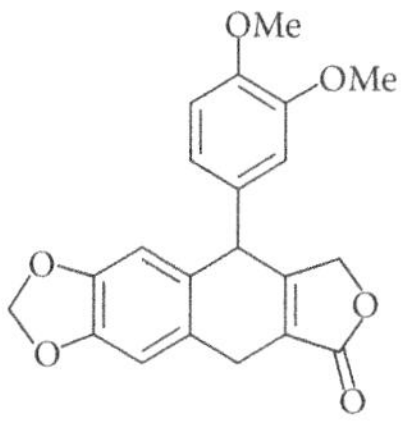

50

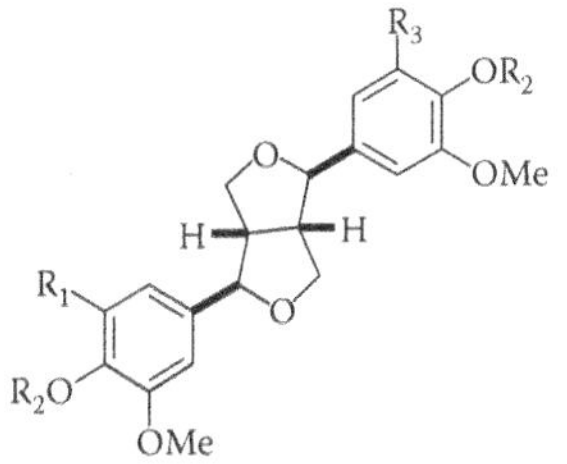

45 R$_1$ = R$_3$ = H R$_2$ = Me (Eudesmin)

46 R$_1$ = R$_2$ = R$_3$ = H (Pinoresinol)

47 R$_1$ = R$_2$ = H R$_3$ = OMe (Medioresinol)

48 R$_1$ = R$_3$ = OMe R$_2$ = H (Syringaresinol)

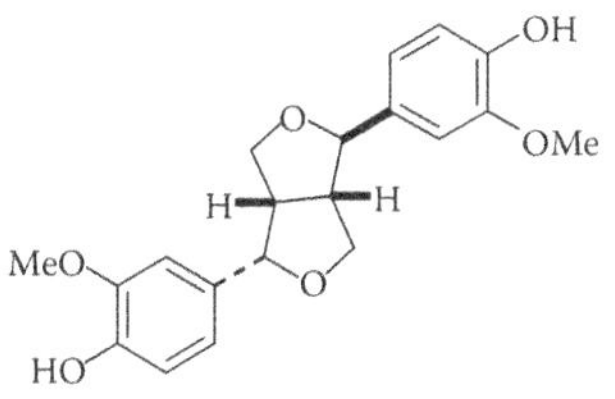

49 (Epipinoresinol)

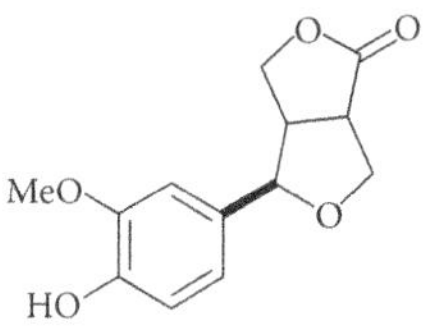

51 (Salicifoliol)

The structural identification of some of them has been facilitated by chemical transformations as shown in Schemes 8.1 through 8.11.

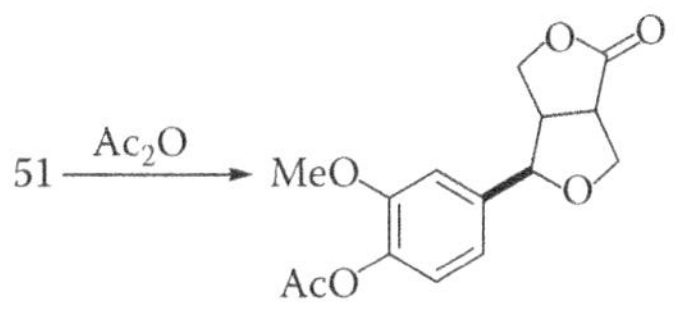

51 $\xrightarrow{\text{Ac}_2\text{O}}$ MeO   AcO   51a

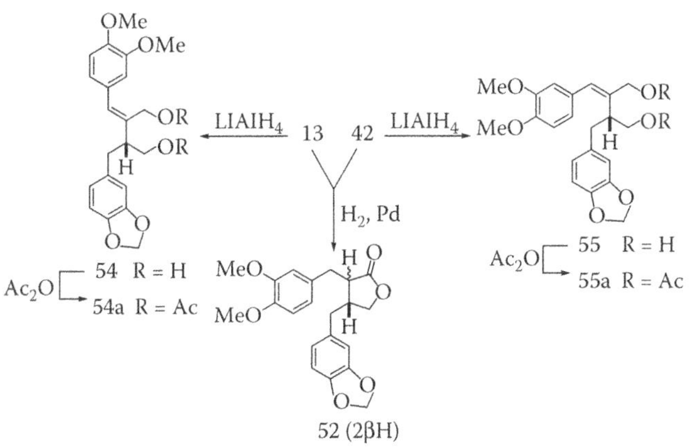

54 R = H
54a R = Ac

$\xrightarrow{\text{Ac}_2\text{O}}$

OR OR OR

$\xrightarrow{\text{LIAIH}_4}$ 13   42 $\xrightarrow{\text{LIAIH}_4}$ MeO   MeO   OR OR

H$_2$, Pd

55 R = H
55a R = Ac

Ac$_2$O

52 (2βH)

53 (2αH)

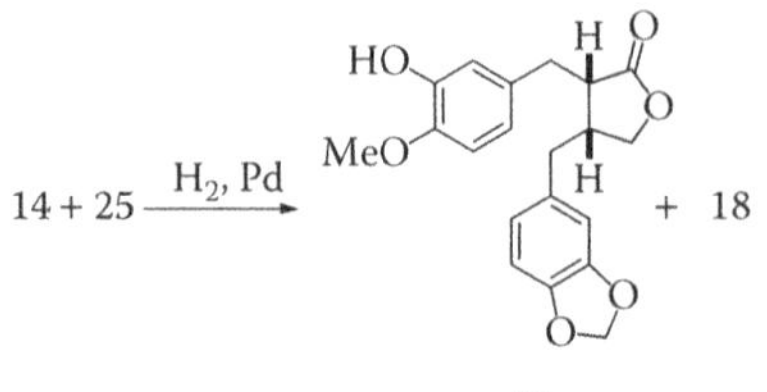

14 + 25 $\xrightarrow{\text{H}_2, \text{Pd}}$ **56** + 18

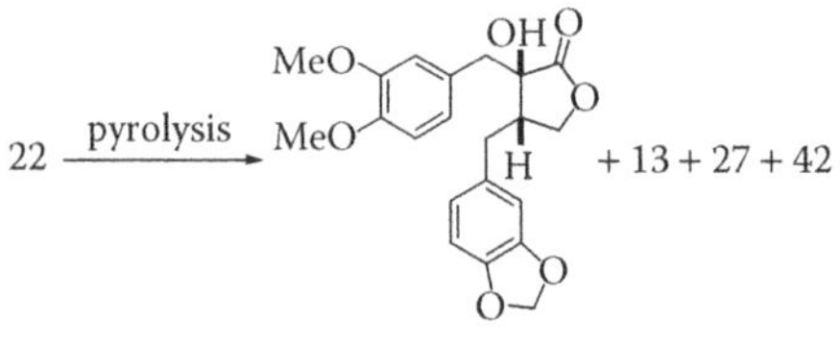

22 $\xrightarrow{\text{pyrolysis}}$ **57** + 13 + 27 + 42

30 , 31 $\xrightarrow{\text{Ac}_2\text{O}}$

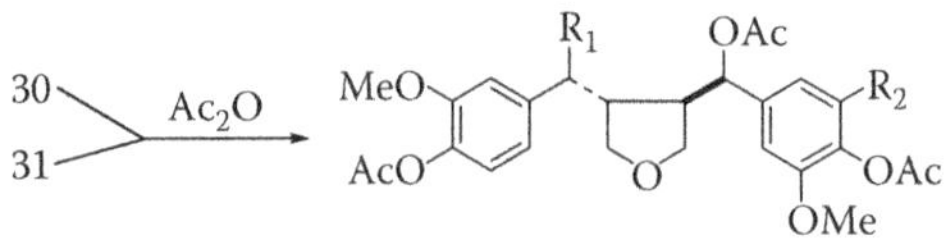

30a $R_1 = H$ $R_2 = OMe$

31a $R_1 = OEt$ $R_2 = H$

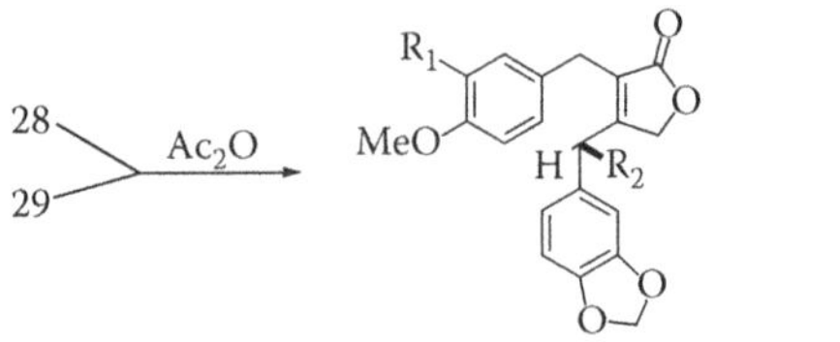

28 , 29 $\xrightarrow{\text{Ac}_2\text{O}}$

28a $R_1 = OMe$ $R_2 = OAc$

29a $R_1 = R_2 = OAc$

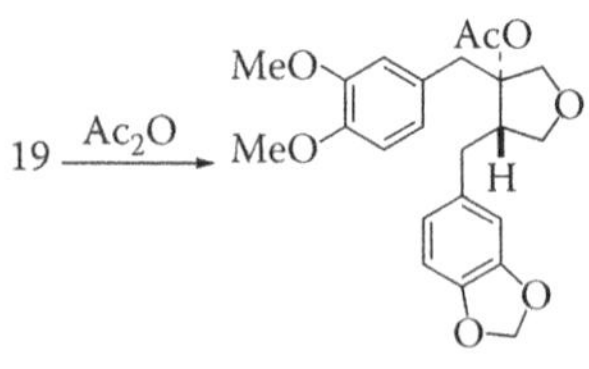

19 $\xrightarrow{\text{Ac}_2\text{O}}$

19a

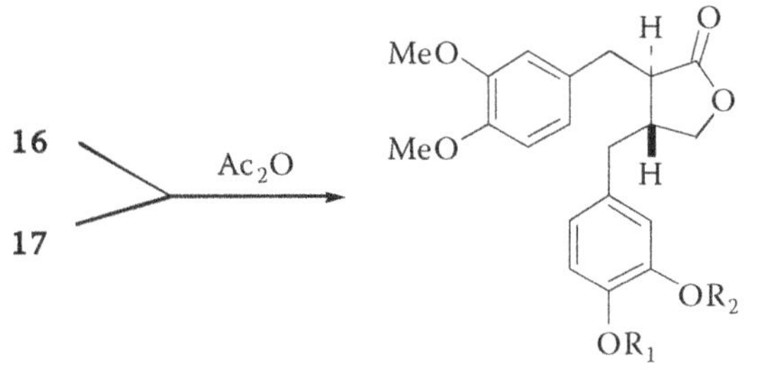

16a   R₁ = Ac R₂ = Me

17a   R₁ = R₂ = Ac

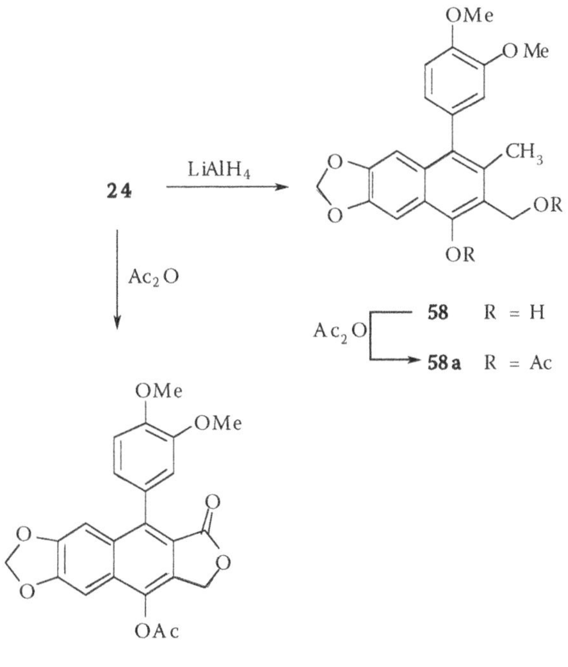

58   R = H

58a   R = Ac

24a

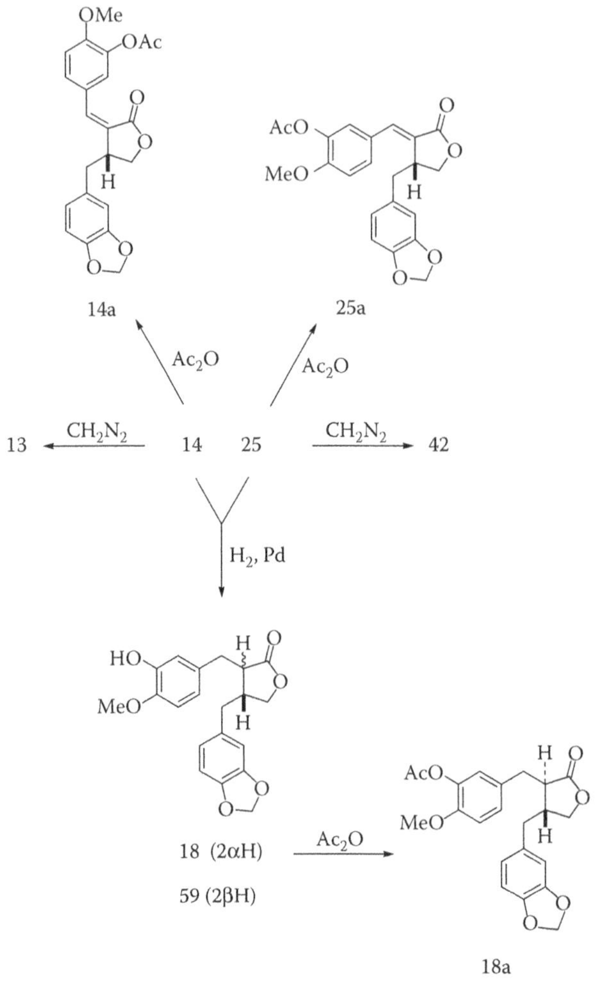
OMe
OAc
O
O
H
AcO
MeO
O
O
H
O
O
O
O
14a
25a
Ac2O
Ac2O
13
CH2N2
14
25
CH2N2
42
H2, Pd
HO
MeO
H
O
O
H
O
O
18 (2αH)
59 (2βH)
Ac2O
AcO
MeO
H
O
O
H
O
O
18a

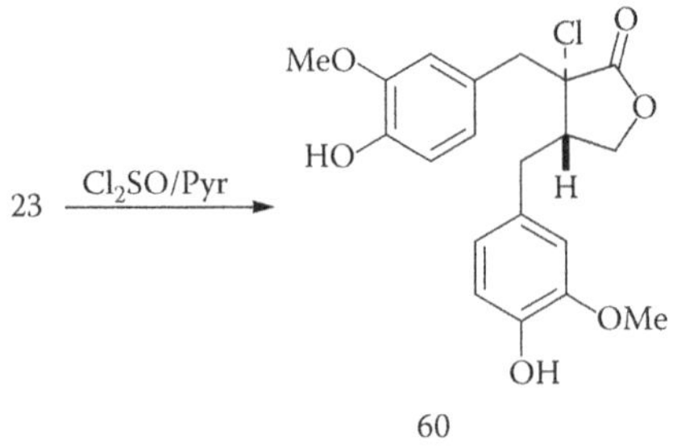
23
Cl2SO/Pyr
MeO
HO
Cl
O
O
H
OMe
OH
60

8.2.3 Flavonoids and Coumarins

Flavonol glycosides 61 through 64 and C-glycoside 65 have been characterized in extracts of *B. acutifolium* (Barrero et al., 2000a) and *B. gibraltaricum* (Mansour, 1998), respectively; 64 is a new natural product.

61   62   R = Me   63   R = H   64

65

66 R_5 = H R_6 = R_7 = R_8 = OMe

67 R_5 = R_8 = H R_6 = R_7 = OMe

68 R_5 = R_8 = H R_6 = OH R_7 = OMe

69 R_5 = R_6 = R_8 = H R_7 = OMe

70 R_5 = R_8 = H R_6 = OMe R_7 = OH

71 R_5 = R_7 = OMe R_6 = R_8 = H

6,7,8-Trimethoxycoumarin (66), scoparone (67), isoscopoletin (68), herniarin (69), scopoletin (70), and limettin (71) have been isolated from *B. fruticescens* (González et al., 1975) and *B. salicifolium* (Estévez-Braun et al., 1994a).

8.2.4 TERPENES AND TRITERPENE SAPONINS

8.2.4.1 Terpenes

Monoterpenes 72 to 79 have been isolated from the hexane extract of *B. gibraltaricum* (Bohlmann et al., 1975; Mansour, 1998; Barrero et al., 1998). Other monoterpenes isolated were also limonene, sabinene, *p*-cymene, *m*-cymene, and terpinen-4-ol (Barrero et al., 1998).

72 R_1 = CH_3 R_2 = Ang R_3 = H

73 R_1 = H R_2 = Ang R_3 = CH_3

74 R_1 = R_2 = H R_3 = CH_3

75 R_1 = H R_2 = Me R_3 = CH_3

76 R_1 = CH_3 R_2 = Ang R_3 = H

77 R_1= H R_2 = Ang R_3 = CH_3

78 R_1 = R_2 = H R_3 = CH_3

79 R_1= H R_2 = Sen R_3 = CH_3

Sesquiterpenes γ-muurolene, α-humulene, γ-calcorene, δ-cadinene, α-muurolene, α-calcorene, *trans*-calamenene, γ-cadinene, β-caryophyllene, α-copaene, ylangene, *cis*-calamenene, germacrene D, α-cubebene, longicyclene, β-bourbonene, β-elemene, valencene, caryophyllene oxide, α-humulene oxide, nerolidol, elemol, α-eudesmol, and guaiol have been identified from *B. acutifolium* (Barrero et al., 1999) and *B. gibraltaricum* (Barrero et al., 1998).

Sterols 81 through 83 together with sandaracopimaradiene (80) have been obtained from *B. gibraltaricum* (Mansour, 1998). Lupeol (84), squalene (85), stigmasterol (86), betulin (87), sterol 82 (spinasterol), and erythrodiol (88) were isolated from *B. acutifolium* (Barrero et al., 1999), *B. salicifolium* (González et al., 1989; Estévez-Braun et al., 1994a) and *B. fruticosum* (Massanet et al., 1997).

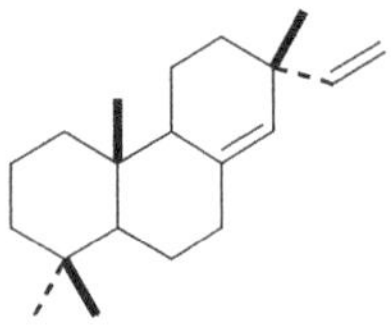

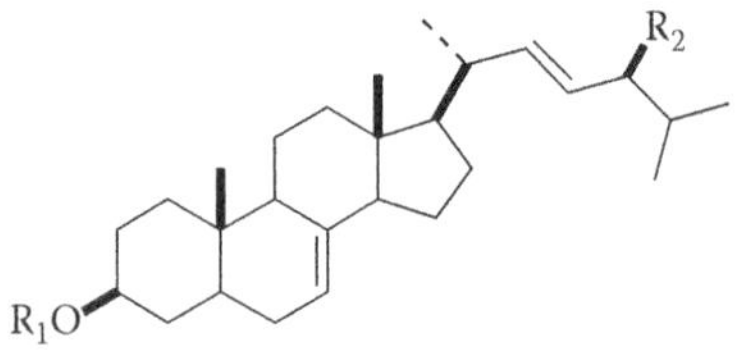

81 R$_1$ = H R$_2$ = CH$_3$
82 R$_1$ = H R$_2$ = CH$_2$CH$_3$
83 R$_1$ = Ac R$_2$ = CH$_2$CH$_3$

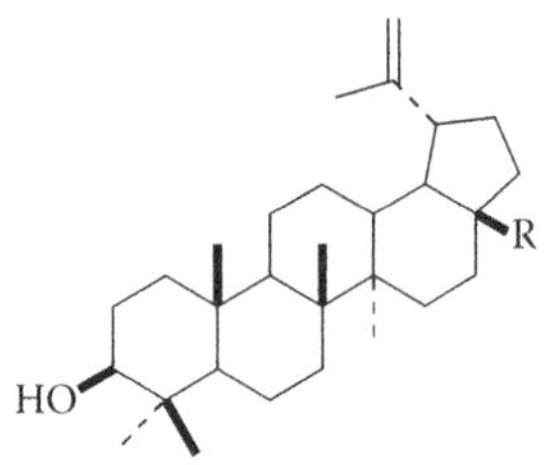

84 R = CH$_3$
87 R = CH$_2$OH

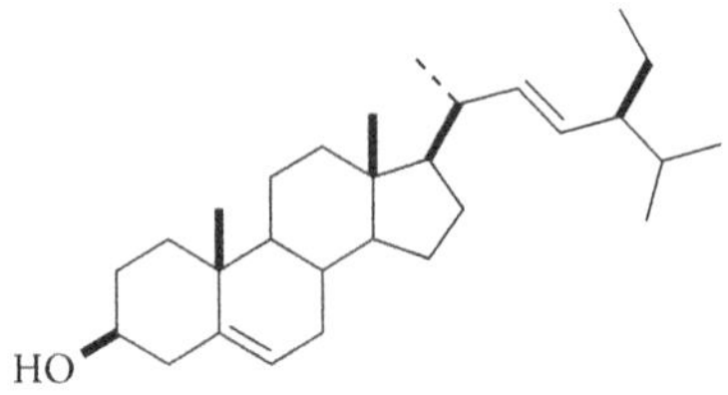

80

86

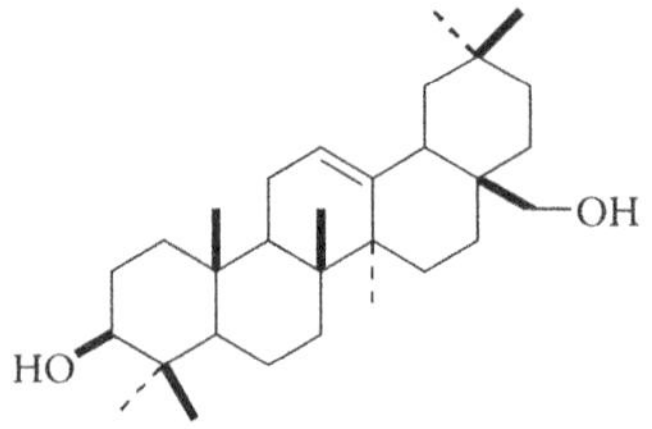

88

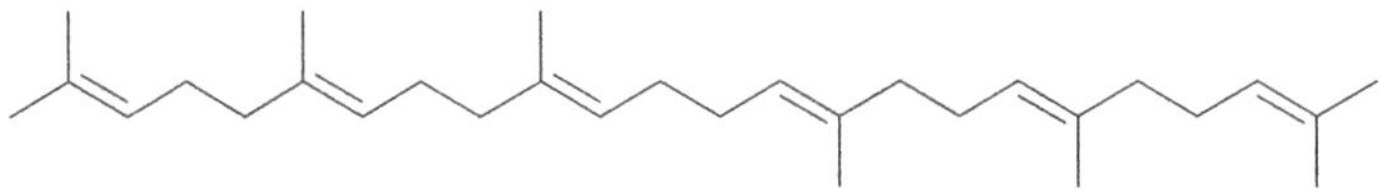

85

The chemical composition of the essential oils from *B. fruticosum* (Lorente et al., 1989), *B. gibraltaricum* (Cabo et al., 1986a, 1986b; Ocete et al., 1989) and *B. fruticescens* (Martín et al., 1993) has been analyzed by gas chromatography/mass spectrometry (GC/MS) (Table 8.3).

TABLE 8.3
Percentage Composition of the Essential Oils of *B. fruticosum* (A), *B. gibraltaricum* (B), and *B. fruticescens*(C)

Compound	A (%)	B (%)	C (%)
α-Pinene	41.2	10.5	16.9
β-Pinene	35.9	4.0	0.9[a]
Sabinene			1.2[b]
3-Carene		33.0	0.9[a]
Myrcene	3.10[c]	3.5	1.2[b]
α-Phellandrene	3.10[c]	4.0	
Limonene	4.1[d]	8.2	2.5
1,8-Cineol	4.1[d]	7.5	
γ-Terpinene	2.5		5.0
p-Cymene	2.9	2.7	4.4
Linalool	t*	t[e]	
Linalyl acetate	t	t[e]	
Bornyl acetate		2.2	
Terpinen-4-ol	t	9.0	0.8
β-Caryophyllene			30.6
Terpinyl acetate		2.5[f]	
Borneol	t	2.5[f]	
Estragol	t	2.5[f]	
α-Humulene			4.9
Carvone		t	
Citral			1.8
δ-Cadinene			6.0
Geraniol			3.4
Anethol		t	
Thymol	t	t	0.9
Carvacrol	1.5	1.2	1.8
Eugenol		1.0	

[a–f]Compounds not resolved for individual quantitation.

* Compositional values less than 0.1 % are denoted as traces (t).

8.2.4.2 Triterpene Saponins

Six new sulfated saikosaponins (89 through 94) together with buddlejasaponin IV (95) were isolated from the aerial parts of *B. rigidum* (Sánchez-Contreras et al., 1998, 2000). Buddlejasaponin IV (95) was also identified in *B. gibraltaricum* (Barrero et al., 2000b) and *B. fruticosum* (Guinea et al., 1994), while saikogenin F (96) was found in *B. fruticosum* (Guinea et al., 1994).

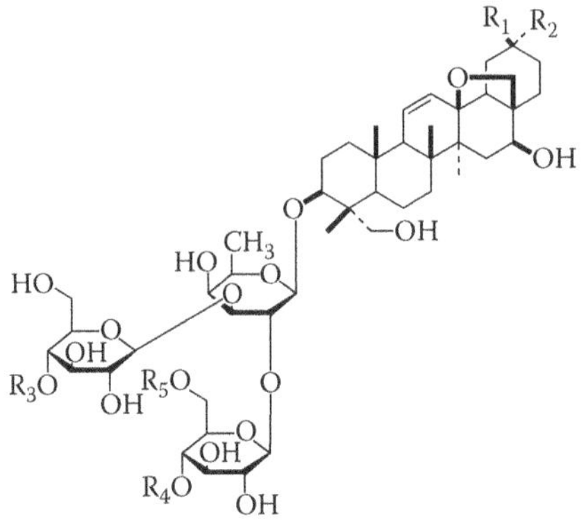

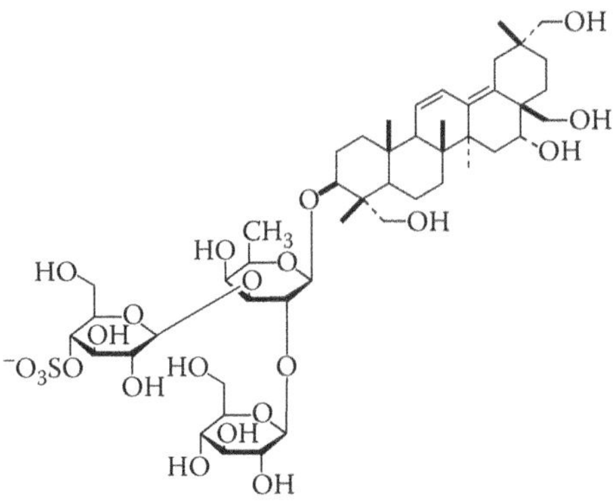

R_1, R_2

94 (Sandrosaponin VI)

89 $R_1 = R_2 = CH_3$ $R_3 = R_5 = H$ $R_4 = SO_3^-$ (Sandrosaponin I)

90 $R_1 = CH_3$ $R_2 = CH_2OH$ $R_3 = SO_3^-$ $R_4 = R_5 = H$ (Sandrosaponin II)

91 $R_1 = CH_2OH$ $R_2 = CH_3$ $R_3 = SO_3^-$ $R_4 = R_5 = H$ (Sandrosaponin V)

92 $R_1 = COOH$ $R_2 = CH_3$ $R_3 = SO_3^-$ $R_4 = R_5 = H$ (Sandrosaponin III)

93 $R_1 = COOH$ $R_2 = CH_2OH$ $R_3 = SO_3^-$ $R_4 = R_5 = H$ (Sandrosaponin IV)

95 $R_1 = R_2 = CH_3$ $R_3 = R_4 = R_5 = H$ (Buddlejasaponin IV)

96 $R_1 = R_2 = CH_3$ $R_3 = R_4 = H$ $R_5 = HOOCCH_2CO^-$ (Saikogenin F)

8.2.5 PHENYLPROPANOIDS

Phenylpropanoids 97 through 105 have been isolated from *B. fruticosum* (Massanet et al., 1997). Eight of them are new natural products. Ferulic acid (106) has been characterized in *B. acutifolium* (Barrero et al., 1999).

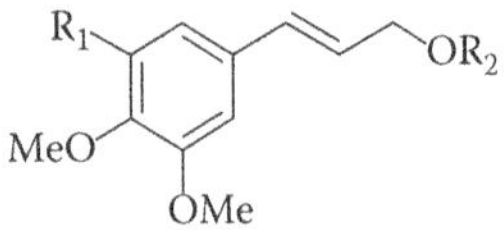

97 $R_1 = OMe$ $R_2 = A$

98 $R_1 = H$ $R_2 = A$

99 $R_1 = OMe$ $R_2 = Et$

100 $R_1 = H$ $R_2 = Et$

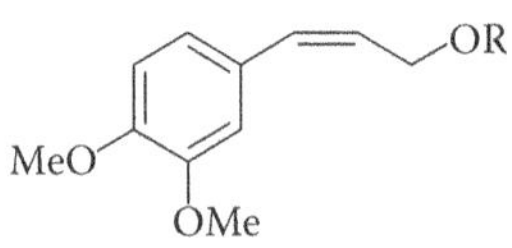

101 R = A

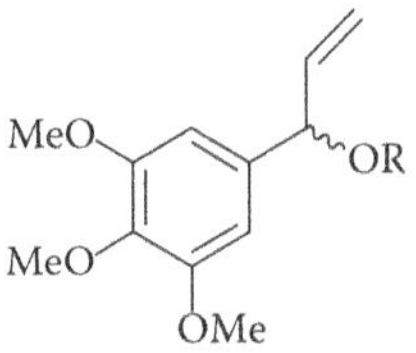

102 R = A

103 R = Et

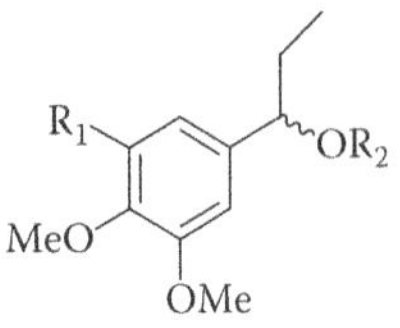

104 $R_1 = OMe$ $R_2 = A$

105 $R_1 = H$ $R_2 = A$

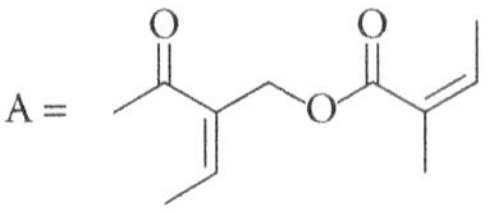

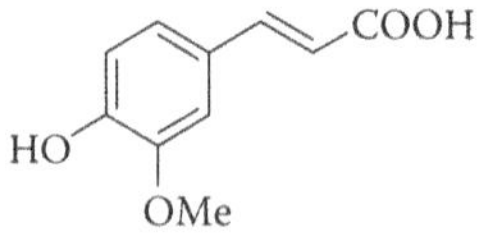

A =

106

TABLE 8.4
Percent Increase in Hindpaw Volume Obtained
with Each Extract Fraction (a dose equivalent
to 150 mg of powdered root/kg body weight)
and with Saikosaponin I Obtained from
Bupleurum gibraltaricum Root

Sample	Time after Carrageenan (5 h)
Ethanolic extract[c]	26.9 ± 0.4[a]
Methanolic fraction[c]	20.3 ± 4.9[b]
Total genins[c]	39.0 ± 13.1
Saikosaponin I	
50 mg/kg[c]	22.4 ± 3.6[b]
100 mg/kg[d]	18.5 ± 2.5[b]
200 mg/kg[d]	15.6 ± 1.4[b]
Untreated control[c]	49.8 ± 3.5
Indomethacin 20 mg/kg[d]	8.4 ± 4.5[b]
Untreated control[d]	42.2 ± 3.5

Note: Tabular values are mean ± SEM.

[a] $p < 0.05$.
[b] $p < 0.01$ Values significantly different from control.
[c] i.p. administration.
[d] p.o. administration.

8.3 BIOLOGICAL ACTIVITY

8.3.1 ANTI-INFLAMMATORY ACTIVITY

The ethanolic extract of *B. gibraltricum* root has been shown to possess an anti-inflammatory activity (Table 8.4). The compound responsible for this activity was a glycoside of saikogenin G containing three sugars (Utrilla et al., 1991).

The essential oil of *B. gibraltaricum*, collected in the Cázulas Mountains, also showed a considerable anti-inflammatory activity (Table 8.5) (Ocete et al., 1989). This activity appeared to be due to 3-carene, the major component of the essential oil (Table 8.6).

Subsequently, Gil et al. (1989) carried out a comparative study of the essential oil extracted from the fruiting apex of *B. gibraltaricum* collected in different areas within the province of Granada, including the Cázulas Mountains, the Balcón de Canales, and the Quéntar Reservoir. All three essential oils were very similar in their chemical composition, consisting mainly of mono-terpenic hydrocarbons (3-carene and α-pinene). When their anti-inflammatory activity was assayed against both acute (carrageenin-induced plantar edema) and subchronic inflammation (granuloma technique), quantitative differences came to light: the essential oil of the Cázulas Mountains population was most active against acute inflammation owing to its high 3-carene content (Table 8.7), whereas the Quéntar Reservoir essential oil of *B. gibraltaricum* was most effective against granuloma-induced inflammation — anti-inflammatory activity (%) 45.14 ± 10.44 vs. -0.49 ± 6.53 for the essential oil from Cázulas Mountains and 15.85 ± 5.65 for the essential oil from the Balcón de Canales.

TABLE 8.5
Percent Increase in Hindpaw Volume with and without Pretreatment with *Bupleurum gibraltaricum* Essential Oil or Indomethacin

Treatment	Dosage (mg/kg)	Time after Carrageenan (5 h)
Control		
i.p.		62.2 ± 9.1
p.o.		61.5 ± 7.4
Essential Oil		
i.p.	200	9.6 ± 3.9[a]
p.o.	3000	29.8 ± 9.4[a]
Indomethacin		
i.p.	20	12.8 ± 1.6[a]
p.o.	20	22.2 ± 3.3[a]

Note: Tabular values = mean ± standard deviation. Significance relative to the control group: [a]$P < 0.001$; N per group = 5.

TABLE 8.6
Percent Increase in Hindpaw Volume in Rats Pretreated i.p. with the Major Components of *Bupleurum gibraltaricum* Essential Oil

Treatment	Dosage (mg/kg)	Time after Carrageenan (5 h)
Control		62.2 ± 9.1
α-Pinene	21	38.4 ± 6.3[a]
β-Pinene	8	30.0 ± 3.5[b]
3-Carene	66	14.1 ± 5.6[c]
Limonene	16	71.3 ± 3.3
1,8-Cineol	15	61.2 ± 2.4
Myrcene	7	50.2 ± 2.5
α-Phellandrene	8	83.1 ± 5.6
Terpinen-4-ol	18	69.0 ± 3.6

Note: Tabular values = mean ± standard deviation. Significance relative to the control group: [a]$P < 0.05$, [b]$P < 0.01$, [c]$P < 0.001$; N per group = 5. Doses approximate the amount of each component to be found in 200 mg/kg of the essential oil.

TABLE 8.7
Anti-Inflammatory Activity (%) of the Essential Oil of *Bupleurum gibraltaricum* and Major Components against Edema Plantar Induced by Carrageenan

Samples	Dosage (mg/kg)	Time after Carrageenan (5 h)
Essential oil (Cázulas)	200	48.60 ± 5.75
Essential oil (Canales)	200	48.54 ± 2.41
Essential oil (Quéntar)	200	31.28 ± 3.52
3-Carene	30	40.54 ± 11.12
α-Pinene	30	27.50 ± 10.27
3-Carene + α-Pinene	30 + 30	10.69 ± 8.88

Note: Mean ± standard deviation.

The essential oil of *B. fruticescens* showed a potent anti-inflammatory activity when it was administered orally, at doses of 500 and 1000 mg/kg, against carrageenin-induced hindpaw edema (Martín et al., 1993). The greatest activity was presented 5 hours after the administration of the phlogogen agent (Table 8.8). The anti-inflammatory activity shown by the essential oil can be attributed to the synergic effect of the two major components, α-pinene and β-caryophyllene. Thus, while the pharmacological action of β-caryophyllene was lower than that shown by the whole essential oil, the activity of a mixture of both components in a relative proportion similar to that found in the oil became comparable to the activity of the whole essential oil (Table 8.8).

TABLE 8.8
Anti-Inflammatory Activity of the Essential Oil of *Bupleurum fruticescens* and Major Components against Plantar Edema Induced by Carrageenin

Sample	Dosage (mg/kg)	Times after Carrageenin (h)	
		1	5
Control		43.6 ± 4.2	72.9 ± 5.3
Essential oil	500	32.8 ± 1.9[a]	16.5 ± 2.6[c]
	1000	27.9 ± 1.7[b]	9.8 ± 3.7[c]
β-Caryophyllene	150	26.8 ± 4.6[a]	52.2 ± 2.8[b]
	300	26.9 ± 2.1[b]	28.8 ± 3.2[c]
β-Caryophyllene + α-Pinene	150 + 90	28.1 ± 2.2[b]	17.7 ± 2.0[c]
Indomethacin	20	32.6 ± 4.9	21.6 ± 3.5[c]

Note: Values are given as mean (% IV) ± s.e.m. ($n = 6$). [a]$p < 0.05$; [b]$p < 0.01$; [c]$p < 0.001$.

TABLE 8.9
Anti-Inflammatory Activity of the Essential Oil of
***Bupleurum fruticosum* and Major Components**
against Plantar Edema Induced by Carrageenin[a]

Sample	Dosage (mg/kg)	Time after Carrageenin (h) 3	Time after Carrageenin (h) 5
Essential oil	200	58.2 ± 10.0	74.5 ± 5.7
α-Pinene	80	26.2 ± 9.1	13.2 ± 3.9
β-Pinene	80	32.2 ± 6.2	31.9 ± 5.7
α-Pinene + β-pinene	80 + 80	34.1 ± 5.7	39.6 ± 1.6
α-Pinene + β-pinene + Thymol + carvacrol	80 + 80 + 1 + 3	62.1 ± 16.7	70.5 ± 15.4

[a] Values are given as mean (A.A.I.) + SEM %A.A.I. = $(I_b - I_x)/I_b \times$ 100, where I_b = % inflammation volume to the control group and I_x = % inflammation volume to the treated group.

Lorente et al. (1989) have studied the anti-inflammatory activity of the essential oil of *B. fruticosum* . The activity of this oil can be attributed to its major components, α–pinene and β-pinene, although the presence of thymol and carvacrol, minor components capable of potentiating the action of these hydrocarbons, was also confirmed (Table 8.9).

8.3.2 ANTISPASMODIC ACTIVITY

The antispasmodic activity of the essential oils of *B. gibraltaricum* (Ocete et al., 1989) and *B. fruticosum* (Lorente et al., 1989) was determined in rat uterus preparations using acetylcholine and oxytocin as agonists. The comparison of the antispasmodic activity against oxytocin shown by both essential oils indicated that the essential oil of *B. gibraltaricum* was able to modify the EC_{50} of the agonist at much lower doses. This activity has been attributed to the major component of the oil, 3-carene, which is lacking in *B. fruticosum* oil. This hydrocarbon was very effective against oxytocin-induced contractions, doses of 1.1 μg/ml and 2.2 μg /ml raised oxytocin EC_{50} by 3.1 and 6.4 times more than control values (Ocete et al., 1989).

8.3.3 ANTIMICROBIAL ACTIVITY

The qualitative antimicrobial activity of the essential oils from the foliar, flowering, and fruiting apex of *B. gibraltaricum* against different microorganisms has been determined (Cabo et al., 1986c). All the essential oils were active against all the microorganisms assayed, although the essential oil from the foliar apex was the least active. The MIC of the essential oil from the flowery apex was also calculated. Among the microorganisms assayed, *Micrococcus luteus* was the most sensitive (minimal inhibitory concentration [MIC] = 0.0031 mg/ml), while *Candida albicans* , *Escherichia coli,* and *Pseudomonas fluorescens* were the most resistant (MIC = 0.0250 mg/ml for the three microorganisms).

Polyacetylene 1 was isolated from *B. salicifolium* and exhibited significant antibiotic activity against the Gram-positive bacteria *Staphylococcus aureus* ATCC 6538 (MIC = 10 μg/ml) and *Bacillus subtilis* CECT 99 (MIC = 10.5 μg/ml). However, it was inactive when tested against Gram-negative bacteria (*E. coli* , *Salmonella* sp., *P. aeuriginosa*) and the yeast *C. albicans* (Estévez-Braun et al., 1994b).

TABLE 8.10
Biological Activity of Secondary Metabolites Isolated from
Bupleurum salicifolium

Compound	Toxicity[a] Mean (% dead)	Antifeedant Activity[b] $FR_{50} \pm MSD^*$	Nematostatic Activity[c] Mean [log $(1 + x)$]
1	100		
14	19.53		
16	26.67	0.74 ± 0.36	1.14898
17	6.67		1.07055
25	56.06		
30	22.69		
31	11.61		
32	50	1.20 ± 0.51	0.84377
33	90		
34		0.60 ± 0.42	0.97771
35	60	0.80 ± 0.41	
36	32.73		
38	16.06		
42	13.33	1.43 ± 0.76	
48	83.33		1.12140
64	36.56		
105	75.15		
106			1.33945
107	26.3		
109	11.5		
Control	6.67		
C1			0.62399
C2			1.26882

[a] Dosage = 100 µg/ml; $LSD_{0.05}$ = 18.692; Error mean square = 128.42.
[b] Dosage = 10 µg/cm²; *Mean standard deviation.
[c] Dosage = 50 µg/ml; $LSD_{0.05}$ = 0.18; Error mean square = 0.08.

8.3.4 TOXICITY ASSAY

Compounds 1, 13 through 17, 25, 30 through 36, 38, 39, 42, 48, 60, 66, 107 through 110 from *Bupleurum salicifolium* were tested against the crustacean *Artemia salina* (González et al., 1995). Polyacetylene 1, lignans 25, 32, 33, 35, 36, 48, and 60, and coumarin 66 killed significantly more larvae of *A. salina* than the control at a concentration of 100 µg/ml, with polyacetylene 1 the most active compound (Table 8.10).

8.3.5 ANTIFEEDANT ACTIVITY

Secondary metabolites (1, 13 through 17, 25, 30 through 36, 38, 39, 42, 48, 60, 66, 107 through 110) from *B. salicifolium* were tested against the insect *Spodoptera littoralis* (González et al., 1995). In this assay, no significant differences were noted in the FR_{50} for the insect when the compounds were tested at 10 µg/cm² (Table 8.10).

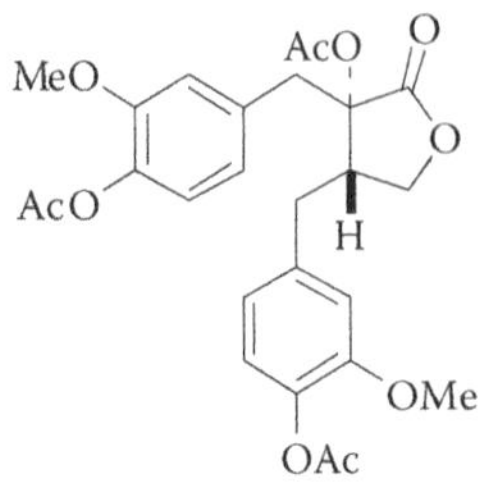

107

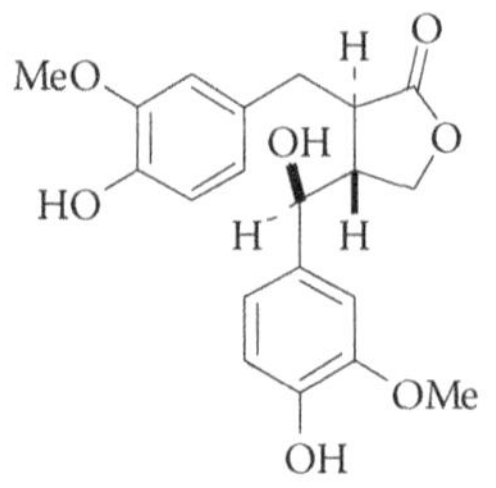

108

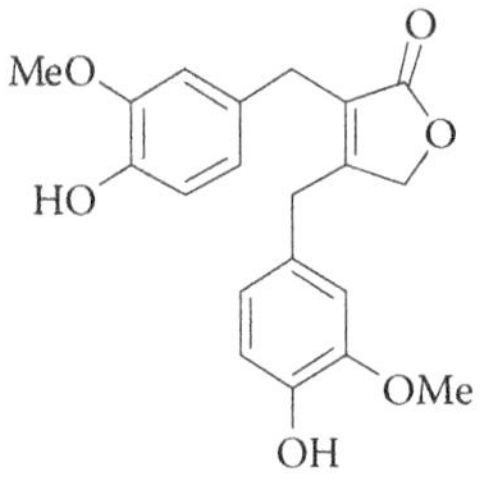

109

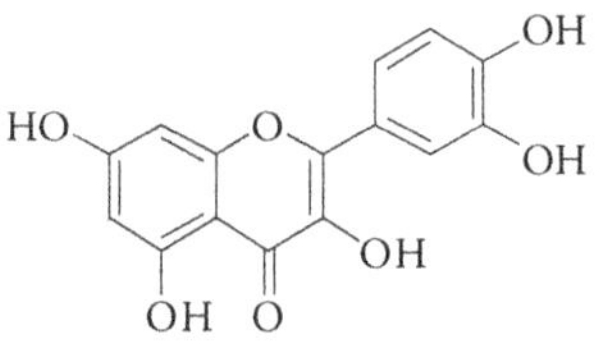

110

8.3.6 NEMATOSTATIC ACTIVITY

A series of lignans (16, 17, 32, 34, 48, and 107) from *B. salicifolium* were tested for nematostatic activity on the cysts and freed second-stage juveniles of the potato cyst nematodes *Glodobera pallida* and *G. rostochiensis* (González et al., 1994, 1995). None of the compounds tested showed nematicidal activity in an *in vitro* analysis with second-stage juveniles, but significant differences were noted when the compounds were assayed for nemostatic activity as cyst-hatching inhibitors. Bursehernin (32) and matairesinol (34) showed the greatest activity, at concentrations of 50 ppm (Table 8.10). Both compounds are the first natural products known to affect the hatching of *G. pallida* and the first lignans ever reported to have an effect on a phytoparasitic nematode.

8.3.7 OTHER ACTIVITIES

Extracts of the root of *B. fructicosum* showed a biological screening hemolytical activity, hepatoprotective, phagocytosis-stimulating effects, and a specific inhibitory activity of leucine aminopeptidase (Guinea et al., 1994). Further monitoring of the fraction with antihepatotoxic activity led to the isolation of a hepatoprotective saikosaponin identified as buddlejasaponin IV (95).

ACKNOWLEDGMENTS

We thank Dr. J. Molero (Departamento de Biología Vegetal, Facultad de Farmacia, Universidad de Granada, Spain) for providing us with the location of the *Bupleurum* species in Spain.

REFERENCES

Barrero, A.F., Haïdour, A., Reyes, F., Sedqui, A., and Mansour, A.I. (1998) Monoterpene aldehydes from *Bupleurum gibraltaricum, J. Nat. Prod.*, 61, 506–507.

Barrero, A.F., Herrador, M.M., Akssira, M., Arteaga, P., and Romera, J.L. (1999) Lignans and polyacetylenes from *Bupleurum acutifolium. J. Nat. Prod.*, 62, 946–948.

Barrero, A.F., Herrador, M.M., Akssira, M., and Arteaga, P. (2000a) Glicosidos flavonoides de *Bupleurum acutifolium. Deuxième Colloque Andalou-Marocain sur la Chemie des Produits Naturels*, Mohammedia, Morocco. Book of Abstracts, p. 31.

Barrero, A.F., Haïdour, A., Sedqui, A., Mansour, A.I., Rodríguez-Garcia, I., López, A. et al. (2000b) Saiko-saponins from roots of *Bupleurum gibraltaricum* and *Bupleurum spinosum, Phytochemistry*, 54, 741–745.

Bohlmann, F., Zdero, C., and Grenz, M. (1975) Notiz über einen weiteren terpenaldehydester aus Umbelliferen, *Chem. Ber.*, 108, 2822–2823.

Cabo, J., Cabo, M.M., Jiménez, J., and Ocete, M.A. (1986a) Essence de *Bupleurum gibraltaricum* Lam. (Ombellifères). I. Études préliminaires, *Plantes Med. Phytother.*, 20, 168–173.

Cabo, J., Cabo, M.M., Jiménez, J., Navarro, C., and Ocete, M.A. (1986b) Essence de *Bupleurum gibraltaricum* Lam. (Ombellifères). III. Étude par GC et GC/MS, *Plantes Med. Phytother.*, 20, 178–182.

Cabo, J., Cabo, M.M., Díaz, R.M., Jiménez, J., Miró, M., and Ocete, M.A. (1986c) Essence de *Bupleurum gibraltaricum* Lam. (Ombellifères). II. Détermination quali- et quantitative de son activité antimicrobienne, *Plantes Med. Phytother.*, 20, 174–177.

Estévez-Braun, A., Estévez-Reyes, R., and González, A.G. (1994a) Structural elucidation and conformational analysis of new lignan butenolides from the leaves of *Bupleurum salicifolium, Tetrahedron*, 50, 5203–5210.

Estévez-Braun, A., Estévez-Reyes, R., Moujir, L.M., Ravelo, A.G., and González, A.G. (1994b) Antibiotic activity and absolute configuration of 8S-heptadeca-2(Z), 9(Z)-diene-4,6-diyne-1,8-diol from *Bupleurum salicifolium, J. Nat. Prod.*, 57, 1178–1182.

Estévez-Braun, A., Estévez-Reyes, R., González-Pérez, J.A., and González, A.G. (1995) Busaliol and Busalicifol, two new tetrahydrofuran lignans from *Bupleurum salicifolium, J. Nat. Prod.*, 58, 887–892.

Estévez-Reyes, R., Estévez-Braun, A., and González, A.G. (1992) Lignanolides from *Bupleurum salicifolium, Phytochemistry*, 31, 2841–2845.

Estévez-Reyes, R., Estévez-Braun, A., and González, A.G. (1993) New lignan butenolides from *Bupleurum salicifolium, J. Nat. Prod.*, 56, 1177–1181.

Gil, M.L., Jiménez, J., Ocete, M.A., Zarzuelo, A., and Cabo, M.M. (1989). Comparative study of different essential oils of *Bupleurum gibraltaricum* Lamarck, *Pharmazie*, 44, 284–287.

González, A.G., Trujillo, J.M., Estévez, R., and Pérez, J.P. (1975) Componentes de Umbelíferas. IV. Lignanos del *Bupleurum fruticescens* L., *An. Quim.*, 71, 109–110.

González, A.G., Estévez-Reyes, R., and Mato, C. (1989) Salicifoliol, a new furolactone-type lignan from *Bupleurum salicifolium, J. Nat. Prod.*, 52, 1139–1142.

González, A.G., Estévez-Reyes, R., Mato, C., and Estévez-Braun, A.M. (1990a) Isokaerophyllin, a butyrolactone from *Bupleurum salicifolium, Phytochemistry*, 29, 675–678.

González, A.G., Estévez-Reyes, R., Mato, C., and Estévez-Braun, A.M. (1990b) Three lignans from *Bupleurum salicifolium, Phytochemistry*, 29, 1981–1983.

González, A.G., Estévez-Reyes, R., and Estévez-Braun, A.M. (1990c) Buplerol and Guayarol, new lignans from the seeds of *Bupleurum salicifolium, J. Chem. Res.*, (S), 220–221.

González, J.A., Estévez-Braun, A., Estévez-Reyes, R., and Ravelo, A.G. (1994) Inhibition of potato cyst nematode hatch by lignans from *Bupleurum salicifolium* (Umbelliferae), *J. Chem. Ecol.*, 20, 517–524.

González, J.A., Estévez-Braun, A., Estévez-Reyes, R., Bazzocchi, I.L., Moujir, L., Jiménez, I.A. et al. (1995) Biological activity of secondary metabolites from *Bupleurum salicifolium* (Umbelliferae), *Experientia*, 51, 35–39.

Guinea, M.C., Parellada, J., Lacaille-Dubois, M.A., and Wagner, H. (1994) Biologically active triterpene saponins from *Bupleurum fruticosum, Planta Med.*, 60, 163–167.

López, H., Valera, A., and Trujillo, J. (1996) Lignans from *Bupleurum handiense, J. Nat. Prod.*, 59, 493–494.

Lorente, I., Ocete, M.A., Zarzuelo, A., Cabo, M.M., and Jiménez, J. (1989) Bioactivity of the essential oil of *Bupleurum fruticosum, J. Nat. Prod.*, 52, 267–272.

Mansour, A.I. (1998) Etude phytochimique du *Bupleurum spinosum* L. et du *Bupleurum gibraltaricum* L. Sc.D. thesis, Faculté des Sciences, Tétouan, Morocco.

Martín, S., Padilla, E., Ocete, M.A., Gálvez, J., Jiménez, J., and Zarzuelo, A. (1993) Anti-inflammatory activity of the essential oil of *Bupleurum fruticescens, Planta Med.,* 59, 533–536.

Massanet, G.M., Guerra, F.M., Jorge, Z.D., and Casalvázquez, L.G. (1997) Phenylpropanoids from *Bupleurum fruticosum, Phytochemistry,* 44, 173–177.

Ocete, M.A., Risco, S., Zarzuelo, A., and Jiménez, J. (1989) Pharmacological activity of the essential oil of *Bupleurum gibraltaricum*: anti-inflammatory activity and effects on isolated rat uteri, *J. Ethnopharmacol.,* 25, 305–313.

Sánchez-Contreras, S., Díaz-Lanza, A.M., Fernández Matellano, L., Bernabé, M., Ollivier, E., Balansard, G. et al. (1998) A sulfated saponin from *Bupleurum rigidum, J. Nat. Prod.,* 61, 1383–1385.

Sánchez-Contreras, S., Díaz-Lanza, A.M., Bartolomé, C., and Bernabé, M. (2000) Minor sulfated saikosaponins from the aerial parts of *Bupleurum rigidum* L., *Phytochemistry,* 54, 783–789.

Utrilla, M.P., Zarzuelo, A., Risco, S., Ocete, M.A., Jiménez, J., and Gámez, M.J. (1991) Isolation of a saikosaponin responsible for the anti-inflammatory activity of *Bupleurum gibraltaricum* Lam. root extract, *Phytotherapy Res.,* 5, 43–45.

9 The Chemistry and Biological Activity of the Genus *Bupleurum* in Italy

Luisa Pistelli

CONTENTS

9.1 1NTRODUCTION

Plants belonging to the genus *Bupleurum* (Umbelliferae) are well-known traditional Chinese drugs and have been accepted for medical use in China for more than 2000 years. The purpose of this chapter is to review the chemistry, pharmacology, and other biological uses of some Italian plants belonging to this genus.

9.2 BOTANY AND GEOGRAPHICAL LOCATION

Species of *Bupleurum* are primarily located in the Northern Hemisphere, Eurasia, and North America. The Italian flora consists of about 15 species, with some restricted endemism (e.g., *B. dianthifolium*, only in Marettimo Island, near Sicily), but others are widely distributed from the Alps to the Apennines. The etymology of the name *Bupleurum* derives from two Greek words: *bous* and *pléuron*, with the meaning of ox and stripes, respectively, referring to the parallel veins evident on the leaves of some *Bupleurum* species. In Italian vernacular language there is no special name for *Bupleurum*, as in Germany (*Hasenoehrchen*), in England (*hare's ear*), or in France (*Oreille de lièvre*), names derived from a translation of the Latin name: *Auricula leporis* (Motta, 1987).

Bupleurum species consist of annual or perennial plants, with herbaceous aspect, sometimes shrubby, with simple, entire, and alternate leaves; the inflorescence is a compound umbel, with flower structures arranged in fives; flowers are small and radial, the petals are yellowish; the fruit is a double achaene. The height of the plants varies from a few decimeters to 1 to 2 m. (Pignatti, 1982; Motta, 1987).

Italian *Bupleurum* species grow on cliffs and stony places, in arid herbous pastures, especially distributed along seacoasts, but are common also in cultivated fields and vineyards. Several species are cultivated as ornamentals in gardens, such as *B. fruticosum* , a perennial shrub with an intense resinous smell when the leaves are rubbed.

Bupleurum fruticosum L., *B. falcatum* L. subsp. *cernum* (Ten.) Arcang. and *B. rotundifolium* L. are the Italian *Bupleurum* species chemically studied to date.

Bupleurum fruticosum L. is an evergreen, glaucous, perennial wild shrub, 1 to 2 m in height. Leaves are elliptic-oblong, coriaceous, subsessile, pinnately nerved. Umbels 7 to 10 cm across; fruits oblong, 5 to 7 mm, vittae 1 in each furrow.

From an ethnobotanical viewpoint in Sardinia *B. fruticosum* is indicated with common name: "*Lau cràbinu* = goats laurel" or "*Linna pùdiga* = fetid wood." These names underline the quality of the aroma which some authors believe to be very unpleasant, goat-like, and also that the wood, i.e., the branches, contain most of the aromatic compounds. One must believe that the repulsion of the animals for this species is due to the presence of these essential oils. However, the plant is not refused, at least the spouts (young shoots) are eaten by goats (Picci et al., 1974). On the contrary, according to Moris (1840), the fragrant and tasty fruits, which remind one of the fennels, although more bitter, have been used as spices. The flavor of this plant is very pleasant, especially after breaking a branch, and it is more bitter in summer.

Bupleurum falcatum L. subsp. *cernum* (Ten.) Arcang. is a perennial herb up to 100 cm high; stem slender, flexuous, basal leaves lanceolate, lower narrowed into a petiole, middle and upper leaves linear to lanceolate, gradually shorter, sessile; fruit oblong 5 mm long, ridges more or less winged.

Bupleurum rotundifolium L. is an annual, erect, glaucous herb, with alternate, entire, amplexicaul leaves, named *Bupleurum* like ox's lung. The edges and veins, which are parallel, are translucent. The flowers are not discernible with the naked eye (up to 0.2 cm wide) and are yellow. They are in a compound umbel with 7 to 12 flowers in each umbel. Blooms first appear in mid spring and continue into late spring.

9.3 MAIN CHEMICAL CONSTITUENTS OF ITALIAN *BUPLEURUM* SPP.

A relatively small number of *Bupleurum* species (about a quarter of the total) have been subjected to phytochemical investigations: the main constituents and the most bioactive components are triterpene glycosides of the oleanane series (named saikosaponins) (Nose et al., 1989; Guinea et al., 1994), but occurrence of polyphenolic compounds, i.e., phenylpropanoids (Massanet et al., 1997), lignanes (Luo et al., 1993; Estévez-Braun et al., 1994b, 1995), coumarins (Gonzalez et al., 1975; Pistelli et al., 1996), several flavonoids (Zhanayeva and Lovanova, 1992), together with polyacetylenes (Popov and Gromov, 1992; Estévez-Braun et al., 1994), polysaccharides, and phytosterols have been reported. The essential oils of genus *Bupleurum* have been extensively studied as well (Peyron and Roubaub, 1970; Lorente et al., 1989; Manunta, 1992; Giamperi et al., 1998; Dugo et al., 2000).

9.3.1 TRITERPENOID SAPONINS

Triterpene glycosides of the oleanane series (the so-called saikosaponins, from the Japanese name "Saiko," the common name of *Bupleurum* spp. used in Kampo medicine) are considered the major bioactive components of *Bupleurum* crude drug, mainly used for its anti-inflammatory and

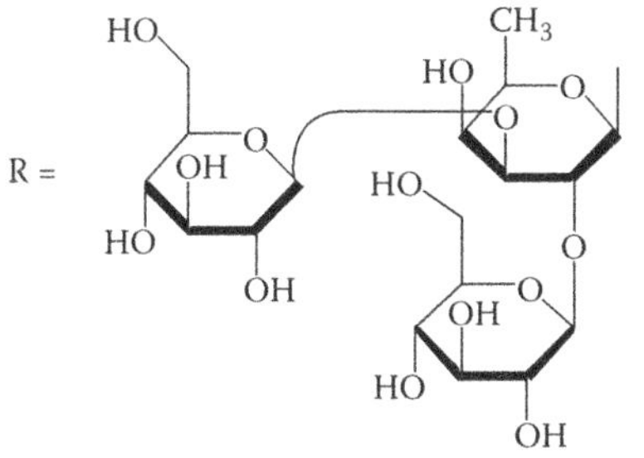

FIGURE 9.1 Sugar moiety of saponins **1** through **4**.

anti-hepatotoxic activity (Yamamoto et al., 1975; Abe et al., 1980). Four novel saponins (Figure 9.1 and Figure 9.2, **1** through **4**) were isolated from the methanolic extract of the roots of *B. fruticosum* , harvested in Sardinia (Italy) (Pistelli et al., 1993a, 1993b, 1996), while the new saponin (see Figure 9.3, **5**), along with the three known saikosaponins b$_2$, b$_3$, and b$_4$, were isolated from whole plants *B. falcatum* subsp. *cernum* , collected in the Marche region of Italy (Pistelli et al., 1993).

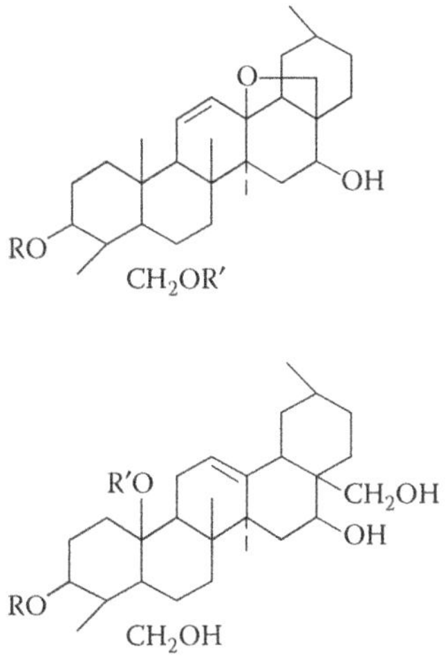

Saponin 1 R′ =
Saponin 2 R′ = COC$_3$H

Saponin 3 R′ = CH$_3$
Saponin 4 R′ = H

FIGURE 9.2 Saponins **1** through **4** isolated from *B. fruticosum*.

Saponin 5

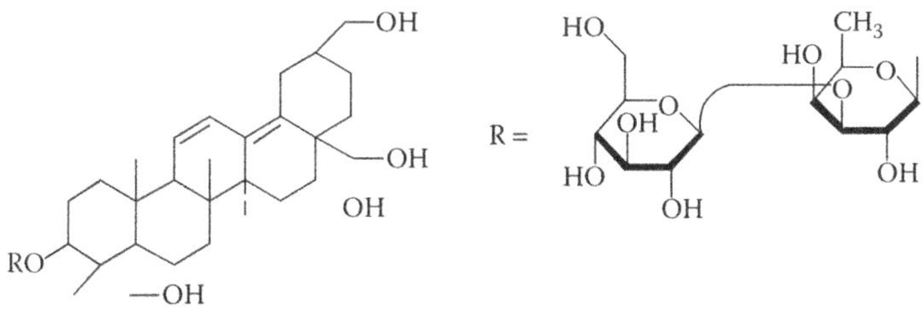

R =

FIGURE 9.3 Saponin **5** from *B. falcatum* subsp. *cernum*.

Saponins (**1** through **4**) are characterized by four different aglycones, but the same sugar moiety: in fact all saponins are monodesmosidic, with the sugar moiety linked to the C-3 of the aglycone to form a trisaccharide, containing sugars such as fucose and glucose linked to each other as in 3-[β-D-glucopyranosyl-(1→2)]-[β-D-glucopyranosyl-(1→3)]-β-D-fucopyranoside (Figure 9.1).

Compound (**1**) has the same aglycone of saikogenin F (with a characteristic 13β,28-oxide ring) (Kubota and Hinoh, 1968), and was also isolated from *Buddleja japonica* with the name buddlejasaponin IV (Yamamoto et al., 1991). Saponin (**2**) presents an acetoxyl function at C-23 position of saikogenin F, while the aglycone of (**3**) is identical to that of saikosaponin b_4, with a methoxyl group in position 11, that becomes a hydroxyl substituent in saponin (**4**) (Figure 9.2).

Saponin (**5**) from *B. falcatum* subsp. *cernum* is a glycoside of an olean-11,13(18)-diene with four hydroxyl groups attached to C-16, C-23, C-28, and C-30. It is a monodesmosidic saponin, in which the disaccharide β-D-glucopyranoyl(1→3)-β-D-fucopyranoside appears linked to C-3. Since no acidic conditions were employed during extraction and isolation, it can be reasonably assumed that compound (**5**), is characterized by a conjugated heteroannular diene in C and D rings, is a primary constituent of the plant, and not an artifact derived from the allyl ether precursor (Pistelli et al., 1993) (Figure 9.3).

Saponins are polar constituents and was purified from the methanolic extract of the dried plants, dissolved in water and then extracted with ethyl acetate and successively *n*-butanol; this latter was subjected first to gel filtration on Sephadex LH 20, then to Lobar RP8 chromatography, eluted with MeOH-H_2O mixture to afford pure compounds. The saponin structure elucidation was performed by spectral analysis (mainly by means of 1D and 2D NMR techniques, which permitted assignment of all ^{1}H and ^{13}C signals), thus providing unambiguous information about the aglycone structure and the nature, position of the glycosidic linkage, and sequence of the monosaccharides in the sugar moiety (Pistelli et al., 1993, 1996).

9.3.2 PHENYLPROPANOIDS

Two novel phenylpropanoids, (*E*)-3-(3,4-dimethoxyphenyl)-2-propen-1-yl (*Z*)-2-[(*Z*)-2-methyl-2-butenoyloxy methyl]butenoate (**6**) and (*E*)-3-(4-methoxyphenyl)-2-propen-1-yl (*Z*)-2-[(*Z*)-2-methyl-2-butenoyloxymethyl]butenoate (**7**), were obtained from the *n*-hexane extract of the leaves of *B. fruticosum* harvested in Dorgali (Sardinia). They were purified after gel filtration on Sephadex LH 20 of the crude hexane extract and subsequently flash chromatographed. 1,2-Dimethoxy-4-(1-methoxy-2-propenyl)benzene (**8**), 1,2-dimethoxy-4-(3-methoxy-1-propenyl)benzene (**9**), and 3,4-dimethoxycinnamaldehyde (**10**) were also found in the same extract. The structures of these phenylpropanoids were established by spectral methods, from ^{1}H and ^{13}C-NMR spectra, also confirmed by ^{1}H-^{1}H, ^{1}H-^{13}C correlations and distortionless enhancement by polarization transfer (DEPT) experiments. The presence and the sequence of the diester moiety were also confirmed from its electron impact mass spectrometry (EIMS) spectrum: the peak at *m/z* 275 [M − 99]$^+$ was due to the loss of fragment angelate, while the peak at *m/z* 193 [M − (99 + 82)]$^+$ arose from the loss of all the diester side chain (Pistelli et al., 1996) (Figure 9.4).

Recently, Massanet et al. (1997) have isolated other similar compounds from the same source, collected in Serrania de Grazalema (Spain), in addition to spinasterol and erytrodiol. The structures of these phenylpropanoids were established by spectroscopic methods too.

9.3.3 COUMARINS

Coumarins are characteristic compounds of the Umbelliferae family (Hegnauer, 1973), so they are typical constituents in *Bupleurum* species as well. Seven coumarins, scopoletin, scoparone, prenyletin, capensin, fraxetin, aesculetin, 7-(3′-methyl-2′-butenyloxy)-6-methoxycoumarin, and two new derivatives. 7-(2′-Hydroxy-3′-methyl-3′-butenyloxy)-6-methoxycoumarin (**11**) and 5,7-dihydroxy-6-methoxy-8-(3′-methyl-2′-butenyl)coumarin (**12**) (Figure 9.5) were isolated, after

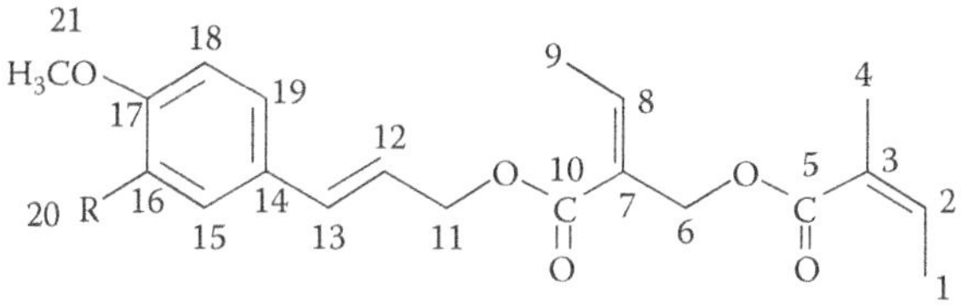

* 6: R = OCH₃
  7: R = H

* The numbering of carbon atoms in structures 6–7 is
not according IUPAC rules.

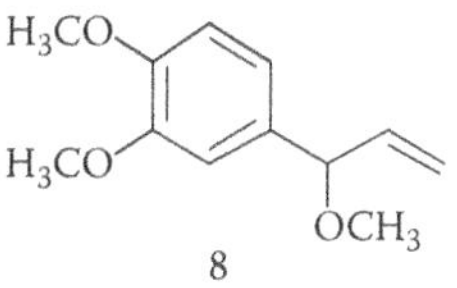

FIGURE 9.4 Structures of phenylpropanoids **6** through **10** from *B. fruticosum*.

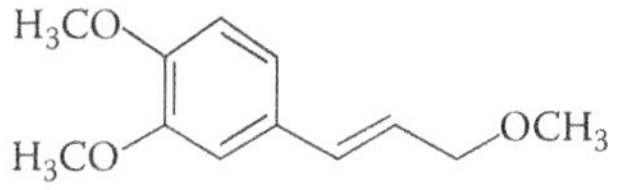

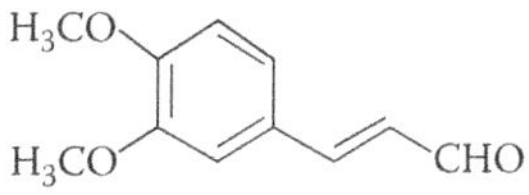

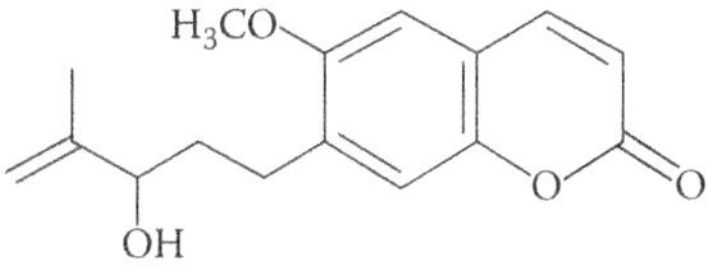

Coumarin 11

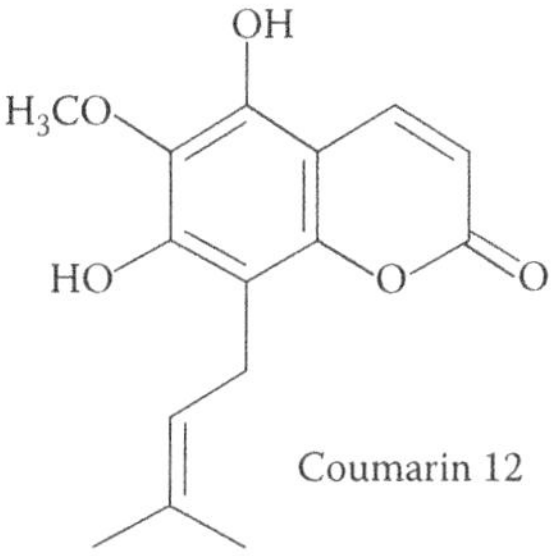

Coumarin 12

FIGURE 9.5 Novel coumarins from *B. fruticosum*.

chromatographic fractionation, from $CHCl_3$ and $CHCl_3$-MeOH of *B. fruticosum* roots. The latter coumarin had not been previously encountered in nature, while 7-(2´-hydroxy-3´-methyl-3´-bute-nyloxy)-6-methoxycoumarin was isolated also from *Pterocaulon virgatum* (Debenedetti et al., 1993). This was the first report of its presence in the genus *Bupleurum* and in the Apiaceae family. The new compounds produced violet coloration on treatment with hydroxylamine and ferric chloride, a reaction typical for coumarins (Feigl, 1960). Their structures were determined by analysis of NMR spectral data including 2D techniques.

9.3.4 FLAVONOIDS

In the course of investigations on the chemical constituents of some *Bupleurum* species of the Italian flora, Pistelli et al. (1996) took into consideration *B. falcatum* L. subsp. *cernum*, from which some flavonoids together with the just mentioned saponins, were isolated. Rutin and two other quercetin glycosides, avicularin (3-α-L-arabinofuranoside) (**13**), and guaijaverin (3-α-L-arabino pyranoside) (**14**), were isolated and identified from the ethyl acetate extract. Their structures were confirmed by NMR spectral analysis and acid hydrolysis and by comparison with the literature data. Both latter compounds were isolated previously from *Andromeda polifolia* L. (Pachaly and Klein, 1987), but this was the first report of their presence in the genus *Bupleurum*.

During phytochemical investigation of *B. fruticosum* aerial parts some other flavonoids were isolated and identified, such as isorhamnetin 3-glucoside, isorhamnetin 3-rutinoside, and rutin; their

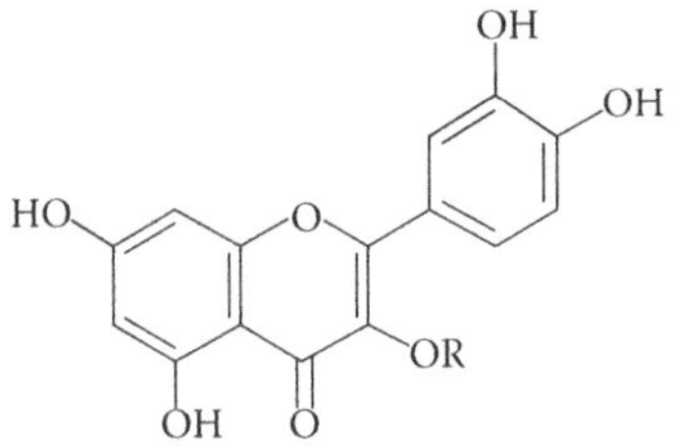

13 R = α-L-Arabino*furanoside*
14 R = α-L-Arabino*pyranoside*

FIGURE 9.6 Avicularin and guaijaverin from *B. falcatum* subsp. *cernum*.

structures were established on the basis of their spectroscopic data in comparison with authentic compounds and references from the literature (data not yet published). These compounds were in good agreement with those reported by Hegnauer (1990) (Figure 9.6).

Bupleurum flavum Forskal, an annual species typical of the eastern regions of Mediterranean area (Bulgaria, Greece, and Turkey), was also investigated in our laboratory. *Bupleurum flavum* is an herbaceous slender, erect plant, 20 to 75 cm (Tutin et al., 1972), that grows on dry rocky places, especially near the sea.

Kaempferol, isokaempferide (3-methoxy-4´,5,7-trihydroxyflavone), quercetin, gossipetin, and luteolin were isolated and identified from the aerial parts of *B. flavum* collected in June 1997 on the Black Sea coast in Bulgaria, together with rutin, isorhamnetin 3-glucoside, isorhamnetin 3-rutinoside. All these compounds are known and have been identified in many other *Bupleurum* species, except for gossipetin, isolated here for the first time. Isorhamnetin as aglycone, quercetin 3-glucoside, kaempferol 3-glucoside, and kaempferol 3-rutinoside were also identified in the extracts of *B. flavum* of the same origin by HPLC profile (Gevrenova, 1997).

9.3.5 ESSENTIAL OIL

Bupleurum is a genus characterized by the presence of a secretory system distributed as a continuous network in the roots, steams, leaves, and umbels; no other independent ducts are evident (Manunta et al., 1992). *Bupleurum fruticosum* has a quite strong aroma especially in the wood, which contains the aromatic compounds in great abundance; therefore the fragrant and tasty fruits have been used as a spice, which reminds one of fennel, although more bitter (Picci et al., 1974a, 1974b). Animals have a certain repulsion for this shrub and some authors believe that this repulsion is due to the presence of the essential oil (1 to 3% v/w).

Research on the essential oil composition of *B. fruticosum* began at the turn of the last century with Francesconi and Sernagiotto (1913), who reported the presence of a terpenic alcohol, named bupleurol (presumed to be a citronellol's isomer, with a characteristic smell of roses) from a species collected in Sardinia.

Successively Peyron and Roubaud (1970) analyzed the essential oil hydrodistilled from flowers of *B. fruticosum* collected in Provence (France) in comparison with the previous oil. They did not detect any trace of bupleurol, and noticed that there were differences in the terpene hydrocarbon content, with β-phellandrene more abundant in the Sardinian oil, while β-pinene was more abundant in the other. Camphene, myrcene, limonene, *cis* - and *trans*-β-ocimene, *p*-cymene, C9-C10 aldehydes, thujone, α-terpineol, and sesquiterpenes were also identified. In 1992, Manunta et al. identified 22 constituents in the oil obtained from the branches of plant material (*B. fruticosum*) grown in the botanical garden of the University of Urbino, but originating from Sardinia (main component γ-terpinene 48.8%), and 14 constituents in the leaf oil (sabinene 39.7%, β-phellandrene 38.7%). The analysis was performed both with GC and GC/MS methods and the presence of citronellol acetate was of particular interest among the constituents identified. More recently, Giamperi et al. (1998) analyzed the composition of the essential oil from the epigean parts of *B. fruticosum* harvested in Cirenaica (Libya), while Dugo G. et al. in 2002 analyzed by HRGC/MS and HRGC/FID the oil of Sicilian *B. fruticosum*, extracted by SDE (Simultaneous Distillation Extraction). Both identified 65 components, which constituted more than 98% of the whole oils, and definitively confirmed that bupleurol must not be considered a naturally occurring compound but rather an artificial one. Table 9.1 reports the essential oil composition of different *B. fruticosum* samples according literature data.

9.3.6 OTHER COMPOUNDS

During the studies conducted by Pistelli et al. cicloeucalenol and lupeol were identified by GC analysis from the unsaponifiable parts of the *n*-hexane extract of *B. fruticosum*, while the main fatty acids in the acidic fraction were linoleic acid (16.24%) and palmitic acid (15.87%) (data unpublished).

Betulin, betulinic acid, lup-20(29)-en-3β,28,30-triol and two unidentified compounds, belonging to the class of lupene derivatives, were isolated and identified in *B. flavum* extracts (data unpublished; Noccioli, 1999). No oleanane derivatives were detected (compounds not stored in the aerial parts but probably in the roots). Nemerosin, named also anhydropodorhizol, a lignan belonging to the benzylidenbenzyl-γ-butirrolactone class, was also isolated and identified (Kamil and Dewick, 1986).

9.4 PHARMACOLOGICAL AND BIOLOGICAL ACTIVITY

9.4.1 TRADITIONAL THERAPEUTIC USES

"Bupleuri radix" (roots of *Bupleurum* spp., Umbelliferae) is a very important crude drug used in Oriental traditional medicine as an anti-inflammatory and hepatoprotective agent, for the treatment of nephrosis syndrome and autoimmune diseases. *Bupleurum* species are officially listed in the *Pharmacopoeia of the People's Republic of China* and in the *Japanese Pharmacopoeia*, mainly *B. falcatum* L., *B. chinense* DC., and *B. scorzonerifolium* Willd. (with the exception of *B. longiradiatum*, considered toxic). *Bupleurum* spp. are not covered by a Commission E monograph and are not on the U.K. General Sale List; however, they are freely available as a "dietary supplement" in the U.S. under DSHEA legislation (Mills and Bone, 2000).

These drugs are not generally used alone, but decocted with several other crude drugs as Oriental herbal formulas (Watanable et al., 1988); liquid extracts and tablets are also used, such as powdered roots.

No *Bupleurum* species is eaten, because the plants are considered toxic if consumed in large amount. In France *B. fruticosum* wood has been used to warm bakers' ovens, and the crushed roots are used for their fish narcotic action in Corsica to fish in rivers (Manunta, 1979). *Bupleurum fruticosum* is also used as an ornamental in Mediterranean gardens, and *B. rotundifolium* is used as a dry plant in ornamental decorations.

Many effects have been referred to *Bupleurum* species in the Mediterranean area, in the Western traditional medicine: *B. fruticosum* L., *B. falcatum* L., *B. rotundifolium* L., *B. opacum* Lange, *B. aristatum* Barth, and *B. odontites* L. are considered as drugs, with a wide range of action (Manunta, 1979).

Bupleurum fruticosum uses:
- Diuretic remedy against urinary retention (roots)
- Laxative, cited in the first edition of French Pharmacopoeia 1818
- antirheumatic, as a root decoction, specially in Sardinia (Ballero and Fresu, 1991)

TABLE 9.1

Percentage Composition of Essential Oils from *B. fruticosum*

| Constituents[a] | Percentage (%) | | | | | | |
	A	B	Br	Le	D	E	F
			C				
α-Pinene	21.66	15.30	—	2.55	—	42.1	t
α-Thujene	0.02	1.20	—	—	—	—	—
Camphene	0.23	0.20	—	—	—	t	—
β-Pinene	13.21	9.10	—	0.40	35.9	—	—
Sabinene	6.74	3.50	12.00	39.74	—	—	—
δ-3-Carene	0.13	—	—	—	—	—	—
α-Phellandrene	0.70	—	12.22	2.30	3.1	—	—
Myrcene	1.98	2.20	—	2.48	3.1	—	—
α-Terpinene	0.13	—	0.83	—	—	—	—
β-Terpinene	—	—	0.87	1.51	—	—	—
Bornylene	—	—	0.46	—	—	—	—
Dihydro-1,8-cineole	t	—	—	—	—	—	—
Limonene	2.00	—	—	5.04	4.1	t	—
1,8-Cineole	—	—	—	—	4.1	—	—
β-Phellandrene	21.29	49.30	—	38.71	—	t	t
γ-Terpinene	2.95	0.10	48.64	—	2.5	—	—
(Z)-β-Ocimene	—	0.10	—	1.33	—	t	—
(E)-β-Ocimene	0.02	—	—	0.31	—	t	—
p-Cymene	—	5.40	—	—	2.9	t	—
Terpinolene	0.08	—	—	—	—	—	—
(Z)-3-Hexenyl acetate	—	0.10	—	—	—	—	—
Amil isovalerate	t	—	—	—	—	—	—
2,6-Dimethyl-5-eptanal	0.51	—	—	—	—	—	—
Nonanal	t	—	—	—	—	—	—
Thujone	—	—	—	—	—	t	—
2,5-Dimethylstirene	0.02	—	—	—	—	—	—
δ-Elemene	0.03	—	—	—	—	—	—
α-Copaene	3.43	0.70	—	—	—	—	—
β-Bourbonene	0.17	1.50	—	—	—	—	—
Linalool	—	—	1.50	—	t	—	—
α-Cubebene	2.41	—	—	—	—	—	—
Linalyl acetate	—	—	—	—	t	—	—
trans-Sabinene-hydrate	t	—	—	—	—	—	—
Calarene	0.05	—	—	—	—	—	—
β-Caryophyllene	0.54	1.50	—	—	—	—	—
Pinocarvone	—	0.20	—	—	—	—	—
Myrtenal	—	0.20	—	—	—	—	—
β-Elemene	0.02	—	—	—	—	—	—
Thymol methylether	t	2.4	—	—	—	—	—
Terpinen-4-ol	0.02	—	1.26	1.79	t	t	—
Isobornyl acetate	—	2.10	—	—	—	—	—
Carvacrol methyl ether	2.93	—	—	—	—	—	—
Longifolene	0.19	—	—	—	—	—	—
α-Humulene	0.40	0.20	—	—	—	—	—
Methyl chavicol	—	—	—	—	t	t	—
trans-Pinocarveol	—	0.20	—	—	—	—	—
Citronellyl acetate	—	0.10	4.20	—	—	—	—

TABLE 9.1 (CONTINUED)
Percentage Composition of Essential Oils from *B. fruticosum*

Constituents[a]	Percentage (%)						
	A	B	C		D	E	F
			Br	Le			
(Z)-Anethole	0.19	—	—	—	—	—	—
Germacrene D	8.74	—	—	—	—	—	—
cis-p-Mentha-2,8-dien-1-ol	—	0.30	—	—	—	—	—
trans-p-Mentha-2,8-dien-1-ol	—	0.40	—	—	—	—	—
trans-Verbenol	—	0.20	—	—	—	—	—
α-Terpineol	0.15	0.30	—	—	—	t	—
Cryptone	—	0.20	—	—	—	—	—
Valencene	0.02	—	—	—	—	—	—
Borneol	—	—	—	—	t	—	t
Dihydro carveol	—	—	5.13	—	—	—	—
Carvone	—	0.40	—	—	—	—	—
Biciclogermacrene	3.03	—	—	—	—	—	—
cis-γ-Cadinene	0.01	—	—	—	—	—	—
δ-Cadinene	1.09	1.10	—	—	—	—	—
Geranyl acetate	—	0.10	—	—	—	—	—
Hexyl isovalerate	—	—	1.58	—	—	—	—
Heptyl acetate	—	—	0.21	—	—	—	—
Octyl acetate	—	—	1.46	—	—	—	—
Bupleurol	—	—	—	—	—	t	—
Nerol	—	—	0.49	—	—	—	—
trans-Piperitol	—	0.10	—	—	—	—	—
Decanol	—	—	1.08	—	—	—	—
trans-Carveol	—	0.21	—	—	—	—	—
(E,E)-Farnesene	0.01	—	—	—	—	—	—
Myrtenol	—	0.10	—	—	—	—	—
cis-Carvyl acetate	—	0.10	—	—	—	—	—
(E)-Anethole	t	—	—	—	—	—	—
Hexyl-2-methylbutyrate	—	0.10	0.33	—	—	—	—
(E)-Cinnamyl valerate	—	—	2.71	—	—	—	—
Thymoquinone methyl ether	—	0.10	—	—	—	—	—
p-Cimen-9-ol	0.07	—	—	—	—	—	—
2,5-Dimethossy-p-cimene	0.40	—	—	—	—	—	—
Cubebol	0.11	—	—	—	—	—	—
Epi-cubebol	0.09	—	—	—	—	—	—
Phenyl,ethyl-2-methylbenzoate	0.03	—	—	—	—	—	—
Phytol acetate	0.06	—	—	—	—	—	—
Phenyl,ethyl-3-methylbutanoate	t	—	—	—	—	—	—
p-Anysaldehyde	t	—	—	—	—	—	—
(E)-Phytol acetate	0.08	—	—	—	—	—	—
Methyl eugenol	—	—	0.64	—	—	—	—
Ledol	t	—	—	—	—	—	—
Cubenol	0.02	—	—	—	—	—	—
1,10-Epicubenol	0.02	—	—	—	—	—	—
Spatulenol	0.01	—	—	—	—	—	—
Myrcenone	t	—	—	—	—	t	—
T-Muurolol	—	t	—	—	—	—	—
Cadinol	0.09	—	—	—	—	—	—

TABLE 9.1 (CONTINUED)
Percentage Composition of Essential Oils from *B. fruticosum*

	Percentage (%)						
			C				
Constituents[a]	A	B	Br	Le	D	E	F
Thymol	—	—	—	—	t	—	—
Carvacrol	0.01	—	—	—	1.47	—	—
α-Cadinol	0.07	t	—	—	—	—	—
Elemicin	0.05	—	1.99	—	—	—	—
Cinnamyl isovalerate	t	—	1.26	0.78	—	—	—
p-Methoxy-cinnamaldehyde	0.01	—	—	—	—	—	—
Benzyle benzoate	0.03	—	—	—	—	—	—
Phytol	0.01	—	—	—	—	—	—
3-(Methoxyphenyl)-2-propen-1-ol	0.12	—	—	—	—	—	—
Salvial-4(14)-en-1-one	—	0.20	—	—	—	—	—

Note: A = Dugo et al. (2000) (15); B = Giamperi et al. (1998) (14); C = Manunta et al (1992) (13); D = Lorente et al. (1989) (11); E = Peyron and Roubaud (1970) (32); F = Francesconi and Sernagiotto (1913) (17). t = traces; Br = branches; Le = leaves.

[a] The compounds are listed in order to retention indices on a polar column.

- emmenagogue (roots and fruits, used in French traditional medicine against amennorhea)
- expectorant and antiasthmatic (root and fruit decoction against asthma and persistent cough)
- antidote against certain animal poisons (especially the fruits)

Bupleurum falcatum use:
- Whole plants (pounded in a mortar) effective as anti-inflammatory against furunculosis

Bupleurum rotundifolium properties:
- Astringent, vulnerary, and stimulant (flowers and leaves)
- Analgesic (leaves boiled in vinegar and applied in hot cataplasm were used in France in the past, to alleviate lymphatic glands pain, to solve hernia, and to eliminate articular aches)
- Febrifuge (leaves infusion, together with *B. falcatum* roots decoction, show activity against fever)

Bupleurum opacum, B. aristatum , and *B. odontites* :
- Leaves are used against toothache

9.4.2 BIOLOGICAL TESTED ACTIVITY

The activity of the essential oil of *B. fruticosum* , the anti-inflammatory effect of the whole oil, and its major components were investigated together with its qualitative and quantitative composition (Lorente et al., 1989). The activity was tested against carrageenan-induced or PGE-induced edema (in the hindpaw of the rat), i.e., in acute exudative inflammation. The oil showed a potent activity when administered both orally and i.p., but the former administration required much higher doses than the latter to produce the same effect. The anti-inflammatory activity can be attributed to the major components of the essential oil, α and β-pinene, that exhibited a clear anti-inflammatory activity at doses equivalent to those of the whole essential oil. Furthermore, *B. fruticosum* essential oil showed a definite antispasmodic activity against acetylcholine- and oxytocin-induced contractions in rat uteri and this behavior varied depending on the agonist tested (Lorente et al., 1989).

Antimicrobic activity of the essential oil obtained from the aerial parts of *B. fruticosum* collected in Sardinia was tested against 13 Gram-positive and Gram-negative bacteria and two fungal species using the aromatogram test (Manunta, 1987). The results showed a strong activity against all tested Gram-positive bacteria (*Streptococcus foecalis*, *Staphylococcus albus*, and *Staphylococcus aureus*) and against *Candida albicans*, and indicated the utilization of this oil in perfumery, aromatherapy, and dermatology. No activity was observed against Gram-negative bacteria.

Since *Bupleurum* spp. show anti-inflammatory, hepatoprotective, antitussive, and diaphoretic actions, and saikosaponins are considered the most biologically active compounds, the triterpenoid saponins isolated from *B. fruticosum* were tested for several *in vitro* activities. In a biological screening, extracts of *B. fruticosum* roots showed hemolytic activity, hepatoprotective and phagocytosis stimulating effects, and a specific inhibitory activity of leucine aminopeptidase (Guinea et al., 1994). The antihepatotoxic activity of the crude saponin fraction and the isolated compounds was monitored against CCl_4 and GalN-cytotoxicity in primary cultured rat hepatocytes: while the crude extract was ineffective in protecting the cells from damage by CCl_4, the same extract showed strong hepatoprotective effect against GalN-cytotoxicity, which was, at a dose of 1 mg/ml, more potent than silybin, a reference natural antihepatotoxic agent. The same effect at the same level was found for the main saponin of this extract, saponin (**1**), i.e., buddlejasaponin IV: it showed a remarkable hepatoprotective effect as compared with silybin against GalN-cytotoxicity. This activity is mainly attributed to 16-OH group in the saikogenin F, aglycone of saikosaponin a of *B. falcatum*, whose hepatoprotection against GalN-cytotoxicity has been confirmed *in vivo*.

Because some triterpene saponins have been reported to exert immunostimulating activities, the effect of crude saponin fraction and compound (**1**) were tested in the *in vitro* granulocyte phagocytosis. The results were in good agreement with that described in *B. falcatum* for the crude saponin fraction, but compound (**1**) was not active. This ineffectiveness could be explained by the fact that its aglycone, saikogenin F, possesses a 16β-OH configuration, like saikosaponin a, which was found to be less effective than saikosaponin d (16α-OH) in the macrophage activation. Like other saikosaponins investigated in the hemolysis test, compound (**1**) showed a strong dose-dependent hemolytic activity (Guinea et al., 1994).

Further, the extracts obtained from the aerial parts and roots of *B. rotundifolium* were subjected to the pharmacological tests to determine the oral and topical anti-inflammatory activities. Root extracts were more active on the carrageenan-induced paw edema test, while aerial part extracts had more action when assayed topically (TPA-induced ear edema). The active constituent of the aerial parts, isolated by the bioassay-directed fractionation, seemed to be a saponin, related to oleanane skeleton, identified here as compound (**1**). This metabolite reduced the edema by 70% at the dose of 0.5 mg/ear, in the same range of indomethacin (Just et al., 1996).

The biological activity of the isolated saponins (**1**), (**3**), (**4**), (**5**), and phenylpropanoid (**6**) from *B. fruticosum* and *B. falcatum* have been prescreened by using *in vitro* cytogenetic assays in human peripheral blood lymphocytes (evaluation of cell toxicity, inhibition of mitotic activity, and induction of micronuclei) (Scarpato et al., 1998a, 1998b). The micronucleus (MN) test relies on the observation of small chromatin bodies in the cytoplasm of interphasic cells passed through one round of cell division, and it is now considered a fast method to detect spontaneous and chemical-induced DNA or mitotic spindle damage (Fenech, 1993). The use of this experimental approach gave information on either general toxicity (cytotoxic assay) and cell cycle arrest ability (antimitotic assay) or mutagenic potential (genotoxic assay) of the plant extracts toward dividing lymphocytes.

Compounds (**1**) and (**6**) were cytotoxic only at elevated dosage causing complete killing of stimulated lymphocytes at 250 μM and 650 μM, respectively. Phenylpropanoid (**6**) showed a marginal sign of cell cycle delay at 260 μM, while no effect was seen for saponin (**1**) at 100 μM. Saponins (**5**) and (**1**) also exhibited a clear dose-related ability to lyse erythrocytes starting from 2.5 and 25 μM, respectively, whereas the other saponins tested showed lower hemolytic activity.

Results from the cytotoxicity as the expression of antimitotic activity, due to interference with the spindle apparatus, showed there was no statistically significant increase in MI (mitotic index) of plant constituents, with the exception of saponin (**4**), which showed a dose-related effect up to 100 µ*M*. However, this effect was present to a very small extent as compared to the potent antimitotic activity displayed by EM (estramustina) and COL (colcemid). Furthermore, the strong depression in MI observed for both compounds (**1**) and (**6**) at the highest concentration tested was the consequence of the severe cytotoxicity previously detected after the 48 h treatment, resulting in a reduction of the number of phytohemagglutinin (PHA)-stimulated lymphocytes.

Saponins (**1**) and (**3**) were also tested with the same methodology for inhibition of genotoxic effects induced by the two well-known DNA-damaging anticancer drugs mitomycin C (MMC) and bleomycin (BLM) (antimutagenesis assay). Differently from the reference compounds EM and MMC, all plant extracts did not significantly increase MN frequencies over the respective spontaneous level after 48 h treatment at all tested concentrations. The absence of genotoxic activity displayed by the triterpenoid saponins is in agreement with other reports showing that several saponins failed to cause point-mutation in the *Salmonella*/microsome assay and chromosome damage *in vitro* in human lymphocytes or *in vivo* in mice (Scarpato et al., 1998).

Saponin (**3**) was able to significantly, and also dose-dependently, either reduce or increase MN induction by MMC or BLM, without affecting cell cycle progression. On the other hand, saponin (**1**) was ineffective toward the genotoxicity of the two anticancer drugs. Interestingly, saponin (**1**) exhibited a significant effect on BLM cytotoxicity causing lymphocyte proliferation to be completely arrested or highly delayed. The 13 β, 28-oxide bridge characteristic of the oleanane-type saponins, the presence of two –OH groups at the C-16 and C-23 positions, or the number of sugar moieties seemed to increase or reduce hemolysis, respectively. Saponin (**1**) proved to be the most cytotoxic among the saponins isolated from *B. fruticosum* . Even though saponin (**5**) from *B. falcatum* presents two sugar molecules at the C-3 oxy residue, its chemical structure resembles that of saponin (**3**). This can explain a behavior against hemolysis and lymphocyte toxicity intermediate between that of saponin (**1**) and the other saponins. The different way the tested saponins modulate the mutagenicity of MMC and BLM may be due to both opening the 13β, 28-oxide bridge and the presence of an O-methyl at carbon atom 11 in saponin (**3**).

Data from this study indicated that the five compounds from *B. falcatum* and *B. fruticosum* were non-genotoxic compounds *in vitro* , as they did not induce MN in human peripheral blood lymphocytes. Only saponin (**1**) and phenylpropanoid (**6**) were shown to be toxic for PHA-stimulated lymphocytes, although at elevated concentrations. However, these compounds did not display antimitotic activity caused by interference with the mitotic apparatus. The protective effect of saponin (**3**) against MMC-induced DNA damage was also demonstrated together with potentiation of the mutagenicity of BLM. Conversely, the related plant extract saponin (**1**) did not affect MN induction of the two anticancers, whereas it enhanced BLM toxicity.

9.4.3 ANTIFEEDANT ACTIVITY

3-Methoxyeugenol, extracted from *B. fruticosum* , showed a strong antifeedant activity to *Mythimna unipunctata* (Muckensturm et al., 1982). Recently, Dodds et al. (1999) reported the antifeedant activity against *Deroceras reticulatum* of 33 species of the plant family Apiaceae by using an electrophysiological recording assay, in which the olfactory sensory epithelium of the posterior tentacle of the slug was exposed to volatile components of the plant extract and the olfactory nerve was recorded. This neurophysiological screening assay combined with the complementary feeding bioassay is an efficient method for the rapid and extensive screening of plant extracts for potentially antifeedant activity. For *B. fruticosum* extract the correlation between electrophysiological and antifeedant activity was not noticeable.

9.5 MICROPROPAGATION OF *BUPLEURUM FRUTICOSUM*

A micropropagation protocol of *B. fruticosum* L. was developed in order to obtain a great number of plants for the production of secondary metabolites. *Bupleurum fruticosum* propagation from seeds has been found to be particularly difficult because seeds germinate with difficulty and lose their viability in a short period of time. Furthermore, propagation from seeds often results in a high variability in the progeny. Micropropagation can give rise to a large number of homogeneous plants, which have the same content of secondary metabolites. No studies on *in vitro* cultures or vegetative propagation via cuttings of this species have been reported until now. Few shoots were obtained in hormone-free MS medium. The best multiplication was obtained with 1.5 mg/l BA and 1.0 mg/l IAA. The *B. fruticosum* shoots produced roots in hormone-free medium. Moreover, triacontanol (a long-chain primary alcohol, which is a component of the epicuticlar waxes of *Medicago sativa*) can be used successfully in *B. fruticosum* micropropagation, either in the multiplication or rooting phases (Fraternale et al., 2002).

REFERENCES

Abe, H., Sakaguchi, M., Yamada, M., Ariki, S., and Odoshima, S. (1980) Pharmacological actions of saiko-saponins isolated from *Bupleurum falcatum*. 1. Effects of saikosaponins on liver function, *Planta Med.*, 40, 366–372.

Ballero, M. and Fresu, I. (1991) Piante officinali impiegate in fitoterapia nel territorio del Marganai (Sardegna Sud Occidentale), *Fitoterapia*, 52(6), 525–531.

Debenedetti, S.L., Nadinic, J.K., Palacios, P.S., Coussio, J.D., Boeykens, M., and De Kimpe, N. (1994) 5-(3-Methyl-2-butenyloxy)-6,7-methylenedioxycoumarin, a 5,6,7-trioxygenated coumarin from *Pterocaulon virgatum*, *J. Nat. Prod.*, 57(11), 1539–1542.

Dodds, C.J., Henderson, I.F., Watson, P., and Leake, L.D. (1999) Action of extracts of Apiaceae on feeding behavior and neurophysiology of the field slug *Deroceras reticulatum*, *J. Chem. Ecol.*, 25(9), 2127–2145.

Dugo, G., Trozzi, A., Verzera, A., and Rapisarda, A. (2000) Essential oils from leaves of typical Mediterranean plants. Note I. *Bupleurum fruticosum*, *Essenze, Derivati Agrumari*, 70(4), 201–204.

Estévez-Braun, A., Estévez-Reyes, R., Moujir, L.M., Ravelo, A.G., and Gonzalez, A.G. (1994a) Antibiotic activity and absolute configuration of *S*-heptadeca-2(Z),9(Z)-diyne-1,8-diol from *Bupleurum salicifolium*, *J. Nat. Prod.*, 57, 1178–1182.

Estévez-Braun, A., Estévez-Reyes, R., and Gonzalez, A.G. (1994b) Structural elucidation and conformational analysis of new lignan butenolides from the leaves of *Bupleurum salicifolium*, *Tetrahedron*, 50, 5203–5210.

Estévez-Braun, R., Gonzalez-Perez, J.A., and Gonzalez, A.G. (1995) Busaliol and busalicifol, two new tetrahydrofuran lignans from *Bupleurum salicifolium*, *J. Nat. Prod.*, 58, 887– 892.

Feigl, (1960) In *Spot Tests in Organic Analysis*. Elsevier, New York, 250.

Fenech, M. (1993) The cytokinesis-block micronucleus technique; a detailed description of the method and its application to genotoxicity studies in human population, *Mutat. Res.*, 285, 35–44.

Francesconi, L. and Sernagiotto, E. (1913) Bupleurol, the alcohol of the essence of *Bupleurum fruticosum*, *Gazz. Chim. Ital.*, 43(1), 153–161.

Fraternale, D., Giamperi, L., Ricci, D., and Rocchi, M.B. (2002) Micropropagation of *Bupleurum fruticosum*: the effect of triacontanol, *Plant Cell Tissue Organ Cult.*, 69, 135–140.

Gevrenova, R., Dimitrova, B., and Asenov, Iv. (1997) Flavonols from *Bupleurum flavum* Forsk.; family Apiaceae, *Farmatsija*, 44(3–4), 9–14.

Giamperi, L., Ricci, D., Fraternale, D., and Manunta, A. (1998) The essential oil from *Bupleurum fruticosum* L. of the Cyrenaica region of eastern Libya and the problem of Bupleurol, *J. Essent. Oil Res.*, 10, 369–374.

Gonzalez, A.G., Trujillo, J.M., Estévez, R., and Péres, J.P. (1975) Componentes de umbeliferas. IV. Lignanos del *Bupleurum fruticescens*), *An. Quim.*, 71,109–110.

Guinea, M.C., Parellada, J., Lacaille-Dubois, M.A., and Wagner, H. (1994) Biologically active triterpene saponins from *Bupleurum fruticosum, Planta Med.*, 60, 163–167.

Hegnauer R. (1973) *Chemotaxonomie der Pflanzen,* Vol. 6. Birkhauser Verlag, Basel, 554.

Hegnauer R. (1990) *Chemotaxonomie der Pflanzen,* Vol. 9. Birkhauser Verlag, Basel, 663.

Just, J., Recio, C., Giner, R., Cuellar, M.J., Manez, S., Rios, J.L., Bilia, A.R., and Morelli, I. (1996) Preliminary study of the pharmacology and phytochemistry of *Bupleurum rotundifolium, Phytother. Res.*, 10, S69–S70.

Kamil, W.M. and Dewick, P.M. (1986) Biosynthetic relationship of aryltetralin lactone lignans to benzylbutyrolactone lignans, *Phytochemistry,* 25(9), 2093–2102.

Kubota, T. and Hinoh, H. (1968) Triterpenoids from *Bupleurum falcatum* L. III. Isolation of genuine sapogenins, saikogenins E, F and G, *Tetrahedron,* 24, 675–686.

Lorente, I., Ocete, M. A., Zarzuelo, A., Cabo, M.M., and Jimenez, J. (1989) Bioactivity of the essential oil of *Bupleurum fruticosum, J. Nat. Prod.*, 52, 267–272.

Luo, S.Q., Lin, L.Z., and Cordell, G.A. (1993) Lignan glycosides from *Bupleurum wenchuanense, Phytochemistry,* 33, 193–196.

Manunta, A. (1979) Note farmaco-botaniche su alcune specie del genere "*Bupleurum* L." Atti delle giornate Herbora, Verona, Italy.

Manunta, A., Morelli, I., and Picci, V. (1987) L'huile essentielle du *Bupleurum fruticosum* L., *Plant. Med. Phytother.*, 21(1), 20–25.

Manunta, A., Tirillini, B., and Fraternale, D. (1992) Secretory tissue and essential oil composition of *Bupleurum fruticosum* L., *J. Essent. Oil Res.*, 4(5), 461–466.

Massanet, G.M., Guerra, F.M., Jorge, Z.D., and Casalvazquez, L.G. (1997) Phenylpropanoids from *Bupleurum fruticosum, Phytochemistry,* 44, 173–177.

Mills, S. and Bone, K. (2000*) Principles and Practice of Phytotherapy — Modernal Herbal Medicine.* Churchill Livingstone, London, 313–318.

Moris, J.H. (1840–1843) *Flora Sardoa, 2.* Taurini, Cagliari.

Motta, F. (1987) *Nel mondo della natura. Enciclopedia Motta di Scienze Naturali.* Motta, Milan, 366–367.

Muckensturm, B., Duplay, D., Mohammadi, F., Moradi, A., Robert, P.C., Simonis, M.T., and Kienlen, J.C. (1982) Role of natural phenylpropanoids as antifeedant agents for insects. *Colloq. INRA 7 (Mediateurs Chim. Agissant Comportement Insectes),* 131–135.

Noccioli, C. (1999) Indagine fitochimica su *Bupleurum flavum* Forskål. Sc.D. thesis, Facoltà di Farmacia, Università degli Studi di Pisa, Pisa, Italy.

Nose, M., Amagaya, S., and Ogihara, Y. (1989) Corticosterone secretion-inducing activity of saikosaponin metabolites formed in the alimentary tract, *Chem. Pharm. Bull.*, 37, 2736–2740.

Pachaly, P. and Klein, M. (1987) Inhaltstoffe von *Andromeda polifolia, Planta Med.,* 442–444.

Peyron, L. and Roubaud, M. (1970) *Bupleurum fruticosum* essential oil, *Plant. Med. Phytother.,* 4(3), 172–175.

Picci, V., Atzei, A., and Manunta, A. (1974a) Content in essential oils in the officinal species of Sardinia. Essential oils in the Umbelliferae of Sardinia. 1. Morphosystematic and chemical notes on *Bupleurum fruticosum, Riv. Ital. EPPOS,* 5, 1–6.

Picci, V., Atzei, A., and Manunta, A. (1974b) Content in essential oil in the officinal species of Sardinia. Essential oils in the Umbelliferae of Sardiniae. 1. Morphosystematic and chemical notes from *Bupleurum fruticosum* Linnaeus, *Riv. Ital. EPPOS,* 56(5), 239–244.

Pignatti, S. (1982) *Flora d'Italia,* Vol. 2. Edagricole, Bologna, 212–217.

Pistelli, L., Bilia, A.R., Marsili, A., De Tommasi, N., and Manunta, A. (1993a). Triterpenoid saponins from *Bupleurum fruticosum, J. Nat. Prod.*, 56, 240–244.

Pistelli, L., Cammilli, A., Manunta, A., Marsili, A., and Morelli, I. (1993b) Triterpenoid saponins and flavonoid glycosides from *Bupleurum falcatum* subsp. *cernuum, Phytochemistry,* 33, 1537–1539.

Pistelli, L., Bilia, A.R., Bertoli, A., Morelli, I., and Marsili, A. (1995) Phenylpropanoids from *Bupleurum fruticosum, J. Nat. Prod.*, 58 (1), 112–116.

Pistelli, L., Bertoli, A., Bilia, A.R., and Morelli, I. (1996). Minor constituents from *Bupleurum fruticosum* roots, *Phytochemistry,* 41, 157–1582.

Pistelli, L., Bertoli, A., Morelli, I., and Scarpato, R. (1998) Consistents of *Bupleurum* spp. from Italian flora: isolation, structure elucidation and their biological activity, *Recent Res. Dev. Phytochem.*, 2, 463–483.

Popov, A.I. and Gromov, K.G. (1992) Analysis of elements in the above-ground part of *Bupleurum longifolium* L., *Rastit. Resur.,* 28(4), 63–66.

Scarpato, R., Bertoli, A., Naccarati, A., Migliore, L., Cocchi, L., Barale, R., and Pistelli, L. (1998a) Different effects of newly isolated saponins on the mutagenicity and cytotoxicity on the anticancer drugs mytomicin C and bleomycin in human lymphocytes, *Mutat. Res.,* 420 (1–3), 49–59.

Scarpato, R., Pistelli, L., Bertoli, A., Nieri, E., and Migliore, L. (1998b) *In vitro* genotoxicity and cytotoxicity of five new chemical compounds of plant origin by means of the human lymphocyte micronucleus assay, *Toxicol. in Vitro,* 12(2), 153–161.

Tutin, G.T., Heywood, V., Burges, N.A., Moore, D.M., Valentine, D.H., Walters, S.M., and Webb, D.A., (1972) *Flora Europaea,* 2. Cambridge University Press, Cambridge, 345–350.

Watanable, K., Fujino, H., Morita, T., Kasai, R., and Tanaka, O. (1988) Solubilization of saponins of Bupleuri radix with ginseng saponins: cooperative effect of dammarane saponins, *Planta Med.,* 405–409.

Yamamoto, A., Miyase, T., Ueno, A., and Maeda, T. (1991) Buddlejasaponins I–IV, four new oleanane triterpene saponins from the aerial parts of *Buddleja japonica* Hemsl., *Chem. Pharm. Bull.,* 39, 2764–2766.

Yamamoto, M., Kumagai, A., and Yamamura, Y. (1975) Structure and action of saikosaponins isolated from *Bupleurum falcatum.* II. Metabolic actions of saikosaponins, specially plasma cholesterol-lowering action, *Arzneim. Forsch. (Drug Res.),* 25(8), 1021–1023.

Zhanayeva, T.A. and Lovanova, I.E. (1992) Extraction of flavonoids from fresh and dried leaves of *Bupleurum multinerve, Rastit. Resur.,* 28, 60–62.

Section IV

Pharmacology

10 The Pharmacological Activity of Chinese "Chaihu" — The Root of *Bupleurum* Species

Xiao-Min Du, Hui Xie, and Yun Kang

CONTENTS

10.1 INTRODUCTION

In Chapter 2 the Chinese medicinal species of *Bupleurum* have been recorded. Under the name of "Chaihu," the root of *Bupleurum* has been used as medicine in China for over 2000 years. The pharmacological activities are described in this chapter, including those of Chinese Chaihu Injection, Chaihu Oral Liquid (see Appendix of Chapter 13 for official definitions etc.), other extracts with water, alcohol, methanol, butanol, petroleum-ether, ether, ethyl acetate, as well as the activities of the essential oil, flavonoids, etc. The toxicity of *B. longiradiatum* is also described.

10.2 PHARMACOLOGICAL ACTIVITY OF *BUPLEURUM*

10.2.1 ANTI-INFLAMMATORY ACTIVITY

Many experiments show that Chaihu has remarkable anti-inflammation activity. Wu et al. (1983) reported that Chaihu injection i.p. with the dose of 5 ml/kg could reduce the increasing of capillary permeability induced by xylene, reduce the high-temperature-induced tumefaction of the hind paw and the growth of granuloma caused by cotton pellets in rabbits. However, the anti-inflammatory activity of aquatic decoction from Chaihu is slight (Ye, 1996).

The essential oil of Chaihu administered i.p. at the dose of 400 mg/kg to rat results in a remarkable reduction in inflammation caused by glair and edema formed with carrageenan in the hind paw (Zhu et al., 1985). The studies showed that the anti-inflammatory activity of the essential oil still existed even if the two adrenal glands were cut. It is suggested that the antiphlogistic effect of essential oil from *Bupleurum* was not altered by the pituitary-adrenal system.

The crude flavone of Chaihu has an anti-inflammatory effect as well, when it is administrated orally (Zheng et al., 1998).

Zhao et al. (1995) reported that when the ether extract from Chaihu was fed to mice i.p. 500 mg/kg/day for 2 days and i.p. 120 mg/kg/day for 4 days it reduced xylene-induced edema of earlaps (Table 10.1) and carrageenan-induced paw edema (Table 10.2). There is a remarkable difference compared with the control group ($p < 0.01$).

The assay data showed Chaihu inhibited the edema caused by carrageenan in the hind paw.

Regarding anti-inflammatory activity, some different results have been reported as well. Studies of Zhou et al. (1979) showed that the essential oil from Chaihu administered to rat with i.p. 240 mg/kg did not reduce inflammation caused by glair and carrageenan-induced edema. Li et al. (1985) studies also showed that the Aqueous Decoction of Chaihu administrated to mice with 4 g/kg did not reduce peritonitis inflammation caused by acetic acid.

TABLE 10.1
Inhibitory Effect of Ether Extract of Chaihu on Xylene-Induced Edema of Earlap in Mice ($X \pm S$) ($n = 10$)

Group	Dose (mg/kg)	Degree of Edema (mg)	*t*-test	Rate of Inhibition (%)
Control	—	13.40 ± 2.88	—	—
Ether extract	500	8.40 ± 2.76	$P < 0.01$	37.31

Note: Control group was administrated an equivalent amount of distilled water.

TABLE 10.2
Effect of Ether Extract of Chaihu on Carrageenan-Induced Edema of the Hind Paw in Mice ($X \pm S$) ($n = 10$)

Group	Dose (mg/kg)	Degree of Edema (mg)	*t*-test	Rate of Inhibition (%)
Control	—	64.90 ± 22.69	—	—
Chaihu	120	35.80 ± 15.29	$P < 0.01$	44.84

Note: Control group was administrated an equivalent amount of distilled water.

TABLE 10.3
Antipyretic Effect of Aqueous Decoction from Chaihu on Typhoid Paratyphoid A and B Triple Vaccine ($X \pm S$) ($n = 10$)

Group	Dose (g/kg)	Normal	1 h	2 h	3 h	4 h	5 h	6 h
					Temperature			
Control	—	39.26 ± 0.18	40.54 ± 0.41	40.68 ± 0.54	40.76 ± 0.39	40.68 ± 0.32	40.47 ± 0.62	39.92 ± 0.45
Aspirin	0.1	39.14 ± 0.26	$39.78 \pm 0.31^{**}$	39.51 ± 0.38	$39.53 \pm 0.29^{**}$	$39.60 \pm 0.41^{**}$	$39.38 \pm 0.33^{**}$	39.31 ± 0.39
Chaihu	10	39.15 ± 0.23	40.30 ± 0.39	$40.18 \pm 0.30^{*}$	$40.04 \pm 0.36^{**}$	$39.81 \pm 0.41^{**}$	$39.63 \pm 0.33^{**}$	39.42 ± 0.22

Note: Compared with control group: $^{*}p < 0.05$; $^{**}p < 0.01$. Control group rabbits were administrated an equivalent amount of distilled water.

10.2.2 ANTIPYRETIC EFFECT

The antipyretic effects of Aqueous Decoction from Chaihu were tested by Gan (1982), Sun (1956), and Li et al. (1992). The results showed that the Aqueous Decoction of Chaihu significantly reduced the rabbit body temperature caused by zymolytic milk, typhoid paratyphoid A, and B triple vaccine. This behavior varied depending on the dose. The antipyretic activity of *B. chinense* DC. was better than that of *B. scorzonerifolium* Willd. (*B. falcatum* L. var. *scorzonerifolium* Ledeb.). And Zhao et al. (1995) also reported that the Aqueous Decoction of Chaihu when administrated to rabbit at a dose of 100 mg/kg significantly reduced rabbit temperature caused by typhoid paratyphoid A and B triple vaccine in 6 hours (Table 10.3).

The antipyretic effects of essential oil from *Bupleurum* have been investigated. Results proved that it significantly reduced rat high temperature in 5 to 8 hours after cerevisiae fermentum and *Bacillus coli* were injected under skin (Zhou et al., 1979, Wang, 1983, Zhu et al., 1985). Zhu et al. (1985) also reported the antipyretic effect can be attributed to r-11-acidylactone, *p*-methoxy acetophenone, engenol, and hexacid.

Wu et al. (1983) reported that Chaihu injection had weaker antipyretic activity. It failed to reduce the rabbit body high temperature induced by injecting typhoid paratyphoid A and B triple vaccine, and only slightly reduced the high temperature induced by injecting cerevisiae fermentum. But it has significant antipyretic effect on the high temperature of rabbit body caused by 20% NaCl solution (Zhang et al., 1989).

10.2.3 EFFECT ON THE CENTRAL NERVOUS SYSTEM

The receptor binding assays indicated that the Chaihu Aqueous Decoction contained the principles acting on the dopamine 2,5-HT1A and γ-amino-*n*-butyric acid (GABA) receptors (Liao et al., 1995).

Gong et al. (1997) studied the anticonvulsant effect of Chaihu injection in rats using the frontal cortical test by direct cortical stimulation. The experiment showed that the anticonvulsant effect of Chaihu is dose-related. Compared to the antiepileptic drug valium, its dose is ten times larger than that of valium. Its change of threshold attains the maximal amount (231 ± 112.53 μA, mean $\pm$ SD) after 3 hours of injection. This increase is significant ($p < 0.05$), and the effect still remains after 6 hours. The experiment also shows that Chaihu injection has no poisonous side effect.

10.2.4 ANODYNIC EFFECT

The anodynic effect of Chaihu Aqueous Decoction was investigated by Wang et al. (1996a). The studies showed that it markedly increased the threshold of pain sensitivity (29.70 to 49.75%) in 3 hours, and the activity could be increased by menthol (Table 10.4).

TABLE 10.4
Anodynic Effect of the Aqueous Decoction from Chaihu in Mice ($X \pm S$) ($n = 10$)

Group	Dose (g/kg)	Normal	Threshold of Pain Sensitivity			
			30 min	60 min	90 min	120 min
Control	—	8.93 ± 3.77	9.35 ± 3.74	9.35 ± 3.71	9.24 ± 3.30	8.71 ± 4.51
			(−0.88 ± 2.34)	(0.42 ± 3.55)	(0.33 ± 3.00)	(−0.22 ± 6.01)
Decoc. Chaihu	10	9.83 ± 1.81	11.95 ± 1.96	12.71 ± 2.50*	13.59 ± 4.61*	14.72 ± 5.31*
			(2.12 ± 1.78**)	(2.93 ± 2.38*)	(3.76 ± 3.63*)	(4.89 ± 4.44*)
Decoc. Chaihu +	10	9.30 ± 3.03	11.16 ± 5.34	14.25 ± 6.13	15.74 ± 3.95***	16.72 ± 7.54*
Menthol	0.5%		(1.86 ± 3.94)	(4.95 ± 5.19)	(6.44 ± 3.46**)	(7.42 ± 7.28*)
Decoc. Chaihu +	10	10.22 ± 2.67	12.10 ± 5.84	11.20 ± 3.88	16.63 ± 8.94	15.18 ± 9.84
Menthol	1.5%		(1.88 ± 3.93)	(0.98 ± 2.25)	(6.41 ± 6.94*)	(4.96 ± 8.25)
Decoc. Chaihu +	10	9.26 ± 2.98	12.14 ± 6.40	16.47 ± 3.60***	18.69 ± 3.28***	18.44 ± 6.89**
Menthol	4.5%		(2.88 ± 5.50)	(7.21 ± 4.76**)[a]	(943 ± 4.00**)[b]	(9.18 ± 4.78**)[a]

Note: Compared with control group: *$p < 0.05$, **$p < 0.01$, ***$p < 0.001$. Compared with Decoc. Chaihu group:
[a] $p < 0.05$, [b] $p < 0.01$. Control group mice were administrated an equivalent amount of distilled water.

The pharmacokinetics studies showed that the lowest dose of anodynic activity of Chaihu was 0.11 g/kg. (Wang et al., 1996b).

10.2.5 HEPATOPROTECTIVE EFFECT

The hepatoprotective effects of Chaihu Aqueous Decoction were tested by Ye (1957), Chen et al. (1994), and Zheng et al. (1998). The results showed that the Aqueous Decoction protected the rabbit liver injury induced by typhoid vaccine, alcohol, and inorganic phosphorus. It significantly reduced serum glutamic-pyruvic transaminase (sGPT) of mice raised by CCl_4 and the liver damage caused by CCl_4 and *Penicillium notatum*.

The Aqueous Decoction protected mouse liver from injury induced by rimifon, but it had no protective effect on rat hepatic fibrosis induced by fresh egg albumen (Jiangsu New Physic College, 1977).

Chen et al. (1998) investigated the effect of Chaihu injection on the hepatocyte apoptosis. The ratio of liver/body weight, hepatic DNA content, morphological changes, and TUNEL reaction (TdT-mediated X-dUTP nick labeling) on the hepatocyte apoptosis caused by Phenobarbital (PB) were observed. The regression of hepatic DNA content and ratio of liver/body weight and typical hepatocyte apoptosis, which occurred in the mice as control after stopping PB, was not found in the mice treated with Chaihu injection, and a negative result of TUNEL assay was presented (Table 10.5). The result showed that Chaihu prevented hepatocyte apoptosis caused by PB in mice.

Wang et al. (2000) established an animal model with the hepatic injury of scarcity of blood by totally interdicting the portal veins of the liver. With the method, Gao et al. (2000) investigated the pathological changes of liver tissue by detecting the zymogram and biochemical parameters at different time courses. The results showed that the Chaihu Aqueous Decoction significantly depressed the activities of ALT, AST, and 5-NT in serum. The morphological changes were also observed with optical and electronic microscopy. The histopathological examination showed that Chaihu could diminish liver degeneration and necrosis, and promote the regenesis ability of hepatocytes after the operation. The degree of liver degeneration and necrosis was significantly lower than that of the control group. The variation in ALT, AST, 5-NT in rat serum is shown in Table 10.6.

Tang et al. (1998) reported the protective effect of Chaihu injection on liver hypoxia-reoxygenation injury. The activity of lactic dehydrogenase (LDH) in liquid, the activity of xanthine

TABLE 10.5
Effect of Chaihu Injection on Hepatocyte Apoptosis in Mice $(X \pm S)$ $(n = 10)$

Group	Dose (g/kg)	DNA (mg/g/BW)	Liver Weight (LW)/ Body Weight (BW)
Normal	—	0.4232 ± 0.0694**	0.0454 ± 0.0036**
TUNEL	—	0.5632 ± 0.0876*	0.0503 ± 0.0024*
Non-TUNEL	—	0.6540 ± 0.0828	0.0569 ± 0.0031
Chaihu injection	12	0.6217 ± 0.0833	0.0644 ± 0.0029*

Note: Compared with non-TUNEL group: *$p < 0.05$; **$p < 0.01$. Chaihu group mice were administrated with Chaihu injection. Normal group mice were administrated an equivalent amount of distilled water. TUNEL and non-TUNEL group mice were administrated an equivalent amount of distilled water (Chen et al., 1998).

TABLE 10.6
Effect of Chaihu Aqueous Decoction on Liver Injury by Scarcity of Blood for the Hepatocyte Enzyme in Rat $(X \pm S)$

After Operation	Group	Animal (n)	ALT (kU/l)	AST (kU/l)	5-Nucleotidase (U/g)
	Normal	8	22 ± 8	26 ± 8	1.65 ± 0.09
Day 1	Control	24	116 ± 18*	192 ± 25*	0.65 ± 0.03*
	Chaihu	24	105 ± 18*	175 ± 23*	0.68 ± 0.04*
Day 4	Control	24	107 ± 15	167 ± 20	0.82 ± 0.04
	Chaihu	24	62 ± 12**	71 ± 14**	1.12 ± 0.07**

Note: Compared with normal group:*$p < 0.05$. Compared with control group: **$p < 0.05$. Chaihu group rats were administrated Chaihu Aqueous Decoction. Normal and control group rats were not administrated Chaihu Aqueous Decoction.

oxidase (XOD), the content of glutathione (GSH) and malondialdehyde (MDA) in liver were investigated at different times (Table 10.7).

The liver pathological changes were observed under optical and electronic microscopy after perfusion. The results implied that Chaihu injection had a significant protective effect on mouse liver injury induced by hypoxia-reoxygenation perfusion. The mechanism of action may be related to the inhibitory formation of free radicals.

The hepatoprotective effect of Chaihu has also been studied in other experiments. The results showed that the mechanism of this kind of effect maybe related to its anti-inflammatory effects, promoting protein assimilation, increasing hepatic glycogen in liver, preventing hyperlipodemia and fatty-liver (Weiguan, 1984).

10.2.6 ANTIBACTERIA AND ANTIVIRUS PROPERTIES

The Aqueous Decoction of Chaihu inhibited the growth of *Mycobacterium tuberculosis in vitro*, it inhibited the falcate leptospira, cowpox virus (Wang, 1983), *Trichophyton rubra, Trichophyton ferrugineum, Microsporum canis*, and pylori spirobacteria (Sun, 1958).

TABLE 10.7
Protective Effect of Chaihu Injection on Hypoxia-Reoxygenation Liver Injury in Mice
(n = 10/liver weight, $X \pm S$)

Perfusion Time	Group	LDH (U/h*g)	GSH (nmol/mg)	XOD (U/g)	MDA (nmol/g)	LW/BW (g/100 g)
60 min	Hypoxia	2564 ± 1294	8.12 ± 1.04	8.75 ± 0.91	20.30 ± 3.98	—
	Chaihu	1113 ± 145**	11.58 ± 0.70**	15.51 ± 0.74**	7.69 ± 1.95**	—
	Reoxygenation	1075 ± 186**	12.38 ± 0.35**	5.33 ± 1.21**	7.27 ± 2.13**	—
120 min	Hypoxia	1507 ± 629	3.64 ± 0.64	6.11 ± 0.64	10.54 ± 1.54	6.52 ± 0.66
	Chaihu	1099 ± 191	10.51 ± 1.02**	12.50 ± 1.20**	11.35 ± 2.51**	4.76 ± 0.45**
	Reoxygenation	941 ± 76	10.91 ± 1.01*	11.75 ± 1.30**	9.17 ± 1.77	4.40 ± 0.30**

Note: Compared with hypoxia group: $*p < 0.05$; $**p < 0.01$. Hypoxia group mouse livers were administrated Krebs-Henseleit perfusion solution with added 95% N_2 and 5%CO_2. Reoxygenation group mouse livers were administrated Krebs-Henseleit perfusion solution with added 95%O_2 and 5% CO_2. Chaihu group mouse livers were administrated Krebs-Henseleit perfusion solution with added Chaihu injection (4 ml/l).

TABLE 10.8
Effect of Chaihu Checked the Pathological
Exudate in Lung Tissue of Mice (n = 20, $X \pm S$)

Group	Lung Index	t-test	Inhibited Rate (%)
Normal	1.68 ± 0.28	—	—
Chaihu	1.18 ± 0.27	$P < 0.05$	29.70
Virazole	1.07 ± 0.17	$P < 0.05$	36.30

Note: Compared with normal group. Normal group mice were administrated an equivalent amount of distilled water. Chaihu group mice were administrated Chaihu. Virazole group mice were administrated virazole.

Wang and Zhao (1998) studied the effect of Chaihu on antivirus. The Aqueous Decoction of Chaihu was fed to mice p.o. 28 g/kg/day for 4 days. Results proved that it checked the pathological exudate in lung tissue (shown in Table 10.8), and decreased the mortality of mice caused by pneumonia virus of murine (shown in Table 10.9), and also significantly inhibited influenza virus A in chicken embryo.

Also it has been reported that the Chaihu injection and essential oils markedly inhibited the grippe virus, cowpox virus, and human skin verruca caused by virus. It slightly inhibited *Staphylococcus aureus* by paper test, but failed to inhibit bacteria such as *Staphylococcus albus, Neisseria, Diplococcus pneumonia*, hemolytic *Streptococcus, Pseudomonas areuginosa in vitro*. Other preparations of Chaihu showed various degrees of inhibition of the organisms (Wu et al., 1983).

10.2.7 EFFECT ON HEART BLOOD VESSEL AND KIDNEY

Wang (1983) reported that the crude flavones of Chaihu significantly reduced blood pressure and slowed heart rate in rabbits. The reduced rate was 48.6% lower than the control group after 5 min of administration, and this effect was maintained for about 20 min.

TABLE 10.9
Effect of Chaihu Decreasing the Mortality of Mice Caused by Pneumonia Virus of Murine ($n = 30$, $X \pm S$)

Group	Died	Exist	Death Rate (%)	X^2-test
Normal	0	30	0	$P < 0.001$
Control	29	1	93.39	—
Chaihu	18	12	60.00	$P < 0.01$

Note: Compared with control group. Normal group mice were administrated an equivalent amount of distilled water. Control group mice were administrated an equivalent amount of distilled water, and injected with the pneumonia virus of murine. Chaihu group mice were administrated Chaihu and injected with the pneumonia virus of murine.

It was also reported that the alcohol extract from Chaihu slightly decreased the blood pressure in anesthetized rabbit, and suppressed heart rate in frog, which could not be reversed by Atropin (Zhang, 1982). But the Chaihu injection had no effect on the blood pressure, breathing, and heart rate in cat.

The protective effect of Chaihu injection on ischemic-reperfusion kidney injury was studied by Dai et al. (1998). The Chaihu injection was injected into Wistar male rat i.p. 2 ml/kg/day, twice a day for 7 days. The modulus of left kidney (left kidney weight/body weight) in rat and the activity of MDA and SOD in kidney were investigated after the operation. The results are shown in Table 10.10 and Table 10.11.

The results proved that Chaihu injection markedly reduced the kidney injury caused by ischemic-reperfusion in rat, increased the activity of SOD, and inhibited the formation of MDA in kidney. And it had a significant protective effect on rat kidney injury induced by ischemic-perfusion. The mechanism of action may be related to its inhibitory effect on the reaction of lipid hyperoxydation (Dai et al., 1998).

TABLE 10.10
Modulus of Left Kidney on Ischemic-Reperfusion Kidney Injury in Rat (left kidney weight/body weight, $X \pm S$)

Group	Animal	Modulus of Left Kidney (g/kg)	t-test
Normal	6	4.07 ± 0.64	$P < 0.01$
Control	8	5.48 ± 0.87	—
Ischemic-reperfusion	9	5.34 ± 0.36	$P < 0.05$
Chaihu	8	4.63 ± 0.68	$P < 0.05$

Note: Compared with control group. Normal group: rat's right kidney was cut and left kidney was undressed in air. Control group: rat's right kidney was cut and left kidney pedicel was clamped for 60 min. Ischemic-reperfusion group: rat's right kidney was cut and left kidney pedicel was clamped for 60 min, and then reperfused for 15 min. Chaihu group: rat's right kidney was cut and left kidney pedicel was clamped for 60 min, and then reperfused for 15 min and injected with Chaihu injection.

TABLE 10.11
Activity of MDA and SOD in Ischemic-Reperfusion Kidney Injury in Rat ($X \pm S$)

Group	Animal	SPD (nu/ml)	MDA (nmpl/g)
Normal	6	453.48 ± 44.48**[a]	94.35 ± 8.05***[a]
Control	8	346.89 ± 33.59[a]	109.56 ± 5.35[a]
Ischemic-reperfusion	9	213.77 ± 55.22	140.12 ± 17.28
Chaihu	8	414.31 ± 38.60**[a]	113.24 ± 8.02[a]

Note: Compared with ischemic group: $**p < 0.01$; $***p < 0.001$. Compared with ischemic-reperfusion group: $^{a}p < 0.01$. Normal group: rat's right kidney was cut and left kidney was undressed in air. Control group: rat's right kidney was cut and left kidney pedicel was clamped for 60 min. Ischemic-reperfusion group: rat's right kidney was cut and left kidney pedicel was clamped for 60 min, and then reperfused for 15 min. Chaihu group: rat's right kidney was cut and left kidney pedicel was clamped for 60 min, and then reperfused for 15 min and injected with Chaihu injection.

Platelet-activating factor (PAF) has been recognized as an important chemical mediator in allergic and inflammatory reactions. Evidence suggests that PAF is deeply involved in the pathogenesis of bronchial asthma, in which PAF induces profound bronchospasms, increased vascular permeability, and eosinophil/neutrophil accumulation in the respiratory tract. It has been shown that the crude extract from Chaihu inhibited production of PAF (Nakamura et al., 1993).

10.2.8 EFFECT ON ACTIVITY OF ENZYMES

The hot water extract from Chaihu reduced the activity of cyclic AMP phosphodiesterase in bull heart; the rate of suppression was 38.1 to 43.1%, and the suppression rate of chloroform extract was 74.1%, but the part of infusibility in chloroform did not reduce the activity of phosphodiesterase in bull (Nikaido, 1981).

The Aqueous Decoction of Chaihu slightly reduced the content of cAMP and increased the content cGMP in mouse liver, but reduced the ratio of cAMP/cGMP significantly (Chen, 1984).

Kanatani (1985) reported the methanol extract from Chaihu significantly increased (170%) the activity of cAMP in the brain of rat. Zhe (1987) reported the butanol extract from Chaihu reduced the activity of sialidase by 94.9%.

The saikosaponins and flavonoids from Chaihu reduced the activities of blood cholinesterase (Zhang et al., 1989). Their ID_{50} concentrations of validity were 44.2 and 30.3 µg/ml. Its ID_{50} concentration of validity was 26.0 µg/ml when the saikosaponins and flavonoids were used together. Both of them exhibited the mixed effect with competed inhibition-noncompeted inhibition. It was also reported by Wang et al. (2000) that the Aqueous Decoction of vinegar roasted Chaihu, vinegar mixed Chaihu, and crude Chaihu significantly reduced the activity of mouse blood cholinesterase.

Polyacetylenes extracted from *B. falcatum* L. are 5-lipoxygenase inhibitor and aldose reductase inhibitors. They could be used for the treatment of inflammation, thrombosis, allergy, asthma, complications of diabetes mellitus, etc. (Kobayashi et al., 1990). Nakajima et al. (1990) reported that saikochromones are 5-lipoxygenase inhibitors and cyclooxygenase inhibitors and are useful for the treatment of diseases and disorders (e.g., allergy, thrombosis, and asthma) caused by abnormal metabolism or arachidonic acids.

The effects of methanol and alcohol extracts from Chaihu on adenylate cyclase in mouse hepatocyte preparation (ACHP) have been studied using five isolated fractions, named CH-1, CH-3,

TABLE 10.12
Reduction in Activity of ACHP in Mice by
CH-7 ($n = 4$; $X \pm S$)

Concentration (µg/ml)	ACHP	Activation of ACHP (%)
1.4	2.5911 ± 0.5853	92.74 ± 8.85
3.5	2.4781 ± 0.7949	83.17 ± 4.22
8.8	2.2113 ± 0.5784	78.16 ± 8.99
21.9	1.8379 ± 0.4009	65.81 ± 7.08
54.9	1.2426 ± 0.2504	44.88 ± 6.09
137.1	0.6389 ± 0.1169	24.38 ± 8.60
342.8	0.2271 ± 0.0617	8.94 ± 3.96
857.1	0.0445 ± 0.0678	1.16 ± 3.50

Note: Activation % = (test value/basic value) × 100%
(Ling et al., 1991).

CH-4, CH-5, and CH-7. These had different effects on the ACHP. The CH-1 caused a reduction at high concentration and an increase at lower concentration. The CH-3 and CH-4 had the same effect on ACHP. There comparative activity changed in 21 to 113% and 56 to 193% according to the concentration. The CH-5 and CH-7 exhibited a clear dose-related ability to inhibit the ACHP. The results for CH-7 are shown in Table 10.12.

10.2.9 EFFECT ON METABOLISM OF GLUCOSE, PROTEIN, AND NUCLEIC ACID

α-Spinasteryl, extracted from Chaihu, could reduce the level of serum cholesterol, increase the cholesterol/phosphorus ratio in rabbit by feeding high-cholesterol food, and reduce the level of serum cholesterol by cutting the thyroid gland. It also could promote a lower rate of basal metabolism and lower activity of glycerophosphate dehydrogenase by feeding thiouracil (Zhang, 1982).

Further, Pan et al. (2002) reported aqueous decoction and extracts from Chaihu could increase blood glucose in rabbit.

10.2.10 EFFECT ON IMMUNOMODULATION

Wang (1983) reported that the extract from *B. chinense* increased the level of serum antibody caused by sheep red blood cells in twice immune mice and increased the inhibition of the leukocyte reproduction. However, it did not affect the formation of antitoxin by tetanus toxin four times immune in rabbit.

Lu and Tuo (1988) proved Chaihu injection could inhibit the E-acceptor of lymphocytes, and decrease the formation of E-rosette by FC-acceptor of celiac macrophage test in mice. The inhibitory activity was raised with increasing concentration. The studies suggested that Chaihu injection had an inhibitory effect on E-rosette by celiac macrophage in mice while the concentration was 1:8, 1:4, and 1:2 (Tuo and Lu, 1985). However, it did not influence the formation of the E-rosette by sheep red blood cells. Chaihu injection has the effect of promoting the humoral immunity reaction, causing the spleen weight and spleen cell to be reduced by adrenal hormone. It also caused adrenal cortical and medullary hyperplasia, with excretion of a lot of glucocorticoid hormone, against the inhibition of feedback by dexamethasone (Zheng et al., 1998).

Four extracts of Chaihu (with 40% Alc., butanol, water, and aqueous decoction of Chaihu residue) were injected into mice i.p. 0.2 ml/mouse/day for 8 days. The results showed that the

TABLE 10.13
Effect of Chaihu Extracts on Antibody-Forming Cells and Multiplication
of the Lymphocytes in the Spleen of Mice ($n = 5$; $X \pm S$)

Group	Dose (mg/kg/d)	PFC (O.D.)	Lymphocyte Multiplication (O.D) Con A	LPS
Normal	—	0.164 ± 0.03	0.030 ± 0.010	0.166 ± 0.006
Sol. in water	50	0.180 ± 0.02	$0.380 \pm 0.059^{**}$	$0.280 \pm 0.051^{**}$
Decoction of residue	5	0.150 ± 0.03	$0.350 \pm 0.021^{***}$	$0.250 \pm 0.008^{***}$
40% Alc. extract	25	0.150 ± 0.01	0.270 ± 0.021	$0.210 \pm 0.018^{***}$
Butanol extract	0.25	0.150 ± 0.03	$0.390 \pm 0.065^{**}$	0.160 ± 0.035

Note: Compared with normal group: $^{**}p < 0.01$; $^{***}p < 0.001$. Normal group mice were injected i.p. with an equivalent amount of distilled water. Sol. in water group mice were injected i.p. with water extract from Chaihu. Decoction of residue group mice were injected i.p. with an aqueous decoction of Chaihu residue. 40% Alc. extract group mice were injected i.p. with alcohol extract from Chaihu. Butanol extract group mice were injected i.p. with butanol extract from Chaihu.

TABLE 10.14
Effect of Four Chaihu Extracts on Celiac Macrophage in Mice
($n = 5$; $X \pm S$)

Group	Dose (mg/kg)	Percentage of Phagocytosis (%)	*t*-test
Normal	—	24.0 ± 3.80	—
Sol. in water	50	46.0 ± 1.90	$P < 0.001$
Decoction of residue	5	48.0 ± 7.30	$P < 0.001$
40% Alc. extract	25	37.0 ± 6.90	$P < 0.05$
Butanol extract	0.25	41.0 ± 4.50	$P < 0.001$

Note: Compared with normal group.

extracts could increase the formation of T cells and B cells (Table 10.13). The alcohol extract could promote the formation of B cells and the activity of celiac macrophage (Table 10.14), but did not influence the formation of the antibody-forming cells in mice. The butanol extract increased the formation of T cells. Furthermore, the aqueous decoction of Chaihu residue activated T cells to release interleukin-2 (IL-2) (Table 10.15).

These results may indicate one of the mechanisms that promote cytoimmunity and the anticancer activity of Chaihu (Chen et al., 1997).

During the immunopharmacological tests on 21 traditional Chinese medicines conducted by Gong (1995), it was discovered that Chaihu could markedly enhance delayed-type hypersensitive reaction (DTH) induced by sheep red blood cells (SRBC), and increase spleen and thymus weights in mice.

The aqueous decoction of Chaihu was fed to mice p.o. 28 g/kg/day for 6 days against dexamethasone-inhibiting activity of celiac macrophage (Table 10.16).

The assay showed Chaihu Decoction was active against the inhibitory activity of macrophages induced by dexamethasone (Wang and Zhao, 1998).

TABLE 10.15
Effect of the Aqueous Decoction of Chaihu Residue on the Activity of T Cells to Release IL-2 in Spleen of Mice Abducted by ConA ($n = 6$; $X \pm S$)

Dose (µg/kg)	IL-2-Released (O.D.)	t-test
0	0.24 ± 0.03	—
62.5	0.32 ± 0.04	$P < 0.01$
15.6	0.35 ± 0.02	$P < 0.001$

Note: Compared with control group (0 µg/kg).

TABLE 10.16
Chaihu Decoction against Dexamethasone-Inhibiting Activity of Celiac Macrophage in Mice ($n = 15$; $X \pm S$)

Group	Phagocytic Index	t-test	Phagocytosis (%)	t-test
Control	0.31 ± 0.09	$P < 0.05$	18.80 ± 3.21	$P < 0.01$
Dexamethasone	0.16 ± 0.10	—	11.23 ± 2.83	—
Chaihu	0.38 ± 0.11	$P < 0.01$	20.35 ± 3.43	$P < 0.01$

Note: Control group mice were injected i.h. with an equivalent amount of distilled water. Dexamethasone group mice were injected i.h. with an equivalent amount of distilled water and i.h. dexamethasone injection 2.5 mg/kg/day for 6 days. Chaihu group mice were injected i.h. with dexamethasone injection 2.5 mg/kg/day and fed p.o. Chaihu Aqueous Decoction 20 ml/kg/day for 6 days.

The therapeutic effects of Chaihu on virus polymyositis in guinea pigs were studied by Chu and Hou (1998). In the study, 25 guinea pigs with polymyositis induced by Coxsackie virus B1 were divided at random into A ($n = 15$) and B ($n = 10$) groups. The mice of A group received Chaihu, while those of B group none. The muscle enzyme spectrum and pathological changes in the two groups were compared. Results are shown in Table 10.17. The conditions of A group mice became better while B group mice showed an aggravated trend ($p < 0.05$).

TABLE 10.17
Therapeutical Effects of Chaihu on Virus Polymyositis in Guinea Pigs (IU/l; $X \pm S$)

Group		CPK	LDH	AST
Normal		91.5 ± 237.5	200.2 ± 93.8	66.4 ± 17.9
Control	Before administration	1175.2 ± 741.2	270.3 ± 64.7	43.44 ± 10.6
	After administration	1593.4 ± 1030.9	432.8 ± 227.3	88.64 ± 41.3
Chaihu	Before administration	1341.7 ± 1361.9	205.3 ± 102.1	83.14 ± 56.9
	After administration	349.8 ± 245.3*	114.1 ± 104.9*	45.30 ± 19.5*

Note: Compared with normal group: *$p < 0.05$.

Result: Chaihu had a therapeutic effect on polymyositis in guinea pigs. The effect may be related with inhibition of free lymphokine, forming IL-2 and inflammation (Chu and Hou, 1998).

10.2.11 EFFECT ON ANTICANCER AND ANTIMUTAGENESIS

The inhibitory effect of some medicines on the expression of viral capsid antigen (VCA) of Epstein–Barr (EBV) virus in B95-8 cells was studied by Pi et al. (1996). There is a close relationship between EBV and nasopharyngeal carcinoma (NPC). Rivavirin, Poly IC, glucurolactone, *Isatis Indigatica*, and Chaihu were added separately to the culture medium of B95-8 cells, which can produce EBV spontaneously. The expression of VCA in EBV under various drug concentrations was studied. Except glucurolactone, all the tested medicines had inhibitory effects on the expression of EBV-VCA. There were powerful inhibitory effects for Rivavirin (10 µg/ml), *Isatis Indigatica* (10 mg/ml), and Chaihu (10 mg/ml); their inhibitory rates were 55.56, 57.89, and 18.75%, respectively. The results show that it may be one of the important ways to control NPC, using medicines that can inhibit duplication and expression of EBV (Pi et al., 1996).

Water extract from Chaihu markedly reduced variants induced by aflatoxin B_1, and markedly reduced the chromosome aberrance evoked by cyclophosphamide in mice (Liu et al., 1990).

The Ames test showed that the extract from Chaihu has antimutagenesis activity to TA98 germ strain. (Yoshimishi, 1988).

10.2.12 EFFECT ON ANTIOXIDATION

Chaihu injection 0.05, 0.1, 0.2, and 0.3 ml (1 g crude herb/ml) were added in 1-ml solution that contained 2.5% liver plasma of mice. The formation of MDA was markedly inhibited in the liver plasma (Table 10.18).

It was also demonstrated that Chaihu injection, *in vitro*, reduced the elevation of serum MDA and free plasma hemoglobin of rabbit caused by H_2O_2. It is suggested that Chaihu injection inhibited lipid peroxidation (Fan et al., 1991).

10.3 SIDE EFFECT OF *BUPLEURUM*

10.3.1 SIDE EFFECTS OF CHAIHU

Chaihu injection was without toxicity when injected into mice i.h. with the dose of 10 ml/kg. It had no influence on the blood pressure, breathing, and heart rate in cat when it was injected i.v. at the dose of 5 ml/kg (Jiangsu New Physic College, 1977).

The LD_{50} of the essential oil of *B. chinense* was 1.19 g ± 0.12 g/kg (Zhou et al., 1979), and the decoction was >6 g/kg to mice (Zhao et al., 1995).

TABLE 10.18
Inhibition of Chaihu to MDA in Mouse Liver Plasma ($n = 5$; $X \pm S$)

Concentration (ml/ml)	MDA (nmol/g liver fresh weight)	t-test
0	436.04 ± 49.04	—
0.05	411.89 ± 32.67	—
0.10	373.52 ± 34.62	$P < 0.05$
0.20	337.31 ± 34.22	$P < 0.01$
0.30	302.78 ± 26.45	$P < 0.01$

The chronic toxicity tests showed that when it was fed to rat p.o. 1.53 g/kg, the extracts from Chaihu increased the pressure of permeability, creatinine, serum -GTP, quantity of kidney albumen, MCHC, NADPH, the activity of LDH, and RBC pigment. The extracts reduced the g-GTP, RBC, proportion of blood cell, serum dissociate TC, general TC, serum GOT, and Cr in liver, UA, K, BUN, and relative weight of hypophysis. There were no marked changes in the common status, spontaneity sport, body weight, dissection, and pathology checks (Zheng et al., 1998).

10.3.2 TOXICITY OF *BUPLEURUM LONGIRADIATUM* TURCZ

The root and rhizome of *B. longiradiatum* are toxic to humans: Patients experience nausea and vomiting, followed by serious twitching and opisthotonus before death. It had been reported that three persons died after administration of powdered root and rhizome of *B. longiradiatum* (Xu and Guo, 1980). The LD_{50}s of the powdered underground organs and four extracts in mice (oral administration) have been investigated by Chen et al. (1981). The LD_{50} of the powder was 0.4994 g/kg, extract with petroleum-ether was 1.708 g/kg, extract with ether was 0.055 g/kg, extract with ethyl acetate was 0.015 g/kg, and extract with alcohol was 0.335 g/kg. Zhao et al (1987) isolated four polyacetylenes from *B. longiradiatum*. Two of them are toxic: bupleurotoxin and acetylbupleurotoxin with an LD_{50} for bupleurotoxin in mice (i.p. injection) of 3.03 and 3.13 mg/kg, respectively. Xu and Guo (1980) revealed that when mice were fed with the powder of *B. longiradiatum* at the dose of 3 g/kg, they began to twitch in 15 min, followed by excitation symptoms such as cauda lifting, jumping, and spinal reflexing. All were dead within 1 hour.

REFERENCES

Chen, D.H., Li, P., Cheng, J.F., Zhong, C.H., He, J.R., Teng, S.B., and He, P. (1998) Effects of radix *Bupleuri* and *Glycyrrhizin* on the hepatocyte apoptisis in mice, *J. Fourth Military Med. Univ.*, 3, 279–280.

Chen, Q.L., Zheng, X.Y., and Huang, X.P. (1994) Effect on processed chaihu for experimental liver injury of mice, *Chin. Trad. Patent Med.*, 3, 22–23.

Chen, S., Chen, F., Zhang, W.R., and Bai, H.Q. (1997) Immuno effect of four extracts of Chaihu on mice, *J. Luzhou Med. Coll.*, 2, 65–67.

Chen, X.S., Liu, X.Z., Li, Z., Sun, M., Chu, D.J., and Sun, Y.L. (1981) Study of toxic principles of *Bupleurum longiradiatum*, *Chin. Pharm. J.*, 5, 318.

Chen, Y.L. (1984) Effects of Chaihu and Shugan-jiantangji on cAMP/cGMP in mouse plasma, liver and thalamencephalon, *J. Hunan Med. Coll.*, 3, 253.

Chu, X.H. and Hou, X.D. (1998) Experimental study on therapeutical effect of Chinese medicine on polymyositis in guinea pigs, *Chin. J. TCM Pharm.*, 1, 12–14.

Dai, X.M., Wu, X.Q., Liu, X.F., and He, Y.H. (1998) Effect of Shenfu, Chaihu injection on hypoblood-reperfusion induced mouse kidney injury, *Jiangsu J. TCM*, 2, 46–47.

Fan, J.R., He, S.L., and Wang, X.K. (1991) Anti-lipid-hyperoxydative effect of Shenfu injection and Chaihu injection, *Chin. Trad. Patent Med.*, 2, 25–26.

Gan, H.H. (1982) A comparison of the quality of the root and the aerial part from *Bupleurum chinense* DC., *J. Chin. Mat. Med.*, 2, 7–8.

Gao, Y., Wang, S., and Zhan, X.H. (2000) Protective effect of Chaihu on liver injury induced by hypoblood, *World Chin. J. Digest.*, 2, 168–170.

Gong, H.Y., Wang, H., Xu, Z., and Liu, G.Z. (1995) Immunopharmacological effects of 21 herbs on mice, *Pharmacol. Clin. Chin. Mat. Med.*, 2, 30–33.

Gong, S.Z., Liao, W.P., and Zheng, D.H. (1997) Study anticonvulsant effect of Chaihu in rats using the method of frontal cortical threshold test, *Acad. J. Guangzhou Med. Coll.*, 1, 24–26.

Jiangsu New Physic College. (1977) *Chinese Traditional Medicine Great Gradus,* Vol. 2. Shanghai Science & Technology, Shanghai, 1832.

Kanatani, H. (1985) Search for adenylate cyclase activator in medicinal plants, *Planta Med.*, 2, 182.

Kobayashi, M., Sato, S., Kaizu, R., and Mihashi, H. (1990) Therapeutic ebromone as Inhibitor of 5-fipoxy-genare and aldose reductase, *Jpn. Kokai Tokkyo Koho JP*, 04 59,773[92 59,773] (Cl.C07D311/22), 26 Feb 1992. Appl. 90/165,696,26 Jun; 7.

Li, L.C., Li, C.Z., and Shi, Y.N.(1985) The pharmacological effect of extract from the aerial part of *Bupleurum chinense* DC., *Chin. Trad. Herbal Drugs*, 5, 32–33.

Li, T.L., Du, X.W., Zhao, J.H., Zhang, D.M., and Chen, C.X. (1992) A comparison of pharmacological effect of *Bupleurum Chinense* DC. and *B. scorzonerifolium* Willd., *Acta Chin. Med. Pharmacol.*, 3, 34–36.

Liao, J.F., Jan, Y.M., Huang, S.Y., Wang, H.H., Yu, L.L., and Chen, C.F. (1995) Evaluation with receptor binding assay on the water extracts of ten CNS-active Chinese herbal drugs, *Proc. Natl. Sci. Counc. Repub. China B*, 3, 151–158.

Ling, M.D., Zeng, X.L., and Hu, B.R. (1991) The effects of the isolated fractions from Chaihu on adenylate cyclase (2), *Pharmacol. Clin. Chin. Met. Med.*, 4, 17–20.

Liu, D.X., Yin, X.J., Wang, H.C., Zhou, Y., and Zhang, Y.H. (1990) Filtered aqueous extracts of 102 herbs for anti-abduction change, *J. Chin. Mat. Med.*, 10, 41–46.

Lu, X.Z. and Tuo, S.W. (1988) Effect of Chaihu injection for E-accepter in human T-lymphocyte, *Chin. J. Clin. Hepatol.*, 3, 17.

Nakajima, K., Morita, M., Sato, S., and Mihashi, H. (Tsumura and Co.). (1990) Polyacetylenes inhibitors of 5-lipoxygenase and cyclooxygenase, *Jpn. Kokai Tokkyo Koho JP*, 02 32,036 [90 32,036].

Nakamura, T., Kuriyama, M., Kosuge, E., Ishihara, K., and Ito, K. (1993) Effects of Saiboku-to (TJ-96) on the production of platelet-activating factor in human neutrophils, *Ann. N.Y. Acad. Sci.*, 23, 685572–685579.

Nikaido, T. (1981) Inhibitors of cyclic AMP phosphodiesterase in medicinal plants, *Planta Med.*, 1, 18.

Pan, S.L., Shun, Q.S., Bai, Q.M., and Bao, X.S. (2002) *The Coloured Atlas of the Medicinal Plants from Genus Bupleurum in China*. Shanghai Science and Technology Literature Publishing, Shanghai, 8.

Pi, Z.M., Zhong, H.S., Huang, Y.Y., Deng, H., and Luo, J.Q. (1996) Inhibitory effect of some medicines on the expression of viral capsid antigen of Epstein–Barr virus in B95-8 cells, *Cancer*, 3, 195–197.

Sun, J. (1958) Study of antifungi effect of some Chinese traditional medicines, *Chin. J. Dermatol.*, 3, 210.

Sun, S.X. (1956) Pharmacological study on antipyretic effect of several Chinese traditional medicines, *Chin. Med. J.*, 10, 964–966.

Tang, B., Wu, Y.R., and Kang, G.F. (1998) Protective effect of Chaiha injection on hypoxia-reoxygenation-induced mouse liver injury, *Chin. Trad. Herbal Drugs*, 12, 814–817.

Tuo, S.W., and Lu, X.Z. (1985) Studies of Chaihu injection to FC-accepter effect of macrophage and T-lymphocyte, *Pharmacol. Clin. Chin. Met. Med.*, 1, 165.

Wang, H., Xu, W.M., and Wang, Z.Y. (1996a) Antipyretic effect of Chaihu, *J. TCM Res.*, 2, 38–39.

Wang, H., Xu, W.M., and Wang, Z.Y. (1996b) Pharmacokinetical study of Chaihu, *Acad. J. Guangzhou Med. Coll.*, 3, 229.

Wang, P. and Chen, Q.L. (2000) Effect of processed Chaihu to activity of acetylcholinesterase in mice blood, *J. Chin. Mat. Med.*, 4, 219–220.

Wang, S., Gao, Y., and Zhan, X.H. (2000) Morphological observation on hepaprotective effect of Chaihu decoctor to liver injury induced by hypoblood, *World Chin. J. Dig.*, 2, 159–161.

Wang, S.C. and Zhao, H.P. (1998) Antipyretic and antiviral effect of Chaihu, *Lishizhen Med. Mat. Med. Res.*, 5, 418–419.

Wang, S.Y. (1958) Inhibition effect on Chinese traditional medicine for growth of mycobacterium tuberculosis, I. *Chin. Sci. Bull.*, 12, 379.

Wang, Y.S. (1983) *Chinese Traditional Medicine Pharmacological Effect and Application*, 1st ed. Beijing Med. & Sanitation Publishing, Beijing, 886.

Weiguan, H. (1984) Pharmacological study of Chinese traditional medicines to chronic hepatitis, *For. Med. Sci. TCM Sec.*, 2, 12.

Wu, K.R. (1983) Effect of several Chinese herbs on the isolated womb of rabbit and of their combined effect, *J. Zhejiang Coll. TCM* (Suppl.), p. 2.

Wu, Z.F., Xiong, C.M., and Zhang, J.B. (1983) Pilot study antipyretic and antiinflammation effect of Chaihu injection. *Chin. J. Pharm. Anal.*, 5, 293–295.

Xu, Z.B. and Guo, X.F. (1980) A study of the toxic principles of *Bupleurum longiradiatum*, *Heilongjiang Med. Pharm.*, 1, 29–32.

Ye, S.L. (1957) Effect of Chaihu and Gancao on liver injury, *New TCM*, 3, 35.

Ye, Z.G. (1996) Study on antiinflammatory activity of medicinal Plant Chaihu. *Foreign Med. Sci. TCM Sec.*, 1, 33–34.

Yoshimishi, S. (1988) Effect on anti-mutation of herb extract, *Foreign Med. Sci. Pharm. Sec.*, 1, 51.

Zhang, B. (1982) The chemical constituents and pharmacological effects of the genus *Bupleurum, World Phytomed.*, 5, 2–9.

Zhang, L.X., Yuan, B.Y., and Li S.Z. (1989) Comparative curative effect of Chaihu injection made by a different technique, *Chin. Trad. Patent Med.*, 12, 7–8.

Zhang, Z.L. and Zhang, D.P. (1989) Study of kinetics on saikosaponin and flavone inhibition of acetycholine-ester-enzyme in plasma, *West Chin. J. Pharm. Sci.*, 1, 48–50.

Zhao, J.F., Guo, Y.Z., and Meng, X.S. (1987) The toxic principles of *Bupleurum longiradiatum, Acta Pharm. Sin.*, 7, 507–511.

Zhao, Y.Z., Tao, S.C., Xing, Y.C., Wang, Y.H., and Xing, S.R. (1995) Study on pharmacological effect of *Bupleurum smithii* Wolff var. *parvifolium* Shan et Y. Li, *J. Chin. Mat. Med.*, 8, 405–408.

Zhe, F.W. (1987) Investigation of Chaihu on reducing the activity of sialidase, *Foreign Med. Sci. TCM Sec.*, 2, 38.

Zheng, H.Z., Dong, Z.H., and Yu, J. (1998) *Modern Study and Application of Chinese Medicines*, Vol. 4. Academy Press, Beijing, 3680–3717.

Zhou, C.C., Zhou, Q.L., and Wang, B.X. (1979) Comparative pharmacological effect of *Bupleurum chinense* DC. and *B. longeradiatum* Turcz., *Chin. Pharm. J.*, 6, 252–253.

Zhu, S.O., Pan, J.Y., and Hu, S. (1985) Effect of Chaihu essential oil on antipyretic and antiinflammatory activity, *Pharmacol. Clin. Chin. Met. Med.*, 1, 150.

11 Pharmacological Activity of Saikosaponins

Byung-Zun Ahn and Dai-Eun Sok

CONTENTS

11.1 INTRODUCTION

Bupleurum species are naturally occurring small shrubs widely distributed in East Asia and the Mediterranean area. This plant has been traditionally used in folk medicine (Lin, 1990; Tang and Eisenbrand, 1992) as anti-inflammatory, antitussive, and antipyretic drugs, and in the treatment of liver disease. In particular, the roots of *Bupleurum* species are listed in the Chinese and Japanese Pharmacopoeias. The crude saponin from this plant possesses a hemolytic activity, and is known to show various activities such as anti-inflammatory, inhibitory effects on chronic hepatitis, immunostimulating effects, and others, in *in vitro* bioassays. Recently, as part of the research for bioactive saponins in the root of *Bupleurum* species, a series of triterpene saponins, such as saikosaponins-a, -b, -c, and -d, and their corresponding prosaikogenins and saikogenins have been isolated, and there have been a number of reports on pharmacological actions of saikosaponins at biochemical or molecular levels.

11.2 STRUCTURE AND BIOTRANSFORMATION

The formulae of the compounds named below have been illustrated in Chapters 7, 8, and 9.

Saikosaponin-a, -d, and -e series are disaccharide glycosides containing the 3-O-β-D-glucopyranosyl ($1 \rightarrow 3$) β-D-fucopyranosyl moiety (Nose et al., 1989). Saikosaponins-a and -d, characterized by an ether linkage between C13 and C28, are epimers at C16 with β-OH and α-OH group, respectively. Saikosaponin-c is a trisaccharide glycoside with a methyl group at C23. Meanwhile, saikosaponin-b_1 and -b_2 with a carbinol function at C28 are epimers at C16 with a β-OH and α-OH group, respectively. Saikosaponin-e is characterized by the presence of fucosylpyranosylglucopy-ranosyl moiety at C3, β-OH at C16, and a methyl group at C4. Metabolism of saikosaponins is expected to follow the general metabolic pathway for saponins. Under gastric condition (Shimizu et al., 1985; Nose et al., 1989), saikosaponin-a and saikosaponin-d are transformed to saikosaponin-b_1 and saikosaponin-b_2, respectively. Further, saikosaponin a yields saikosaponin-g, which possesses a homoannular diene moiety at C9 (11), 12 under the same acidic condition. In intestinal contents, saikosaponins are converted to corresponding prosaikogenins, containing one sugar, by the cleavage of β-D-glucopyranosyl-β-D-fucopyranosyl moiety due to the existence of intestinal microflora, and in turn, each prosaikogenin is converted to the corresponding saikogenin, an aglycone of saikosa-ponin. From human intestinal bacterium, *Eubacterium* sp. A-44, two glycosidases, capable of hydrolyzing saikosaponins to saikogenins, were isolated and characterized as saikosaponin-hydro-lyzing β-D-glucosidase and prosaikogenin-hydrolyzing β-D-fucosidase (Shimizu et al., 1985; Kida et al., 1998).

11.3 TOXICITY (HEMOLYTIC ACTION)

It is well known that a number of plant saponins can induce hemolysis by binding to plasma membranes of red blood cells (Nose et al., 1989). Interestingly, some saponins were observed to exhibit pharmacological actions by changing the electrostatic properties of cell surface polysaccha-rides, altering morphological states, or by unknown mechanisms.

Moreover, the hemolytic action of saikosaponins differed according to the structure of the saikosaponin in the following order: saikosaponin-d > saikosaponin-a > saikosaponin-b_1. Of saikosaponin-d metabolites, prosaikogenin G was similar to saikosaponin-d in potency, but saikogenin G was devoid of any remarkable hemolytic action. The importance of the configu-ration of hydroxyl function at C16 is suggested from the higher potency of saikosaponin-d and its metabolites, compared to saikosaponin-a and its metabolites. In addition, the existence of the ether ring is essential for the hemolytic action; the hemolytic activities were reduced in saikosaponin-b_2 and its monoglycoside form, prosaikogenin D, where the ether ring was cleaved to give a carbinol function at C28. Thus, in addition to the sugar moiety, the configuration of the hydroxyl group at C16 and the ether linkage are recognized as important for the hemolytic activity, although the structure–activity relationship of saikosaponin metabolites cannot be explained fully in terms of these factors. Noteworthy, the adsorbability of these compounds to red blood cell membranes appeared to closely parallel their degree of hemolytic activity. The affinity of saikosaponins for the cell membrane is well evidenced by the change of membrane fluidity of erythrocytes monitored by electron spin resonance spectroscopy (Abe et al., 1978). Overall, various bioactivities of saikosaponins might be related primarily to their interaction with biomembranes of cells. Noteworthy, saikosaponin-d with a β-hydroxyl group was more potent than saikosaponin-a possessing an α-hydroxyl group.

11.4 THE PHARMACOLOGICAL ACTIVITY OF SAIKOSAPONINS

11.4.1 IMMUNOREGULATORY ACTION

Saikosaponins have been demonstrated to cause the activation of immunological functions of macrophages, a parameter of immune potentiation, and to modify immune responses of T and B cells. A significant increase of phorbol myristate acetate–induced chemiluminescence in peritoneal macrophage was expressed by saikosaponin-d at a low concentration, suggestive of the activation of peritoneal macrophages (Kumazawa et al., 1989; Ushio and Abe, 1991). In this activity, saiko-saponin-d was more potent than ginsenoside Rg1 or glycyrrhizin. In modifying the immune responses of T and B cells (Kato et al., 1995), saikosaponin-d appeared to show a cell type-dependent immunomodulatory action; saikosaponin-d downregulated the DNA synthesis and growth response of thymocytes stimulated by anti-CD3mAb, while increasing that of spleen cells. On the other hand, saikosaponin-d greatly upregulated the growth response and intereukin-2/4 production induced through a receptor-bypassed pathway, while slightly enhancing them in spleen cells. Since saikosaponins have a common steroid-like structure, the downregulation of lymphocyte response by saikosaponin was supposed to be due to glucocorticoid-induced apoptotic action. Seemingly consistent with this, saikosaponin-d at relatively higher concentrations induced the apoptosis of human CEM lymphocytes, accompanied by the necrosis (Hsu et al., 2000). Especially, the apoptotic action of saikosaponin at 10^{-5} M is associated with the change of c-myc, p53, and bcl-2 mRNA levels, but not caspase activity. In this regard, the biochemical mechanism for apoptotic action of saikosaponin-d is different from that of dexamethasone.

11.4.2 ANTI-INFLAMMATORY AND ANTIALLERGIC ACTION

Anti-inflammatory actions of *Bupleurum* saponins were suggested from the suppressive effect of crude saponin fraction, containing saikosaponins a and d, on dextran-induced edema of rat paw. Furthermore, the saponin fraction showed a protective effect on histamine-shocked guinea pigs (Takagi and Shibata, 1969b; Yamamoto et al., 1975). Because saikosaponins have a common steroid-like structure, they are expected to have some steroid-related anti-inflammatory action. One of the mechanisms responsible for the inflammation may involve the arachidonic acid cascade pathway; arachidonic acid is released from phospholipase A_2-catalyzed hydrolysis of phospholipids, and then free arachidonic acid is enzymatically converted to prostaglandins and leukotrienes, inflammation mediators. A recent study (Bermejo Benito et al., 1998) shows that buddlejasaponin I, and saikosaponin 1 and 2 exert a potent *in vitro* anti-inflammatory effect on PMA-induced edema of mouse ear. In comparison, saikosaponins a and d are more potent than other saikosaponins, with saikosaponin-d more potent than saikosaponin-a. Since most saikosaponins showed a significant inhibitory effect on the formation of cyclooxygenase metabolites, prostaglandin E and thromboxane, and lipoxygenase metabolite, leukotriene C, the putative antiphlogistic activity of saikosaponins was ascribed to the inhibition of arachidonic acid metabolism. Separately, an independent study indicates that saikosaponin-a significantly inhibited the passive cutaneous anaphylaxis reaction in rats and asthmatic bronchoconstriction in sensitized guinea pigs. It is suggested that the inhibition of allergic mediators as well as the antagonism of histamine action may account for the antiallergic action of saikosaponin (Park et al., 2002).

11.4.3 ANODYNIC AND SEDATIVE ACTION

Glucocorticoid hormone enables the body to respond to a stress, especially a long-term stress. Oral administration of corticosterone acetate together with the *Bupleurum* root extract to rats markedly elevated the hepatic tyrosine transaminase activity as an indicator of corticosterone activity (Hashimoto et al., 1985; Tang and Eisenbrand, 1992). In corticosterone secretion-inducing activity, saikosaponin-d and its metabolite, prosaikogenin G, were about four times more potent than saikogenin-a and prosaikogenin F, respectively. Moreover, intracerebroventricular administration of saikosaponin-d increased plasma adrenocorticotropic hormone (ACTH) and corticosterone levels in the rat (Dobashi et al., 1995). Further study indicates that saikosaponin-d stimulates both corticotropin-releasing factor (CRF) gene expression and CRF release from hypothalamus, which in turn increases ACTH release in the anterior pituitary. Taken together, saikosaponins may exert anti-stress action by causing the elevation of ACTH level, followed by the increase of corticosterone level. Although a further study on the mode of action in the stimulation of CRF neurons was not performed, the activity–structure relationship for the stimulation of CRF neurons appears to parallel with that for the hemolytic activity. Therefore, it is more likely that the stimulatory effect of saikosaponin-d on CRF neurons expression might be related partially to its direct effect on the cell membrane.

11.4.4 HEPATOPROTECTIVE ACTION

The crude saponins from *Bupleurum* species were reported to normalize the liver dysfunction, as indicated by serum alkaline phosphatase or glutamate pyruvate transaminase (GPT) level (Tang and Eisenbrand, 1992). Treatment of rats with crude saponins prevented the increase in serum GOT and GPT levels induced by D-galactosamine, but not CCl_4, which was confirmed by other observers (Guinea et al., 1994). Nevertheless, saikosaponin-a expressed a positive antihepatotoxic action against CCl_4-hepatotoxicity enhanced by phenobarbitone (Abe et al., 1985). Major principles responsible for the reduction of sGOT and sGPT activities in rats intoxicated with D-galactosamine are saikosaponins a and d (Guinea et al., 1994; Yen et al., 1994). In addition, buddlejasaponin IV and malonylbuddlejasaponin IV, possessing three saccharides, also showed a hepatoprotective activity against the cytotoxicity of galactosamine in primary cultured rat hepatocytes, but not the CCl_4 cytotoxicity (Guinea et al., 1994). Noteworthy, these saikosaponins were more potent than silybin, a representative natural antihepatotoxic agent. Although the mechanisms for the hepatoprotection are not clear, one is supposed to be the prevention of lipid peroxidation in microsomal compartment of cells.

11.4.5 ANTITUMOR ACTION

"Sho-saiko-to," one of the Chinese antitumorigenic herbal drugs, has been known to play a chemopreventive role in the development of hepatocellular carcinoma in patients with cirrhosis (Shimizu, 2000). In inhibiting the cell growth of human hepatoma cell line (Motoo and Sawabu, 1994), the order for the efficacy of saikosaponins was as follows; saikosaponin-d > saikosaponin-a > saikosaponin-b$_2$. A possible mechanism for the saikosaponin-a was suggested to be necrosis rather than apoptosis, because of the appearance of the sub-G$_1$ peak and the non-ladder type degradation of nuclear DNA in the early cell death stage (Qian et al., 1995). Subsequently, saikosaponins, in combination with other natural products, as exemplified in the traditional Chinese anticancer drug, Bu-Zhong-Yi-Qi-Tang (Kao et al., 2001), appeared to remarkably inhibit the proliferation of hepatoma cell lines, by probably inducing apoptosis via G$_0$/G$_1$ arrest. Separately, the antiproliferation effect of saikosaponin-d on HL60 cells was supposed to be due to the inhibition of HL60 cells through the arrest at G$_0$/G$_1$ phase, accompanied by upregulation in expression of glucocorticoid receptor (GR) mRNA (Bu et al., 1999). However, the relation of the upregulation of GR mRNA to apoptosis was not clarified further. Recently (Wu and Hsu, 2001), the molecular mechanism of saikosaponin-a in the inhibition of HepG2 growth was suggested to be due to the induction of cyclin-dependent kinases, which are known to phosphorylate retinoblastoma (Rb) protein, leading to the release of transcriptionally active E2F, a transcription factor. Especially, saikosaponin-a induced both mRNA and protein of CDK inhibitors, p-15[INK4b] and p-16[INK4b], supposedly mediating the inhibition of cell growth through the arrest of cell cycle at the sub-G$_1$ peak. Independently, the anti-cell adhesive effects of saikosaponins on some solid tumor cells were reported (Ahn et al., 1998). The mechanism for the alteration of cell adhesion was suggested to be due to the metabolic alterations in tumor cell surface oligosaccharides, consistent with earlier observation that natural products, which modify cell surface oligosaccharides, consequently affect the adhesive properties of murine B16 melanoma cells. The structure–activity relationship for the anti-adhesive activity of saikosaponins indicates that there is a good relationship between anti-cell adhesive property of saikosaponins and their hemolytic activity. Nevertheless, the anti-cell adhesive action of saikosaponins could not be fully explained by the mechanism of their hemolytic action; saikosaponin-d, less potent in the hemolytic action, expressed a much greater anti-cell adhesive action than saikosaponin-e. Therefore, it is supposed that in addition to the adsorption to cell membrane, the biochemical alteration of components of cell membrane may be also implicated in the anti-cell adhesive bioactivity of saikosaponins.

11.4.6 ANTIBACTERIAL AND ANTIVIRAL ACTIVITIES

Saikosaponins and sapogenins, administered i.p., i.v., or s.c., showed nonspecific resistance against *Pseudomonas aeroginosa* and *Listeria monocytogenes* infections in mice (Kumazawa et al., 1990); the most effective resistance was observed with i.p. administration of saikosaponin-d 1 day before the infection with *P. aeroginosa*. Effector cells participating in the enhanced protection induced by saikosaponin-d were suggested to be macrophages, a major component of peritoneal cells. The intracellular activity of peritoneal macrophages against *P. aeroginosa* was suggested to be responsible for the antibacterial activity of saikosaponins. In a recent study (Bermejo et al., 2002) of the antiviral activity of saikosaponins, buddlejasaponin IV exhibited antiviral activity against vesicular stomatitis virus (RNA virus), but not herpes simplex type I, at concentrations ranging from 20 to 25 µg/ml without a cytotoxic effect.

11.4.7 SECRETAGOGUE ACTION

It was found that *Bupleurum* saikosaponins had a significant promoting effect on the secretion of enzyme in rat pancreatic acini, suggesting a secretagogue-like role of saikosaponin (Yu et al., 2002). In rat pancreatic acinar cells, saikosaponin I at a low concentration (1 to 10 µM) enhanced the secretion of amylase preceded by the increase of intracellular Ca^{2+}, consistent with Ca^{2+}-induced exocytosis. The time-dependent course for amylase secretion and enhancement of intracellular Ca^{2+}, and the antagonism of saikosaponin action by CCK-8 receptor antagonist, imply a receptor-mediated selective action of saikosaponin. Besides (Yang et al., 2001), the inhibitory effect of GDP on saikosaponin-induced secretion of amylase and elevation of intracellular Ca^{2+} may support the involvement of G protein signaling in a higher potency action of saikosaponin. This finding may attract much attention, since a selective interaction between saikosaponins and target proteins may be implicated. A further study to provide positive evidence for the binding of saikosaponin molecule to target protein remains to be carried out.

11.5 INDUCTION OF DIFFERENTIATION

Induction of differentiation without inhibitory effect on the cell growth was expressed by saikosaponin-b$_2$ (Zong et al., 1998); the treatment of B16 melanoma cells with saikosaponin-b$_2$ induced the differentiation of B16 melanoma cells without growth inhibition or cytotoxicity under conditions of a low dose (5 µM) and a long-term treatment (30 days). The effect of saikosaponin-b$_2$ was suggested to be due to the downregulation of protein kinase C activity. Another example for the differentiation action of saikosaponin is well provided by the enhancing effect of saikosaponin-d on the activities of glutamine synthetase and 2′,3′-cyclic nucleotide 3′-phosphohydrolase in C6 glioma cells (Tsai et al., 2002); saikosaponin-a enhanced the activities of glutamine synthetase and 2′,3′-cyclic nucleotide 3′-phosphohydrolase, indicative of the differentiation into astrocytes and oligodendrocytes, while saikosaponin-d showed an increase of glutamine synthetase activity only, suggesting the differentiation into astrocytes. The selective effect of saikosaponins on the differentiation of neural cells needs further studies.

11.6 FUTURE PERSPECTIVES

It is of interest to observe that saikosaponins have various pharmacological actions. Recent studies reveal that saikosaponins express biological effects on various types of cells. Although the bioactivities of saikosaponins appear to be primarily due to their interaction with cell membranes, various pharmacological actions of saikosaponins may not be explained fully by the membrane effect. Therefore, the selective binding of saikosaponins to targets, such as membrane proteins, is to be examined to understand the exact mechanism for actions of saikosaponins in specific cells. For this purpose, further investigations employing a selective assay of protein binding, such as the radioligand binding assay, which possess the potential to selectively identify molecular targets of saikosaponin, and elucidate its responsive mechanism, may be required. In addition, the delivery of saikosaponins containing sugar moiety to target membranes or proteins through gastrointestinal tracts is to be monitored to provide supportive data for the evaluation of pharmacological efficacy of saikosaponins. Finally, the toxicity of saikosaponins is to be considered for the choice of saikosaponins in the clinical use, where the membrane effect such as hemolytic action should be reduced or minimized. In conclusion, an attempt to induce the selective expression of pharmacological action of saikosaponins, while decreasing the nonspecific membrane effect, is worthy of much attention in the near future.

REFERENCES

Abe, H., Odashima, S., and Arichi, S. (1978) The effect of saikosaponins on biological membranes, *Planta Med.*, 34, 287–290.

Abe, H., Orita, M., Konishi, H., Arichi, S., and Odashima, S. (1985) Effects of saikosaponin-d on enhanced CCl_4-hepatotoxicity by phenobarbitone, *J. Pharm. Pharmacol.*, 37, 555–559.

Ahn, B-Z., Yoon, Y.-D., Lee, Y.H., Kim, B.-H., and Sok, D.-E. (1998) Inhibitory effect of Bupleuri radix saponins on adhesion of some solid tumor cells and relation to hemolytic action: screening of 232 herbal drugs for anti-cell adhesion, *Planta Med.*, 64, 220–224.

Bermejo Benito, P., Abad Martinez, M.J., Silvan Sen, A.M., Sanz Gomez, A., Fernandez Matellano, L., Sanchez Contreras, S., and Diaz Lanza, A.M. (1998) *In vivo* and *in vitro* antiinflammatory activity of saikosaponins, *Life Sci.*, 63, 1147–1156.

Bermejo, P., Abad, M.J., Diaz, A.M., Fernandez, L., Santos, J.D., Sanchez, S., Villaescusa, L., Carrasco, L., and Irurzun, A. (2002) Antiviral activity of seven iridoids, three saikosaponins and one phenylpropanoid glycoside extracted from *Bupleurum rigidum* and *Scrophularia scorodonia*, *Planta Med.*, 68, 106–110.

Brunetti, M., Martelli, N., Colasante, A., Piantelli, M., Musiani, P., and Aiello, F.B. (1995) Spontaneous and glucocorticoid-induced apoptosis in human mature T lymphocytes, *Blood*, 86, 4199–4205.

Bu, S., Xu, J., and Sun J. (1999) Saikosaponin-d up-regulates GR mRNA expression and induces apoptosis in HL-60 cells, *Zhonghua Xue Ye Xue Za Zhi* (abstract), 20, 354–356.

Dobashi, I., Tozawa, F., Horiba, N., Sakai, Y., Sakai, K., and Suda, T. (1995) Central administration of saikosaponin-d increases corticotropin-releasing factor mRNA levels in the rat hypothalamus, *Neurosci. Lett.*, 197, 235–238.

Guinea, M.C., Parellada, J., Lacaille-Dubois, M.A., and Wagner, H. (1994) Biologically active triterpene saponins from *Bupleuri fruticosum*, *Planta Med.*, 60, 163–167.

Hashimoto, M., Inada, K., Ohminami, H., Kimura, Y., Ochuda, H., and Arichi, S. (1985) Effects of saikosaponins on liver tyrosine aminotransferase activity induced by cortisone in adrenalectomized rats, *Planta Med.*, 41, 401–403.

Hsu, M.-J., Cheng, J.-S., and Huang, H.-C. (2000) Effect of saikosaponin, a triterpene saponin, on apoptosis in lymphocytes: association with c-myc, p53, and bcl-2 mRNA. *Br. J. Pharmacol.*, 131, 1285–1293.

Kao, S.-T., Yeh, C.-C., Hsieh, C.-C., Yang, M.-D., Lee, M.-R., Liu, H.-S., and Lin, J.-G. (2001) The Chinese medicine Bu-Zhong-Yi-Qi-Tang inhibited proliferation of hepatoma cell lines by inducing apoptosis via G0/G1 arrest, *Life Sci.*, 69, 1485–1496.

Kato, M., Pu, M., Isobe, K.-I., Hattori, T., Yanagita, N., and Nakashima, I. (1995) Cell type-oriented differential modulatory actions of saikosaponin-d on growth responses and DNA fragmentation of lymphocytes triggered by receptor-mediated and receptor-bypassed pathways, *Immunopharmacology*, 29, 207–213.

Kida, H., Akao, T., Meselhy, M.R., and Hattori, M. (1998) Metabolism and pharmacokinetics of orally administered saikosaponin b1 in conventional, germ-free and *Eubacterium* sp. A-44-infected gnotobiote rats, *Biol. Pharm. Bull.*, 21, 588–593.

Kumazawa, Y., Takimoto, H., Nishimura, C., Kawakita, T., and Nomoto, K. (1989) Activation of murine peritoneal macrophages by saikosaponin a, saikosaponin d and saikogenin d, *Int. J. Immunopharmacol.*, 11, 21–28.

Kumazawa, Y., Kawakita, T., Takimoto, H., and Nomoto, K. (1990) Protective effect of saikosaponin A, saikosaponin D and saikogenin D against *Pseudomonas aeruginosa* infection in mice, *Int. J. Immunopharmacol.*, 12, 531–537.

Lin, C.-C. (1990) *Crude Bupleurum and Bupleurum-Containing Prescriptions.* Kaohsiung, Taiwan, China, 43–71.

Motoo, Y. and Sawabu, N. (1949) Antitumor effects of saikosaponins, baicalin and baicalein on human hepatoma cell lines, *Cancer Lett.*, 86, 91–95.

Nose, M., Amagaya, S., and Ogihara, Y. (1989) Effects of saikosaponin metabolites on the hemolysis of red blood cells and their adsorbability on the cell membrane, *Chem. Pharm. Bull.*, 37, 3306–3310.

Park, K.H., Park, J., Koh, D., and Lim, Y. (2002) Effect of saikosaponin-A, a triterpenoid glycoside, isolated from *Bupleurum falcatum* on experimental allergic asthma, *Phytother. Res.*, 16, 359–363.

Qian, L., Murakami, T., Kimura, Y., Takahashi, M., and Okita, K. (1995) Saikosaponin A-induced cell death of a human hepatoma cell line (HuH-7): the significance of the "sub-G1 peak" in a DNA histogram, *Pathol. Int.*, 45, 207–214.

Shimizu, I. (2000) Sho-saiko-to: Japanese herbal medicine for protection against hepatic fibrosis and carcinoma, *J. Gastroenterol. Hepatol.*, 15(Suppl.), D84–90.

Shimizu, K., Amagaya, S., and Ogihara, Y. (1985) Structural transformation of saikosaponins by gastric juice and intestinal flora, *J. Pharmacobiodyn.*, 8, 718–725.

Takagi, K. and Shibata, M. (1969a) Pharmacological studies on *Bupleurum falcatum*. I. Acute toxicity and central depressant action of crude saikosides, *Yakugaku Zasshi*, 89, 712–720.

Takagi, K. and Shibata, M. (1969b) Pharmacological studies on *Bupleurum falcatum*. II. Antiinflammatory and other pharmacological actions of crude saikosides, *Yakugaku Zasshi*, 89, 1367–1378.

Tang, W. and Eisenbrand, G. (1992) *Chinese Drugs of Plant Origin.* Springer-Verlag, Hong Kong, 222–232.

Tsai, Y.J., Chen, I.L., Horng, L.Y., and Wu, R.T. (2002) Induction of differentiation in rat C6 glioma cells with saikosaponins, *Phytother. Res.*, 16, 117–121.

Ushio, Y. and Abe, H. (1991) Effects of saikosaponin-d on the functions and morphology of macrophages, *Int. J. Immunopharmacol.*, 13, 493–499.

Wu, W.-S. and Hsu, H.-Y. (2001) Involvement of p-15[INK4b] and p-16[INK4a] gene expression in saikosaponin a and TPA-induced growth inhibition of HepG2 cells, *Biochem. Biophys. Res. Commun.*, 285, 183–187.

Yamamoto, M., Kumagai, A., and Yamamura, Y. (1975) Structure and actions of saikosaponins isolated from *Bupleurum falcatum*. I. Antiinflammatory action of saikosaponins, *Arzneimittelforschung*, 25, 1021–1023.

Yang, W.X., Yu, Y., Zhang, W.Z., Wang, H., Li, X.D., Zhao, Y.Y., and Liang, H. (2001) Inhibitory role of GDP on saikosaponin(I) stimulated enzyme secretion and rising of [Ca^{2+}]i in rat pancreatic acini, *Acta Pharmacol. Sin.*, 22, 669–672.

Yen, M.-H., Lin, C.-C., Chuang, C.-H., and Lin, S.-C. (1994) Anti-inflammatory and hepatoprotective activity of saikosaponin-f and the root extract of *Bupleurum kaoi*, *Fitoterapia*, 65, 409–417.

Yu, Y., Yang, W.-X., Wang, H., Zhang, W.-Z., Liu, B.-H., and Dong, Z.-Y. (2002) Characteristics and mechanism of enzyme secretion and increase in [Ca^{2+}]i in saikosaponin (I) stimulated rat pancreatic acinar cells, *World J. Gastroenterol.*, 15, 524–527.

Zong, Z.-P., Fujikawa-Yamamoto, K., Ota, T., Guan, X., Murakami, M., Li, A.-l., Yamaguchi, N., Tanino, M., and Odashima, S. (1998) Saikosaponin b$_2$ induces differentiation without growth inhibition in cultured B16 melanoma cells, *Cell Struct. Funct.*, 23, 265–272.

12 Mitogenic Substances of Bupleuri Radix

Naohito Ohno and Toshiro Yadomae

CONTENTS

12.1 INTRODUCTION

During the period of rapid growth in the latter half of the 1980s, many enterprises entered the biotechnology industry, with one of their targets being the development of immunomodulatory substances. The new immunomodulators have inspired us to dream of contributing to various medical procedures including phylaxis, enhancement of immunity to cancer, mitigation of the adverse effects of carcinostatics, transplants, modulation of autoimmune response, and slowing of the process of aging. All of the ailments/conditions mentioned above have been the major causes of death to this day. There were two factors that supported the numerous new entries into this industry: In Japan, Krestin, a carcinostatic, the main mechanism of which is the activation of the immune system, was showing strong sales, and Maruyama vaccine made from tubercle bacillus was one of the most exciting means of immunotherapy against cancer. Around the same time, in the area of basic immunology, the crystal structure of the histocompatibility antigen was discovered, and as a result, the functions of the T cell, one of the immunocompetent cells, were being explained at both the clonal level and the molecular level. This clarified the mechanism of self/non-self discrimination, and immunology, which previously was a science that was mainly based on hypothesis, rapidly transformed itself into a science of real substances. In addition, with the discovery of the $\gamma\delta$ T cell, the specificity of the immune system of the mucous membrane was explained. The remarkable advancement in genetic and cellular engineering technologies supported the development of basic science. Thus, expectations were high for immunology to contribute to both basic science and industry. With the number of new research groups increasing, investment in this industry skyrocketed. In the 21st century, some of the biotechnological products that were developed in the 1980s are being clinically applied as pharmaceuticals and used for treating patients.

The effort to scientifically explain the effects of Chinese herbal medicine has a long history. One objective of such effort is to understand the effects of Chinese herbal medicine from a scientific or Occidental-medicinal viewpoint. Another is to develop new pharmaceuticals from the components of Chinese herbal medicine. There are many Chinese herbal medicines that contain Bupleuri radix (see Chapters 13 and 16) and, therefore, analysis of this crude drug is significant for the analysis of a model crude drug. Moreover, Chinese herbal medicines are ethical drugs that are listed in the NHI (National Health Insurance) Price Standards of Japan, and therefore, the afore-mentioned analysis is also important in terms of the appropriate use of medical expenses.

Mitogens induce lymphoblastogenesis, and bacterial endotoxin lipopolysaccharide (LPS) and concanavalin A, a plant agglutinin, are known to be typical mitogens. When these substances are added to a suspension of splenic cells in an *in vitro* culture system, lymphocytes in the stationary phase undergo blastogenesis and DNA synthesis. Antigens activate only single clones and therefore, their specificity is high but their sensitivity is low. In contrast, mitogen induces polyclonal blasto-genesis of lymphocytes, enabling high-sensitivity detection. The incubation period is 2 to 3 days. Bacterial endotoxins that show this activity are also septic shock inducers; therefore, various analyses have been conducted to modify these substances and develop new and useful pharmaceu-ticals from them. These are being used as the prototypical substances today. Although mitogen induces polyclonal blastogenesis, some substances activated have unique characteristics. Bacterial endotoxins mainly act as B cell mitogens, and activate macrophages as well. On the other hand, concanavalin A is a T-cell mitogen. Among the exotoxins of pathogenic microorganisms are the super antigens that activate specific groups of T cells to the oligoclonal state. In many cases, mitogen exhibits activity in other immunity evaluation systems. For example, bacterial endotoxins demon-strate adjuvant activity, antitumor activity, metastatis-repressing activity, macrophage activation, complement activation, and cytokine generation; in fact, they seem to demonstrate all the immune activities imaginable. This indicates that using mitogenic activity as the index for screening active substances may lead to discoveries of various immunological activities. Today, a number of eval-uation systems have been established, but in the 1980s, there were only a limited number of systems, and mitogenic activity was widely used. We used this activity as the index for searching active substances.

Before we studied Bupleuri radix mitogen, we attempted to fractionate and purify mitogens from ascomycetes (of fungi *Peziza vesiculosa* and *Sclerotinia sclerotiorum*), and mitogens origi-nating from the crude drug Dang Gui (Tohki in Japanese, the root of *Angelica actiloba*) (Ohno et al., 1983, 1984, 1985, 1986a, 1986b; Mimura et al., 1985; Suzuki et al., 1985; Shinohara et al., 1991a, 1991b, 1992). Because we were also interested in the immunomodulatory activities of polysaccharides, we determined the structure of the pneumococcal capsular polysaccharide (Yadomae et al., 1979; Ohno et al., 1982), isolated D-glucan from various mycetes, and analyzed their structures and activities (Ohno et al., 1986, 1987, 2000, 2001; Cirelli et al., 1989; Suzuki et al., 1989, 2002; Kurachi et al., 1990; Sakurai et al., 1992; Tokunaka et al., 2000). When D-glucan was fractionated using the *in vivo* antitumor activity against transplanted tumor in mouse as the index, we found that 6-branched 1,3-D-glucan could be relatively easily purified. Mitogen could also be heat-extracted; therefore, it is a thermostable component, and the active component must be a polysaccharide. However, there were significant difficulties in the purification and structural analysis of the active component. For example, the active component of *P. vesiculosa* showed an extremely wide molecular weight distribution and strong adsorbability by hydrophobic chromatog-raphy, lost its activity in alkaline media, and generally demonstrated qualities that contrasted to the known qualities of polysaccharides (Ohno et al., 1984, 1986). On the other hand, the active component of *S. sclerotiorum* is a protein that we named sclerogen, but it showed activity only after thermal polymerization (Shinohara et al., 1991, 1992). Dang Gui was obtained together with its main component, pectin, but its activity was maintained even after hydrolysis by pectinase; therefore, the component was unlikely to be a simple polysaccharide (Ohno et al., 1983). Because the crude hot-water extract of Bupleuri radix demonstrated mitogenic activity, we attempted to isolate mitogen from it. As most Chinese herbal medicines are orally administered, our objective was to isolate a low-molecular-weight component that could be easily absorbed. This was in line with our primary objective of utilizing the component as a future pharmaceutical after structural

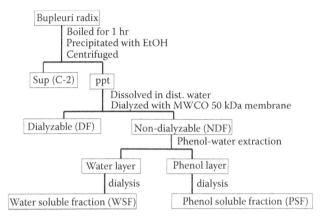

FIGURE 12.1 Fractionation scheme of Bupleuri radix.

analysis and modification. However, as explained below, we were unable to find a component that meets this goal. Instead, we were able to obtain a macromolecular active component.

12.2 FRACTIONATION

Root of *Bupleurum chinense* DC. imported from China, cut into thin slices, was provided by Kanebo Co., Ltd. (Osaka). After much trial and error, we found that the most efficient fractionation method for the active component from the hot-water extract was dialysis based on molecular weight cutoff, followed by phenol extraction (Figure 12.1) (Oka et al., 1995; Izumi et al., 1997). Table 12.1 and Figure 12.2 show the yield and composition and the corresponding activities. The macromolecular fraction (NDF) exhibited strong activity, and NDF was fractionated into the water-soluble fraction (WSF) and the phenol-soluble fraction (PSF) by phenol-water extraction. As is explained later, the oxidation of these fractions by $NaClO_2$ suggested that WSF contained the active component with polysaccharide qualities, while PSF contained the active component with lignin-like qualities. By examining possible immunostimulating properties using WSF and PSF, we observed, in addition to mitogenic activity, the ability to increase B lymphocyte surface immunoglobulin (sIg) (Table 12.2), the production of nitric oxide (NO) by macrophages (Figure 12.3), the production of acid phosphatase (data not shown), and the production of interleukin-6 (IL-6) (Figure 12.4). In all cases, PSF showed stronger activity than WSF. In this study, we initially assumed that the thermostable active component must be a polysaccharide; however, the primary active component was obtained from substances that did not seem to be polysaccharides. Bacterial endotoxins, the most extensively

TABLE 12.1
Yield and Physicochemical Properties of High-Molecular-Weight Fractions

	Yield (mg/100 g radix)	Protein/Polyphenol (%)	Neutral Sugar (%)	Uronic Acid (%)	Elemental Analysis (%)		
					C	H	N
NDF	1230 ± 98	27 ± 3.7	40 ± 3.7	24 ± 3.2	39.8	5.9	1.1
PSF	71 ± 21	48 ± 5.6	27 ± 3.5	2.2 ± 1.7	46	6.1	4.7
WSF	551 ± 71	2.8 ± 1.3	37 ± 4.7	38 ± 5.5	39.5	5.5	0.4

Note: Concentration of protein and/or polyphenol, neutral sugar, and uronic acid were determined by BCA kit, phenol-sulfuric acid, and *m*-hydroxydiphenyl methods, respectively, using bovine serum albumin, glucose, and galacturonic acid as the standards.

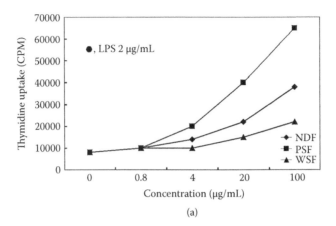

(a)

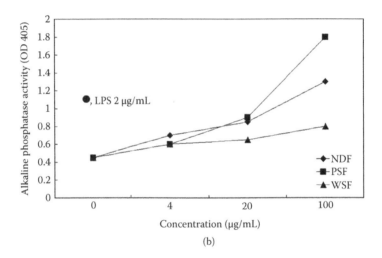

(b)

FIGURE 12.2 Mitogenic activity of high-molecular-weight fractions of Bupleuri radix extracts. Indicated concentration of each fraction was added to murine (male C3H/HeN) spleen cell suspension and cultured for 3 days in CO_2 incubator. (a) Proliferation of leukocytes was measured by adding tracer amount of ^{3}H-TdR. (b) Resulting culture supernatants were collected and measured alkaline phosphatase activity to monitor leukocyte proliferation and differentiation. Bacterial LPS was used as standard.

analyzed active components, were obtained from WSF by phenol-water extraction, suggesting that the active components have at least a novelty. Some may find the mention of bacterial endotoxins unusual; however, these endotoxins demonstrated most of the known actions to activate the immune system, they are widely distributed in nature, and some plants live in symbiosis with microorganisms (Dziarski and Gupta, 2000; Beutler, 2002). Therefore, we believe that the endotoxins are worth mentioning for the sake of comparison. This is an important point that requires special attention in our search for immunostimulating components.

We further fractionated PSF by ion-exchange chromatography, and found that the active fraction adsorbed strongly to DEAE-Cellulofine (Figure 12.5 through Figure 12.7, Table 12.3). The stronger the adsorption, the stronger the activity of the fraction. In terms of molecular weight distribution, using different dialysis membranes with different cutoff molecular weights, we further fractionated PSF into 1 to 3.5 kDa, 3.5 to 10 kDa, 10 to 50 kDa, and >50 kDa fractions (Figure 12.8, Table 12.4). Comparison of these fractions revealed that mitogen activity was observed in all of them,

TABLE 12.2
Expression of Surface Immunoglobulins by High-Molecular-Weight Fractions

	Concentration (µg/ml)	Positive Cell (%)	
		sIgM	sIgG
Control		20.1	14.2
LPS	10	69.3	50.1
	2	58.2	45.4
PSF	100	45.5	40.6
WSF	100	30	26.7

Note: Spleen cells (1.25×10^6cells/well) were cultured for 72 h with each material. The resulting cells were collected and stained with FITC conjugated anti-mouse IgM or anti-mouse IgG. Values were analyzed by flow cytometer.

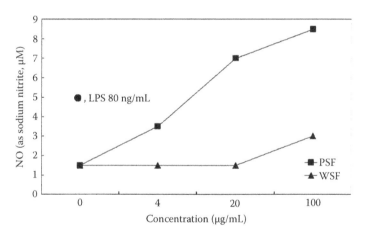

FIGURE 12.3 Nitric oxide synthesis of murine monophage RAW264.7 by Bupleuri radix extracts. Each fraction was added to RAW 264.7 cell suspension and cultured for 1 day in CO_2 incubator. Resulting supernatants were collected and measured nitric oxide by Griess reagent.

suggesting that the active component is extremely diverse in terms of molecular weight (Figure 12.9). However, the activity was dependent on the molecular weight, and the larger the molecule, the stronger the activity.

The above-described fractionation revealed that the active component was found in the high-molecular-weight fraction, and its specific activity was much higher than that of the crude extract. This suggests that an immunosuppressive component may coexist in the crude extract. We therefore tested crude extract with LPS, a representative immunostimulator. The results showed that the ethanol-soluble fraction C-2 strongly suppressed mitogenic activity (Figure 12.10). We did not study this active component further; however, it is likely to be a low-molecular-weight component, and is likely to exhibit some effect *in vivo* .

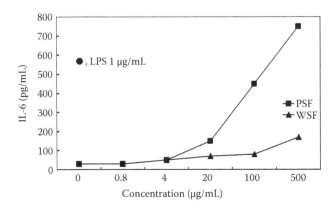

FIGURE 12.4 Interleukin-6 synthesis of murine peritoneal macrophage by Bupleuri radix extracts. Each fraction was added to peritoneal macrophages, elicited by proteose peptone, and cultured for 1 day in CO_2 incubator. Resulting supernatants were collected and measured IL-6 by ELISA.

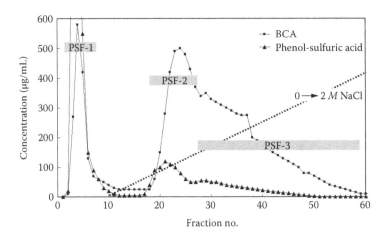

FIGURE 12.5 Further fractionation of mitogenic fraction, PSF, by DEAE-cellulofine A-500m. PSF dissolved in distilled water was applied to DEAE-cellulofine, and extensively washed with distilled water (PSF-1). The column was eluted with a linear gradient of 0 to 2 M NaCl and fractionated. Protein (BCA) and carbohydrate (phenol sulfuric acid) were measured and plotted. Adsorbed fractions were pooled as weakly acidic (PSF-2) and strongly acidic (PSF-3) fractions. PSF-1, -2, and -3 were extensively dialyzed and lyophilized.

12.3 STRUCTURAL ANALYSIS

The above-described results strongly suggested that the primary active component was not a simple polysaccharide. To identify the active component or components, we conducted enzymolysis and chemical modification to check if the activity disappeared. The activity did not disappear upon the addition of protease or glycosidic enzymes. The activity was suppressed upon exposure to acid or base. This tendency was especially conspicuous with alkali treatment. Also, the activity disappeared after oxidation by sodium chlorite ($NaClO_2$), which is a lignin degradation method (Figure 12.11) (Kurakata et al., 1989; Fukuchi et al., 1989; Sakagami et al., 1999).

Lignin is one of the main structural components of the xylem of plants, and the possibility that lignin possesses the activity is undeniable. To compare the solid-state properties of lignin with those of commercially available alkali-treated lignin as control, we conducted various instrumental analyses. Ultraviolet (UV) analysis revealed maximum absorbances at 198, 244, 277, 316, 367,

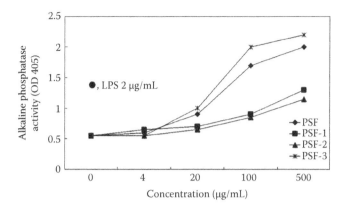

FIGURE 12.6 Mitogenic activity of subfractions of PSF. Indicated concentration of each fraction was added to murine (male C3H/HeN) spleen cell suspension and cultured for 3 days in CO_2 incubator. Resulting culture supernatants were collected and measured alkaline phosphatase activity to monitor leukocyte proliferation and differentiation. Bacterial LPS was used as standard.

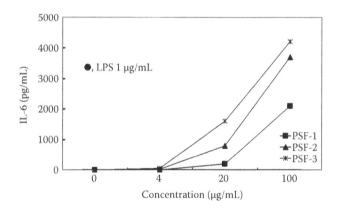

FIGURE 12.7 Interleukin-6 synthesis of murine peritoneal macrophage by subfractions of PSF. Each fraction was added to peritoneal macrophages, elicited by proteose peptone, and cultured for 1 day in CO_2 incubator. Resulting supernatants were collected and measured IL-6 by ELISA.

TABLE 12.3
Yield and Physicochemical Properties of Subfractions of PSF Separated by DEAE-Cellulofine A-500m

	Yield (%)	Protein/Polyphenol (%)	Neutral Sugar (%)	Uronic Acid (%)	Elemental Analysis (%)		
					C	H	N
PSF	100	48.0 ± 5.6	27.0 ± 3.5	2.2 ± 1.7	46	6.1	4.7
PSF-1	22.6 ± 2.0	14.1 ± 3.6	49.9 ± 11.7	1.7 ± 0.8	40.0 ± 1.3	5.7 ± 0.2	1.6 ± 0.4
PSF-2	12.2 ± 3.9	41.1 ± 9.7	20.9 ± 4.3	5.7 ± 4.5	44.6 ± 1.0	5.8 ± 0.1	5.5 ± 0.7
PSF-3	21.1 ± 4.5	63.4 ± 5.8	13.2 ± 1.3	3.2 ± 2.2	43.6 ± 2.5	5.4 ± 0.3	5.5 ± 0.2

Note: Components were determined by the methods shown in Table 12.1 note.

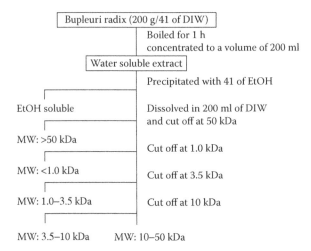

FIGURE 12.8 Fractionation of Bupleuri radix mitogen by means of molecular weight. Molecular weight separation was done by the dialysis membrane having appropriate molecular weight cutoff size.

TABLE 12.4
Physicochemical Properties of Subfractions of Bupleuri Radix by Means of Molecular Weight Fractionation

MW (kDa)	<1.0	1.0–3.5	3.5–10	10–50	>50
Yield (g) from 200 g Bupleuri radix	7.04 ± 0.98	0.28 ± 0.11	0.55 ± 0.26	0.59 ± 0.11	2.46 ± 0.2
BCA (%)	1.5	4.9	4.8	4.1	Not done
Phenol-sulfuric acid (%)	10.2	23.2	28.1	29.8	Not done
R.I. value (ESR)	0.1687	0.989	1.0536	1.5017	Not done
g value (ESR)	2.0055	2.0053	2.0055	2.0054	Not done
After NaClO$_2$ treatment					
Yield (%)	Not done	20	20	38	Not done
BCA (%)	Not done	1.6	1.4	1.1	Not done
Phenol-sulfuric acid (%)	Not done	18.3	16.7	34.9	Not done
R.I. value (ESR)	Not done	0.1613	0.2787	0.2592	Not done
g value (ESR)	Not done	2.0055	2.0051	2.0053	Not done

Note: Subfractions were prepared as shown in Figure 12.8. R.I. and g values were measured in solid state by ESR.

and 404 nm, similar to those of alkali-treated lignin. These peaks were shifted to the lower wavelength region under acidic conditions, again similar to the case of alkali-treated lignin. Electron spin resonance (ESR) showed that the stable radical of the lignin was found at $g = 2.005$, and this property was also similar between the two (Ohtsu et al., 1997; Sakagami et al., 1998). Infrared (IR) and nuclear magnetic resonance (NMR) analyses also showed that the signals of the two substances were similar. Since the substance was still a mixture, structural analyses could not be conducted, but the activity strongly suggested that it was a product of the partial degradation of lignin.

12.4 PEROXIDASES

To prove the presence of lignin, we studied the peroxidases (PODs) that are closely related to the synthesis and degradation of lignin. In general, Bupleuri radix and other crude drugs of plant origin

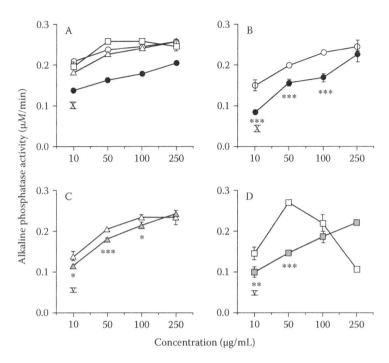

FIGURE 12.9 Mitogenic activity of subfractions of Bupleuri radix extracts by means of molecular weight and chemical modification. (A): <10 kDa, ●: 1.0 to 3.5 kDa, ○: 3.5 to 10 kDa, △: 10 to 50 kDa, □. (B to D) Effect of NaClO₂ treatment. (B) <10 kDa: before, ○, after, ●. (C) 1.0 to 3.5 kDa: before, △, after, ▲. (D) 10 to 50 kDa: before, □, after, ■. The significance was evaluated by Student's t-test against the corresponding parent sample. $*p < 0.05$; $**p < 0.01$, $***p < 0.001$.

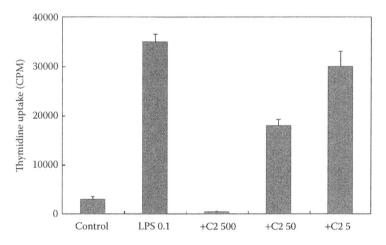

FIGURE 12.10 Effect of ethanol soluble subfraction, C-2, on mitogenic activity of LPS. A solution of LPS (0.1 µg/ml) was mixed with various concentration of C-2 (500, 50, or 5 µg/ml) and added to the spleen cell culture. Proliferation of leukocytes were measured by adding tracer amount of ³H-TdR.

are dried under appropriate conditions before use. It is believed that many plant PODs are more stable than other enzymes and their activities are retained after collection (Kolattukudy et al., 1992; Nicolas et al., 1994; Fujiyama et al., 1995; Wojtaszek, 1997; Piontek et al., 2001; Gajhede, 2001). One such generally used enzyme is horseradish peroxidase (HRP), which is essential for various immunochemical analyses.

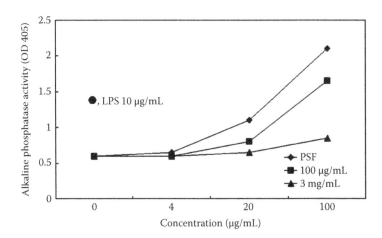

FIGURE 12.11 Effect of $NaClO_2$ treatment on mitogenic activity of PSF. A solution of PSF was treated with 100 μg/ml or 3 mg/ml of $NaClO_2$ at 75°C for 5 min. After extensive dialysis, the mitogenic activity of the resulting materials was measured.

We discovered by chance that the commercially available thinly sliced Bupleuri radix retained this enzymatic activity. To identify the mitogen, we deemed it necessary to prepare synthetic lignin by utilizing this enzyme and to compare the activity. For this purpose, we attempted to isolate the enzyme (Figure 12.12). As is shown in the scheme, we obtained the crude extract at 4°C from the thinly sliced Bupleuri radix by PBS, then purified it to an almost single protein band by dialysis, ion-exchange chromatography, and affinity chromatography using Con A agarose. The table indicates the purification process (Table 12.5). We performed Western blotting using commercially available anti-HRP antibody, and observed a distinct reaction (data not shown). The final purification product also showed the reaction. Interestingly, in the case of the crude extract, multiple bands were stained by the antibody, but as the purification progressed, the number of stained bands decreased. Many higher plants have POD isozymes, and it is known that their occurrence is controlled tissue-specifically. There are reports that 42 types of isozymes coexist in commercially available HRP. Considering the above, there is a high possibility of multiple PODs existing in Bupleuri radix, and they are similar to HRP in terms of protein chemical composition.

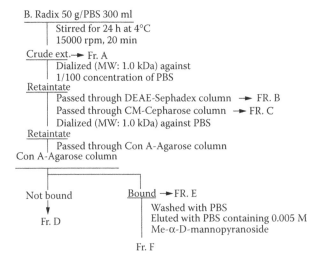

FIGURE 12.12 Purification of peroxidase from Bupleuri radix.

TABLE 12.5
Purification of Peroxidase from Bupleuri Radix

Fraction	Peroxidase (U/ml)	Total Activity (U)	Protein (mg/ml)	Total Protein (mg)	Specific Activity (U/mg)
A	0.26	53.5	7.8	1590	0.03
B	0.12	34.1	1	302	0.12
C	0.11	32.3	0.61	180	0.18
D	0.0062	1.6	0.17	43.4	0.04
E	0.0038	1.9	0.016	8	0.24
F	0.2	2	0.048	0.48	4.2

Note: Peroxidase of Bupleuri radix was purified by the method shown in Figure 12.12. Peroxidase activity was measured by the tetrametnylbenzidine substrate system. Unit was calculated in comparison with that of HRP.

12.5 SYNTHESIZED LIGNIN

Using HRP and Bupleuri radix POD purified as described above, and using also three types of phenyl propanoids — caffeic acid (CA), *trans*-ferulic acid (FA), *p*-coumaric acid (pCA) — as precursors, we performed the enzymatic synthesis of the lignin-like macromolecular component. The basic synthetic method was similar to that by Sakagami et al. (Sakagami et al., 1995, 1998, 1999; Fukuchi et al., 1989; Kurakata et al., 1989, 1990; Abe et al., 1989; Kikuchi et al., 1991). The yield and analytical data are shown in Table 12.6. The yield or quality was not uniform, perhaps because the synthesis was performed under a single reaction condition. The synthesized lignin also showed characteristic ESR signals. We used them to assess mitogenic activity. As a result, the macromolecular component exhibited strong mitogenic activity (Figure 12.13).

We attempted the same process as above with Bupleuri radix POD. The yield and analytical data are shown in Table 12.7. The yield of the macromolecular fraction by using Bupleuri radix POD was not as high as that using HRP, perhaps due to an insufficient amount of the enzyme. Furthermore, the macromolecular component obtained by using CA as precursor indicated similar activities between Bupleuri radix POD and HRP (Figure 12.14). With these synthesized lignins, however, macrophage activation was not observed, which suggested that the active component was not formed only by simple enzymatic synthesis. As was mentioned before, multiple POD isozymes existed in Bupleuri radix as well. We used only the fraction that adsorbed to Con A agarose for enzymatic synthesis. The possibility of different isozymes forming different polymer structures remains and should be studied in the future.

12.6 INTERACTION WITH LOW-MOLECULAR-WEIGHT COMPONENT

As discussed, the active component of *S. sclerotiorum* was formed only after thermal denaturation of the protein (Shinohara et al., 1991). Since Chinese herbal medicines are prepared by hot-water extraction, it is possible that the active component is formed, enhanced, lost, or otherwise modified in the process. We obtained anti-Bupleuri radix antiserum by immunizing rabbits against the hot-water extract of the Bupleuri radix macromolecular fraction. We added this antiserum to the cold-water extract of Bupleuri radix. Multiple protein bands were stained by Western blotting. On the other hand, in the case of the hot-water extract, we observed the reaction of an ultrahigh-molecular-weight component that did not get into the PAGE gel. These results suggested that protein

TABLE 12.6
Yield and Properties of Polymerized Phenylpropanoids Catalyzed by HRP

Phenylpropanoid	Molecular Weight Range (kDa)	Endwise Polymerization			Bulk Polymerization		
		1.0–10	10–50	>50	1.0–10	10–50	>50
Caffeic acid	Yield (g)	0.35	0.88	0.49	0.25	1.31	0.41
(CA)	Recovery (%)	17.3	44	24.3	12.6	65.4	20.7
	R.I. value	3.04	3.41	3.28	3.2	3.25	3.26
	g value	2.0068	2.0054	2.0053	2.0061	2.0053	2.0053
trans-Ferulic acid	Yield (g)	0.06	0.02	1.65	0.14	0.04	1.6
(FA)	Recovery (%)	3.2	1.1	82.5	7.2	2.2	80
	R.I. value	2.4	1.86	1.94	2.34	2.52	2.51
	g value	2.0057	2.0056	2.0055	2.0056	2.0056	2.0055
p-Coumaric acid	Yield (g)	0.11	0.05	1.07	0.16	0.06	1.7
(pCA)	Recovery (%)	5.6	2.5	53.6	8.1	2.8	85.1
	R.I. value	0.73	0.77	1.33	1.32	1.34	1.33
	g value	2.0055	2.0058	2.0057	2.0056	2.0057	2.0058
Mixture	Yield (g)	0.11	0.05	1.26	0.05	0.03	1.48
(Co-polymer)	Recovery (%)	6.5	3.1	77.7	3.3	2.1	91.8
	R.I. value	3.04	2.56	2.59	2.3	1.78	2.35
	g value	2.0065	2.0067	2.0063	2.0055	2.0055	2.0056

Note: HRP: horseradish peroxidase. Corresponding phenylpropanoid was added gradually for 1 h period in the case of endwise polymerization. R.I. and g values were obtained in solid state by ESR measurement.

denaturation and polymerization occurred during the hot-water extraction of Bupleuri radix, and that it had some relation to the formation of the active component.

Based on this observation, we analyzed the possible formation and modification of the active component through the extraction and purification process from several points of view. First, we checked the possibility of the transformation of low-molecular-weight components into macromolecular components. We added amino acid and sugar labeled with trace amounts of isotope, and then prepared extract from Bupleuri radix (Figure 12.15). The amino acid and sugar used were arginine and glucose, respectively, because they were found in the largest amounts in Bupleuri radix. Then, we fractionated the extracts to ethanol-soluble and ethanol-insoluble fractions. The results showed that in Bupleuri radix most of the arginine in the extracts was found in the ethanol-insoluble fraction, whereas most of the glucose remained in the ethanol-soluble fraction (Table 12.8). Next, we heated the ethanol-soluble fraction of Bupleuri radix containing arginine, in an attempt to form the insoluble macromolecule. The results showed that the larger the amount of arginine added, the larger the amount of macromolecule formed, and the macromolecule demonstrated mitogenic activity. This indicated that a component that did not originally have the activity was transformed into an active component by heat treatment.

12.7 CONCLUSIONS

We discovered that a lignin-like macromolecule, polysaccharides, and products of heat denaturation contribute to the mitogenic activity of Bupleuri radix. In particular, the lignin-like macromolecule was proved to have the strongest mitogenic activity, as confirmed by enzymatic synthesis using POD.

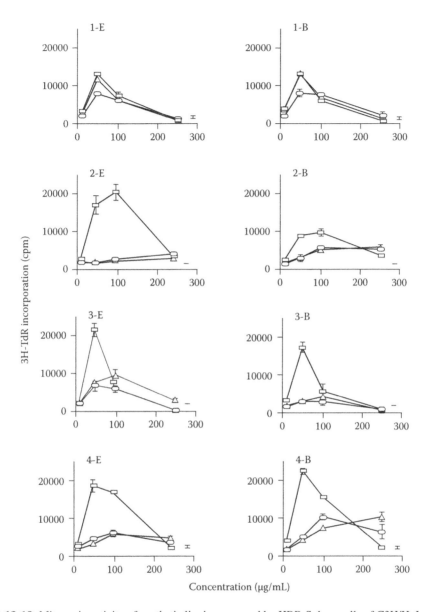

FIGURE 12.13 Mitogenic activity of synthetic lignins prepared by HRP. Spleen cells of C3H/HeJ mice were cultured with various concentrations of synthetic lignins shown in Table 12.6. Mitogenic activity was measured by ^{3}H-TdR incorporation. 1: caffeic acid, 2: *trans*-ferulic acid, 3: *p*-coumaric acid, 4: co-polymer; E: endwise polymerization; B: bulk polymerization; 1.0 to 10 kDa, ○; 10 to 50 kDa, △; >50 kDa, □.

Known examples of the immunomodulating activity of the lignin-like macromolecule originating from natural sources include the pinecone lignin and the shiitake mushroom LEM (Kurakata et al., 1990; Bolwell et al., 1995; Wojtaszek 1997). Sakagami et al. systematically analyzed the antimicrobial and pharmacological actions of synthetic lignin (Sakagami et al., 1995, 1998, 1999; Fukuchi et al., 1989; Kurakata et al., 1989, 1990; Abe et al., 1989; Kikuchi et al., 1991). Bupleuri radix mitogen is expected to belong to the same category. However, the crude drug contains various polyphenols, and their quality as well as quantity varies widely from one crude drug to another. There is no doubt that the microstructure of the product of enzymatic synthesis depends strongly on the type of polyphenol present at the time of synthesis of the lignin-like substance. The structure

TABLE 12.7
Yield and Properties of Polymerized
Phenylpropanoids Catalyzed by Peroxidase
from Bupleuri Radix

Phenylpropanoid		Endwise	Bulk
Caffeic acid	Yield (mg)	66	100
(CA)	Recovery (%)	33	50
	R.I. value	1.55	1.68
trans-Ferulic acid	Yield (g)	45	67
(FA)	Recovery (%)	22.5	33.5
	R.I. value	1.22	1.61
p-Coumaric acid	Yield (g)	17	18
(pCA)	Recovery (%)	8.5	9.
	R.I. value	0.94	0.79

Note: Polymerization was performed by a method similar to that shown in Table 12.6. Peroxidase of Bupleuri radix was used for polymerization.

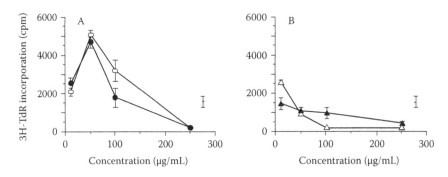

FIGURE 12.14 Mitogenic activity of synthetic lignins prepared by peroxidase of Bupleuri radix. Spleen cells of C3H/HeJ mice were cultured with various concentrations of synthetic lignins shown in Table 12.7. Mitogenic activity was measured by ^{3}H-TdR incorporation. (A) Caffeic acid; (B) *trans*-ferulic acid; endwise polymerization, ○, △; bulk polymerization, ●, ▲.

and activity of the lignin-like macromolecule of individual crude drugs should be studied further. In this study, we were able to confirm the mitogenic activity of the synthesized lignin on B cells; however, macrophage activation was not reproduced. This may be explained by the difference in the precursor involved in enzymatic synthesis, and the heat treatment procedure.

Various receptors involved in natural immunity are found to exist in immunocompetent cells. Each of the more than ten types of Toll-like receptors recognizes bacterial endotoxins, peptidoglycans, lipoproteins, flagellae, or DNAs, and differentiates and activates each immunocompetent cell (Means et al., 2000; Akira, 2001; Beutler, 2002; Kaisho and Akira, 2002; Henneke and Golenbock, 2002). The bacterial endotoxin that drew the greatest attention initially was the CD 14 molecule as a receptor (Henneke and Golenbock, 2002). In addition, the importance of the TLR4-MD2 complex is slowly gaining recognition (Dziarski and Gupta, 2000; Henneke and Golenbock, 2002). It is difficult to analyze the mechanism of even a single immunostimulating component. Regarding

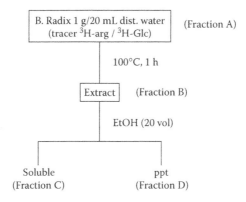

FIGURE 12.15 Incorporation of arginine and glucose into polymer fractions by hot water extraction of Bupleuri radix assessed by tritiated tracers.

TABLE 12.8
Recovery of Radioactivity in Subfractions of the Hot Water Extract of Bupleuri Radix

	Subfraction			
	A	B	C	D
^{3}H-Arginine (%)	100	95.1	38.7	57.8
^{3}H-Glucose (%)	100	90.9	83.6	9.1

Subfractions were prepared as shown in Figure 12.15.

	Subfraction (molecular weight)			
	<1.0	1.0–3.5	3.5–10	>10
^{3}H-Arginine (%)	92.7	2.7	0.7	1.4
Weight (mg)	29.4	3.6	2.3	25.9
BCA (µg)	214	32	36	758
Phenol-sulfuric acid (mg)	4.3	0.5	0.4	12

From 1 g Bupleuri radix. Subfraction D was further separated by dialysis membrane.

the primary immunostimulating component, the mechanisms involved in activating cells through receptors have been clarified, but many other secondary immunostimulating components have been overlooked. Of course, some of these mechanisms are difficult to explain because of their complexity, despite strenuous effort to analyze them. We need to exert more effort than ever in the detailed and multidimensional analyses of the lignin-like macromolecule. As the lignin-like macromolecule is expected to have molecular diversity, considerable effort will be needed to analyze it in detail.

As discussed in other chapters of this book, Bupleuri radix contains various immunomodulatory substances. We discovered that the methanol-soluble fraction considerably lowers the activity of bacterial endotoxins. This means that immunostimulating and immunosuppressing components coexist in Bupleuri radix. This study mainly focused on the immunostimulating components; however, considering that most of the Chinese herbal medicines are administered orally, we may be required to think that the effects of the macromolecular components should be optimized. Recent advances in immunology have revealed that approximately half of the lymphocytes in the body are concentrated in the digestive tract. The lymphocytes of the digestive tract are found on the surface of mucous membranes, where contact with the external environment is facilitated (Mayer, 1997; Duchmann et al., 1997; Owen, 1999; Zarzaur and Kudsk, 2001; Chodosh and Kennedy, 2002). In addition, Peyer's patches are found on the inner surface of the digestive tract, to obtain information directly from within the digestive tract. The active component of mitogen induces lymphoblasto-genesis on the Peyer's patches, thereby possibly activating the host's immune system *in vivo* through gastrointestinal immunity.

It has been proved that the immune system works in coordination with the nervous and endocrine systems. As was explained before, the lignin-like substance commonly exists in plants around us, and it is highly possible that we are ingesting it daily as food. The maintenance of the immune mechanism is dependent not solely on specific drugs, but also on clothing, eating, and living habits, as well as on other aspects of human life. The processing of food by enterobacteria, and the products that the enterobacteria themselves produce must not be overlooked either. We hope that the use-fulness of Chinese herbal medicine will be clarified in detail in the near future.

ACKNOWLEDGMENTS

We are grateful to Professor Kikuo Nomoto, Professor emeritus, Kyusyu University, and Dr. Takuya Kawakita, Kanebo Co., Ltd. for scientific discussions, advice, and valuable reagents; Dr. Shigeru Izumi, Hideki Oka, Shogo Iwanaga, and Sadanori Ohtsu for their contributions in fractionation, cell culture, and instrumental analyses.

REFERENCES

Abe, M., Okamoto, K., Konno, K., and Sakagami, H. (1989) Induction of antiparasite activity by pine cone lignin-related substances, *In Vivo*, 3, 359–362.

Akira, S. (2001) Toll-like receptors and innate immunity, *Adv. Immunol.*, 78, 1–56.

Beutler, B. (2002) Toll-like receptors: how they work and what they do,. *Curr. Opin. Hematol.*, 9, 2–10.

Bolwell, G.P., Butt, V.S., Davies, D.R., and Zimmerlin, A. (1995) The origin of the oxidative burst in plants, *Free Radic. Res.*, 23, 517–532.

Chodosh, J. and Kennedy R.C. (2002) The conjunctival lymphoid follicle in mucosal immunology, *DNA Cell Biol.*, 21, 421–433.

Cirelli, A.F., Covian, J.A., Ohno, N., Adachi, Y., and Yadomae, T. (1989) Effect of sulfation on the biological activity of beta-$(1\rightarrow3)$-glucans from the tree fungus *Cyttaria harioti* Fischer, *Carbohydr. Res.*, 190, 329–337.

Duchmann, R., Neurath, M., Marker, Hermann, E., Meyer, Z., and Buschenfelde, K.H. (1997) Immune responses towards intestinal bacteria—current concepts and future perspectives, *Z. Gastroenterol.*, 35, 337–346.

Dziarski, R. and Gupta, D. (2000) Role of MD-2 in TLR2- and TLR4-mediated recognition of Gram-negative and Gram-positive bacteria and activation of chemokine genes, *J. Endotoxin Res.*, 6, 401–405.

Fujiyama, K., Intapruk, C., and Shinmyo, A. (1995) Gene structures of peroxidase isoenzymes in horseradish and Arabidopsis thaliana and their expression, *Biochem. Soc. Trans.*, 23, 245–246.

Fukuchi, K., Sakagami, H., Ikeda, M., Kawazoe, Y., Oh Hara, T., Konno, K., Ichikawa, S., Hata, N., Kondo, H., and Nonoyama, M. (1989) Inhibition of herpes simplex virus infection by pine cone antitumor substances, *Anticancer Res.*, 9, 313–317.

Gajhede, M. (2001) Plant peroxidases: substrate complexes with mechanistic implications, *Biochem. Soc. Trans.*, 29, 91–98.

Henneke, P. and Golenbock, D.T. (2002) Innate immune recognition of lipopolysaccharide by endothelial cells, *Crit. Care Med.*, 30, S207–213.

Izumi, S., Ohno, N., Kawakita, T., Nomoto, K., and Yadomae, T. (1997) Wide range of molecular weight distribution of mitogenic substance(s) in the hot water extract of a Chinese herbal medicine, *Bupleurum chinense*, *Biol. Pharm. Bull.*, 20, 759–764.

Kaisho, T. and Akira, S. (2002) Toll-like receptors as adjuvant receptors, *Biochim. Biophys. Acta,* 1589, 1–13.

Kikuchi, K., Sakagami, H., Fujinaga, S., Kawazoe, Y., Oh Hara, T., Ichikawa, S., Kurakata, Y., Takeda, M., and Sato, T. (1991) Stimulation of mouse peritoneal macrophages by lignin-related substances, *Anticancer Res.,* 11, 841–845.

Kolattukudy, P.E., Mohan, R., Bajar, M.A., and Sherf, B.A. (1992) Plant peroxidase gene expression and function, *Biochem. Soc. Trans.,* 20, 333–337.

Kurachi, K., Ohno, N., and Yadomae, T. (1990) Preparation and antitumor activity of hydroxyethylated derivatives of 6-branched (1→3)-beta-D-glucan, SSG, obtained from the culture filtrate of *Sclerotinia sclerotiorum* IFO 9395, *Chem. Pharm. Bull* (Tokyo), 38, 2527–2531.

Kurakata, Y., Sakagami, H., Takeda, M., Konno, K., Kitajima, K., Ichikawa, S., Hata, N., and Sato, T. (1989) Mitogenic activity of pine cone extracts against cultured splenocytes from normal and tumor-bearing animals, *Anticancer Res.,* 9, 961–966.

Kurakata, Y., Sakagami, H., Oh Hara, T., Kawazoe, Y., Asano, K., Fujinaga, S., Takeda, M., and Sato, T. (1990) Mitogenic activity of natural and synthetic lignins against cultured splenocytes, *In Vivo,* 4, 377–380.

Mayer, L. (1997) Review article: Local and systemic regulation of mucosal immunity, *Aliment. Pharmacol. Ther.,* 11(Suppl. 3), 81–85.

Means, T.K., Golenbock, D.T., and Fenton, M.J. (2000) The biology of Toll-like receptors, *Cytokine Growth Factor Rev.,* 11, 219–232.

Mimura, H., Ohno, N., Suzuki, I., and Yadomae, T. (1985) Purification, antitumor activity, and structural characterization of beta-1,3-glucan from *Peziza vesiculosa, Chem. Pharm. Bull.* (Tokyo), 33, 5096–5099.

Nicolas, J.J., Richard Forget, F.C., Goupy, P.M., Amiot, M.J., and Aubert, S.Y. (1994) Enzymatic browning reactions in apple and apple products, *Crit. Rev. Food Sci. Nutr.,* 34, 109–157.

Ohno, N., Yadomae, T., and Miyazaki, T. (1982) Characterization of type XIX capsular polysaccharide from *Streptococcus pneumoniae* IID 559, *Microbiol. Immunol.,* 26, 523–530.

Ohno, N., Matsumoto, S., Suzuki, I., Miyazaki, T., Kumazawa, Y., Otsuka, Y., and Yadomae, T. (1983) Biochemical and physicochemical characterization of a mitogen obtained from an oriental crude drug, Tohki (*Angelica actiloba* Kitagawa), *J. Pharmacobiodyn.,* 6, 903–912.

Ohno, N., Suzuki, I., Miyazaki, T., and Yadomae, T. (1984) Requirement of anionic groups for the mitogenicity of a fungal mitogen, vesiculogen, *Microbiol. Immunol.,* 28, 821–830.

Ohno, N., Mimura, H., Suzuki, I., and Yadomae, T. (1985) Antitumor activity and structural characterization of polysaccharide fractions extracted with cold alkali from a fungus, *Peziza vesiculosa, Chem. Pharm. Bull.* (Tokyo), 33, 2564–2568.

Ohno, N., Mimura, H., Suzuki, I., and Yadomae, T. (1986a) Chemical characterization of a fungal B-cell mitogen obtained from the fruit body of *Peziza vesiculosa, Chem. Pharm. Bull.* (Tokyo), 34, 2112–2117.

Ohno, N., Suzuki, I., and Yadomae, T. (1986b) Structure and antitumor activity of a beta-1,3-glucan isolated from the culture filtrate of *Sclerotinia sclerotiorum* IFO 9395, *Chem. Pharm. Bull.* (Tokyo), 34, 1362–1365.

Ohno, N., Kurachi, K., and Yadomae, T. (1987) Antitumor activity of a highly branched (1→3)-beta-D-glucan, SSG, obtained from *Sclerotinia sclerotiorum* IFO 9395, *J. Pharmacobiodyn.,* 10, 478–486.

Ohno, N., Miura, N.N., Nakajima, M., and Yadomae, T. (2000) Antitumor 1,3-beta-glucan from cultured fruit body of *Sparassis crispa, Biol. Pharm. Bull.,* 23, 866–872.

Ohno, N., Furukawa, M., Miura, N.N., Adachi, Y., Motoi, M., and Yadomae, T. (2001) Antitumor beta glucan from the cultured fruit body of *Agaricus blazei, Biol. Pharm. Bull.,* 24, 820–828.

Ohtsu, S., Izumi, S., Iwanaga, S., Ohno, N., and Yadomae, T. (1997) Analysis of mitogenic substances in *Bupleurum chinese* by ESR spectroscopy, *Biol. Pharm. Bull.,* 20, 97–100.

Oka, H., Ohno, N., Iwanaga, S., Izumi, S., Kawakita, T., Nomoto, K., and Yadomae, T. (1995) Characterization of mitogenic substances in the hot water extracts of bupleuri radix, *Biol. Pharm. Bull.,* 18, 757–765.

Owen, R.L. (1999) Uptake and transport of intestinal macromolecules and microorganisms by M cells in Peyer's patches — a personal and historical perspective, *Semin. Immunol.,* 11, 157–163.

Piontek, K., Smith, A.T., and Blodig, W. (2001) Lignin peroxidase structure and function, *Biochem. Soc. Trans.,* 29, 111–116.

Sakagami, H., Sakagami, T., Yoshida, H., Omata, T., Shiota, F., Takahashi, H., Kawazoe, Y., and Takeda, M. (1995) Hypochlorite scavenging activity of polyphenols, *Anticancer Res.,* 15, 917–921.

Sakagami, H., Kashimata, M., Toguchi, M., Satoh, K., Odanaka, Y., Ida, Y., Premanathan, M., Arakaki, R., Kathiresan, K., Nakashima, H., Komatsu, N., Fujimaki, M., and Yoshihara, M. (1998) Radical modulation activity of lignins from a mangrove plant, *Ceriops decandra* (Griff.) Ding Hou, *In Vivo*, 12, 327–332.

Sakagami, H., Satoh, K., Ida, Y., Koyama, N., Premanathan, M., Arakaki, R., Nakashima, H., Hatano, T., Okuda, T., and Yoshida, T. (1999) Induction of apoptosis and anti-HIV activity by tannin- and lignin-related substances, *Basic Life Sci.*, 66, 595–611.

Sakurai, T., Hashimoto, K., Suzuki, I., Ohno, N., Oikawa, S., Masuda, A., and Yadomae, T. (1992) Enhancement of murine alveolar macrophage functions by orally administered beta-glucan, *Int. J. Immunopharmacol.*, 14, 821–830.

Shinohara, H., Ohno, N., and Yadomae, T. (1991a) Distribution of the mitogenic protein, sclerogen, in extracts from *Sclerotinia sclerotiorum* IFO 9395 assessed by using immunochemical analysis, *J. Pharmacobiodyn.*, 14, 215–221.

Shinohara, H., Ohno, N., and Yadomae, T. (1991b) Isolation of mitogenic substance from sclerotia of *Sclerotinia sclerotiorum* IFO 9395 extracted with phosphate buffer, *Chem. Pharm. Bull.* (Tokyo), 39, 1258–1262.

Shinohara, H., Ohno, N., and Yadomae, T. (1992) Heat induced conformational changes generate mitogenicity to splenocytes by sclerogen from Sclerotinia sclerotiorum IFO 9395, *Chem. Pharm. Bull.* (Tokyo), 40, 2562–2564.

Suzuki, I., Yonekubo, H., Ohno, N., Miyazaki, T., and Yadomae, T. (1985) Effect of a B cell mitogen extracted from a fungus Peziza vesiculosa on antibody production in mice, *J. Pharmacobiodyn.*, 8, 494–502.

Suzuki, I., Hashimoto, K., Ohno, N., Tanaka, H., and Yadomae, T. (1989) Immunomodulation by orally administered beta-glucan in mice, *Int. J. Immunopharmacol.*, 11, 761–769.

Suzuki, T., Tsuzuki, A., Ohno, N., Ohshima, Y., Adachi, Y., and Yadomae, T. (2002) Synergistic action of beta-glucan and platelets on interleukin-8 production by human peripheral blood leukocytes, *Biol. Pharm. Bull.*, 25, 140–144.

Tokunaka, K., Ohno, N., Adachi, Y., Tanaka, S., Tamura, H., and Yadomae, T. (2000) Immunopharmacological and immunotoxicological activities of a water-soluble $(1\rightarrow3)$-beta-D-glucan, CSBG from Candida spp., *Int. J. Immunopharmacol.*, 22, 383–394.

Wojtaszek, P. (1997) Oxidative burst: an early plant response to pathogen infection, *Biochem. J.*, 322, 681–692.

Yadomae, T., Ohno, N., and Miyazaki, T. (1979) On the phosphate linkages and the structure of a disaccharide unit of the type-specific polysaccharide of *Pneumococcus* type XIX, *Carbohydr. Res.*, 75, 191–198.

Zarzaur, B.L. and Kudsk, K.A. (2001) The mucosa-associated lymphoid tissue structure, function, and derangements, *Shock*, 15, 411–420.

Section V

Clinical Application

13 Clinical Applications of Prescriptions Containing *Bupleurum* Root

Bai-Can Yang and Jun Wang

CONTENTS

13.1 INTRODUCTION

Bupleuri radix was first recorded in *Shen-Nong's Herbal*, the earliest professional work describing Chinese materia medica. It includes *Bupleurum* root and covers the root's property, flavor, effects, and clinical applications as follows:

Property, Flavor, and Channel Tropism: Bitter and pungent flavor, slightly cold property, and acting on the lung, spleen, liver and gallbladder channels.

Effects/Properties and Indications:
- Expelling pathogenic factors from the exterior to reduce fever: There are two sides to its effectiveness: it can disperse the exterior evil of wind-cold and then remove the fever so caused. It can disperse the exterior evil of wind-heat and then again remove the fever. It also can expel exterior pathogenic factors, clear away the semi-exterior and semi-interior evil, and then heal the alternate spells of chills and fever. Thus, *Bupleurum* root is widely used in all kinds of fever syndromes.
- Soothing the depressed liver: It is used where stagnation of the liver-qi is diagnosed. Its effect is very significant, and it is regarded as a principal drug having been used

widely for very many years and in clinics today for irregular menstruation, epigastric pain, pain of swollen breast, depression, hypochondriac pain, etc.

* Invigorating the spleen-yang: The root is used in diseases due to deficiency and sinking of qi such as proctoptosis, hysteroptosis, gastroptosis, and chronic diarrhea, for their symptomatic treatment as an essential medicine (Lin, 1998).

Dosage and administration: Generally speaking, the dosage cannot be too large, but kept between 1.5 and 15 g a day. For expelling pathogenic factors from the exterior to reduce fever, the crude drug should be used, while for other purposes, a preparation of the root at a little lower dose is justified.

13.2 REPRESENTATIVE PRESCRIPTIONS

Because several effects of *Bupleurum* root are very significant, and the clinical application is also very effective, its use with other drugs has become very important. Many prescriptions include *Bupleurum* root whether or not it acts as the principal drug. These prescriptions are widely used today and are very effective; there are even some new applications. This chapter introduces several representative prescriptions and their major clinical applications.

13.2.1 Xiao-Chaihu-Tang (Sho-Saiko-To in Japanese) (Minor Decoction of *Bupleurum*)

Source: *Treatise on Febrile Diseases,* by Z.J. Zhang

Ingredients: Radix Bupleuri, Radix Scutellariae, Rhizoma Pinelliae, Fresh ginger, Ginseng, Radix Ginseng, Fructus Ziziphi Fujubae, Prepared licorice root, Radix Glycyrrhizae Praeparata

Effects and Indications: Treating shaoyang disease by mediation, strengthening healthy qi to eliminate pathogenic factors, regulating stomach to lower adverse flow qi; used in shaoyang diseases, malaria, jaundice, etc.

Clinical Applications: This prescription is one of the most widely used, particularly for a number of diseases.

13.2.1.1 Liver, Gallbladder, and Digestive Diseases

13.2.1.1.1 Hepatitis

When using the recipe/prescription as the principal drug in the treatment of chronic active hepatitis, one dose a day is given; the shortest efficacious time is within 2 months, the longest is 3 years. The result was that among 16 cases, the patients' serum glutamic-pyruvic transaminase (SGPT) and serum glutamic-oxaloacetic transaminase (SGOT) became normal. Liver function recovered more significantly in 6 patients with positive hepatitis B core antigen (HbsAg). In 45 other cases of chronic active hepatitis when the Xiao-Chaihu-Tang was administered with prednisone, for 2 to 6 months, it had no effect or a negative effect. Omitting the hormone, the auto-symptoms, physical signs, and liver function improved significantly. Administering the extract of Xiao-Chaihu-Tang to 23 cases of non-A non-B hepatitis and 7 cases of hepatitis B for 6 months, the clinical parameter of the patients was improved by about 46.7% and the patients' SGPT decreased significantly (Xiao, 1986).

13.2.1.1.2 Choler Reflex Gastritis

The modified recipe (Li et al., 1983) was used to treat 36 cases of choler reflex gastritis using one dose a day for 30 days, when the symptoms reduced or disappeared. Various degrees of improvement were observed by gastrofiberscope.

13.2.1.1.3 Acute Dropsy Pancreatitis

The combined application of the modified recipe, acupuncture, moxibustion therapy, and atropine was used to treat 50 cases of acute dropsy pancreatitis. After 3 to 14 doses of the recipe the average time for a complete cure time was 6 to 8 days (Li, 1982).

13.2.1.1.4 Reflex Esophagitis

When using the modified recipe to treat 78 cases of reflex esophagusitis, the result was that 69 cases were completely cured, 6 cases were improving, 3 cases had no effect. The whole effective rate was 96.2% (Fu, 1992).

13.2.1.2 Infection and Inflammatory Diseases

Use of Xiao-Chaihu-Tang as the principal drug can treat many infectious diseases.

13.2.1.2.1 Chronic Bronchitis

When using the modified recipe to treat 88 cases for 3 to 6 days, 50 cases were cured completely, and the cough of other patients had improved. (X.X. Wang, 1986).

13.2.1.2.2 Vestibulitis

When using the modified recipe to treat 23 cases of this disease for about 1 week, patients' symptoms completely disappeared; the cured rate was 100%.

The modified recipe was also used to treat acute parotitis with testitis, chronic urinary infection, and viral myocarditis, etc. (Gong, 1984; Sun, 1986).

13.2.1.3 Fever Diseases

The modified recipe could also be used to treat many fever diseases. For example, in treatment of 3 patients with unclear cause, 16 patients suffering with the common cold, and 15 children whose fever appeared at night, all had remarkable effects. In addition, with fevers caused by infection of the biliary tract, pneumonia, influenza, leptospiral infection, and immunopathy, where temperatures were between 38 to 40°C, people took many medicines such as antibiotics, antipyretic drugs, and analgesic with no effect, whereas after administration with Xiao-Chaihu-Tang, their fever decreased in 2 to 10 days.

13.2.1.4 Allergic Skin-Deep Diseases

When using Xiao-Chaihu-Tang to treat acute eczema, chronic urticaria, and abnormal acne, the significant effect was 13% and the effect was 73% (Liang and Dong, 1994).

13.2.1.5 Pernicious Vomiting

When using the recipe to treat 320 cases of pernicious vomiting, the whole effective rate was 88% (C.S. Wang, 1986)

13.2.1.6 Primary Dysmenorrhea

When using Xiao-Chaihu-Tang to treat 57 cases of primary dysmenorrhea, taking the recipe at the first day of menstrual cycle, one dose a day, continuing 10 days, 3 months for a medical process, the result was that 28 cases (49.1%) were completely cured, 22 cases (38.6%) were significantly effective, 5 cases (8.8%) were remarkably improved, only 2 cases had no effect. The whole effective rate was 96.5% (Xie and Liu, 2003).

13.2.1.7 Epilepsy

When using the modified recipe to treat 107 cases of epilepsy, the whole effective rate was 93.5%, among this the completely cured was 31.8% (Wang, 1988).

In addition, minor decoction of *Bupleurum* can be applied to the treatment of such diseases as climacteric syndrome, nephritis, systemic lupus erythematosus (SLE), and others.

13.2.2 DA-CHAIHU-TANG (DAI-SAIKO-TO, MAJOR DECOCTION OF *BUPLEURUM*)

Source: Synopsis of Prescription of the Golden Chamber by Z.J. Zhang.

Ingredients: Radix Bupleuri, Radix Scutellariae, Radix et Rhizoma Rhei, Fructus Aurantii Immature Praeparata, Radix Paeoniae Alba, Rhizoma Pinelliae, Fresh ginger, Fructus Ziziphi Fujubae

Effects and Indications: In traditional Chinese medicine (TCM), Da-Chaihu-Tang has the function of treating shaoyang diseases by mediation, purging away internal stasis of heat. Its indications in shaoyang and yangming diseases are complex, marked by alternate attacks of chills and fever, fullness and oppression in the chest, hypochondriac discomfort, dysphoria, retching, distension and fullness in the chest and abdomen, constipation. Modern pharmacological research has proved that the recipe had the effect of protecting the liver, promoting the function of gallbladder, removing calculus stone, resisting inflammation, bringing down the fever, resisting platelet collecting, and preventing atherosclerosis. At present we often use the recipe to treat liver and gallbladder diseases, acute pancreatitis, and higher fever.

13.2.2.1 Hepatitis

Use of the modified recipe to treat acute icterohepatitis and acute or chronic hepatitis is effective. It can reduce symptoms, reduce abnormal biochemical tests, and improve physical signs (Fang, 1988).

13.2.2.2 Cholelithiasis, Biliary Colic, and Infection of the Biliary Tract

A good effect is achieved using Da-Chaihu-Tang to treat these diseases. When using the modified recipe to treat 26 cases that had residual calculus stone after the operation of the biliary tract, the result was that in 18 cases (69.2%) the calculus stone was removed. Among the 18 cases, the recipe was stopped and the patients visited irregularly during 3 years. In 16 cases, symptoms never reappeared. In treating 20 cases of chronic cholecystitis with cholelithiasis, the calculus stone removal rate was 65%. In treating 324 cases of biliary colic with the prescription, 94.5% of the patients had reduced pain with complete removal of calculus stone, a rate of 46.1%. In treating 40 cases of acute cholecystitis, 35 cases were completely cured, 5 cases significantly improved and recovered to normal within 72 hours. In the treatment of 88 cases of chronic cholecystitis, the whole effective rate was 96.5% (C.C. Wang, 1986).

13.2.2.3 Acute Pancreatitis

The recipe is commonly used in clinics to treat acute pancreatitis. In 132 cases of acute dropsy pancreatitis, all except 3 cases (97.7%) of acute necrotic pancreatitis were completely cured in 1 to 7 days of their abdominal pain, urinary amylase, and others symptoms. When using the recipe to treat 50 cases of pediatric pancreatitis, all the patients were completely cured (Cai, 1986).

13.2.2.4 Higher Fever

Common cold with higher fever and fever without clear cause can be treated with the recipe, which may have an ideal effect. When using Da-Chaihu-Tang to treat 39 cases of pediatric higher fever that had not responded to antibiotics, 37 patients were healed after taking the recipe for 1 to 6 doses (Zhang, 1990).

In addition, the use of Da-Chaihu-Tang to treat Menière's diseases, distortion of stomach, nephritis, and acute or chronic gastritis resulted in various degrees of effectiveness.

13.2.3 CHAIHU-GUIZHI-TANG (SAIKO-KEISHI-TO, DECOCTION OF *BUPLEURUM* AND CINNAMON TWIG)

> **Source:** *Treatise on Febrile Diseases* by Z.J. Zhang
>
> **Ingredients:** Radix Bupleuri, Ramulus Cinnamoni, Radix Paeoniaet, Radix Scutellariae, Radix Ginseng, Prepared licorice root, Radix Glycyrrhizae Praeparata, Pinellia tuber, Rhizoma Pinelliae, Fructus Ziziphi Fujubae, Fresh ginger
>
> **Effects and Indications:** This recipe has the functions of treating shaoyang disease by mediation and dispersing the exterior evil; the special indications are fever with aversion to cold, arthralgia of limbs, vomiting, etc. Modern research has confirmed that the recipe has the effects of local anesthesia, resisting syncope due to fright, improving immunity, and resisting ulcer. At present, it is mainly used to prevent or treat epilepsy, peptic ulcer, chronic pancreatitis, arrhythmia, and exogenous fever.

13.2.3.1 Epilepsy

When using the recipe to treat 433 cases of epilepsy, 25 cases were completely cured, 78 cases were significantly reduced in frequency (Zeng, 1990).

13.2.3.2 Treatment and Preventing of Peptic Ulcer

When using the recipe to treat peptic ulcer, including duodenal ulcer and gastric ulcer, it not only can heal them significantly, but also can prevent the ulcers from recurring (Qu and Han, 1991).

13.2.3.3 Hepatitis and Its Syndrome

When using the recipe to treat 116 cases of hepatitis and its syndrome, after 3 weeks, 87 cases were cured completely, 2 cases were effective, 8 cases had no effect. The effect was significantly better than that in the controlled trial (Liu and Wang, 1991).

13.2.3.4 Arrhythmia

When using the modified recipe to treat 24 cases of various arrhythmias, 16 cases were completely cured, 4 cases were improved, and 4 cases had no effect (Beijing An'ding Hospital, 1982).

13.2.3.5 Fever

When using the modified recipe to treat 112 cases of fever caused by viral infection, 85 cases were completely cured, 13 cases were improved, 14 cases had no effect.

When using the recipe to treat neurasthenia, nephritis, and other diseases, all had varying degrees of effectiveness.

13.2.4 XIAO-YAO-WAN (PILL FOR EASE)

Ingredients: Radix Bupleuri, Radix Paeoniae Alba, Radix Angelicae Sinensis, Poria, Rhizoma Atractylodis Macrocephalae, Radix Glycyrrhizae Praeparata, Herba Menthae, Roasted ginger

Effects and Indications: This recipe has the functions of soothing the liver to disperse the depressed qi, and invigorating the spleen to nourish the blood. Its indications are stagnation of liver-qi and disharmony between liver and spleen marked by hypochondriac pain, headache, dizziness, mental weariness and poor appetite, irregular menstruation, distension, and pain in the breast. Modern pharmacological research has proved that the recipe had the effects of coordinating the endocrine and central nervous system, nourishing the liver, promoting peristalsis of intestines. At present, it is mainly used to treat emotional psychosis, nipple adenoidism, gynecomastism, hypergalatonemia, obstructive postpartum lactation, chronic adnexitis and ovarian cyst, dysmenorrhea, inflammation of pelvis, climacteric syndrome, senile trembles, hepatitis, cholecystitis and cholelithiasis, syndrome of retina and optic nerve, hyperlipidemia, diabetes, etc.

13.2.4.1 Emotional Psychosis

When using the recipe to treat 26 cases of emotional psychosis, 16 cases were remarkably improved, 7 cases were improved, and 3 cases had no effect. In treating 14 cases of schizophrenia, a satisfactory effect was achieved (Wang, 1984).

13.2.4.2 Nipple Adenoidism

When using the modified recipe to treat 182 cases of udder adenoidism, the result was that 75 cases were completely cured, 78 cases were significantly effective, 20 cases were improving, 8 cases had no effect; the completely cured and effective rate was 84.1% (Zhou, 1994).

13.2.4.3 Gynecomastism

When using the recipe to treat 62 cases of gynecomastism for 1 to 5 medical processes, the result was that 52 cases were completely cured, 7 cases were remarkably effective, and 3 cases had no effect.

13.2.4.4 Hypergalatonemia

The modified recipe was used to treat 54 cases of hypergalatonemia, stopping it during the menstruation period. When the Prolactin (PRL) became normal, the dose was stopped. If the PRL was not reduced after taking 30 doses, it was considered to be ineffective. Among 54 cases, there were 49 cases whose PRL reduced to normal after taking the recipe for 8 to 54 days with the rate of 90.2%. In others (9.3%) the PRL was reduced but did not reach normal (Li et al., 1991).

13.2.4.5 Obstructive Postpartum Lactation

When using the modified recipe to treat 30 such cases with 7 days for a medical process, the result was that 20 cases were completely cured, 7 improved, 2 cases showed no effect; the whole effective rate was 93.3%.

13.2.4.6 Chronic Adnexitis and Ovarian Cyst

When using the recipe to treat 46 cases of chronic adnexitis and ovarian cyst, 32 cases were completely cured, 13 cases improved, and 1 case showed no effect. Among 30 cases of ovarian cyst, constantly taking the recipe for 3 months resulted in 24 cases completely cured, 3 with effective results, and 3 with no effect.

13.2.4.7 Primary Dysmenorrhea

The recipe was used to treat 52 cases of primary dysmenorrhea, beginning to take the medicine 3 to 5 days prior to menstruation and with 5 to 7 doses for a medical process. In the clinic, 14 cases were completely cured, 32 cases improved; the effective rate was 88.4% (Gong et al., 1985).

13.2.4.8 Hepatitis

When using the modified recipe to treat 253 cases of anicteric hepatitis, the whole effective rate was 68.8%. There were 36 cases whose liver function became normal, while 136 cases improved. In treating 75 cases of chronic hepatitis, 1 month for a medical process and generally using 2 medical processes, 30 cases were remarkably effective, 36 were effective, 9 had no effect; the whole effective rate was 88%. When using the recipe to treat 20 cases of metastatic hepatitis, 67 cases of chronic hepatitis, and 1 case of hepatocirrhosis, the whole quantity was 88. Results: 75 cases were completely cured, 4 were significantly effective, and 8 improved better. When using the modified recipe to treat 30 cases of hepatitis B, after 1 to 3 months, there were 29 cases in which it had a remarkable effect, and 1 case had no effect. In treating 100 cases of hepatocirrhosis with ascites, 46 cases were completely cured, 47 improved, and 7 showed no effect (Gong et al., 1985).

13.2.4.9 Ophthalmopathy

When using the recipe to treat 16 eyes of 15 cases of central retinitis for 1 to 3 months, the result was that 10 eyes were completely cured, 1 eye was significantly improved, 2 eyes showed no effect. To treat 120 cases of central serous choroidretina diseases, 74 cases were remarkably cured, 38 were effective, 8 had no effect. In treating 48 pediatric cases caused by acute pyreticosis, 44 cases were completely cured, 3 cases improved (He, 1985).

13.2.4.10 Hyperlipidemia

When using the recipe to treat 84 cases of hyperlipidemia, as far as reducing cholesterol was concerned, 60 cases were significantly effective, 16 were effective, 6 had no effect. As far as reducing triglyceride was concerned, 57 cases were significantly effective, 16 were effective, 11 had no effect (Yang et al., 1995).

13.2.4.11 Diabetes

When using the modified recipe to treat 60 such cases, the result was that 22 cases were completely cured, 18 were remarkably effective, 14 improved, 6 cases showed no effect; the whole effective rate was 90% (Liu, 1993).

In addition, Xiao-Yao-Wan also has significant effects in treating many diseases such as singers' nodes, cholecystitis, cholelithiasis, climacteric syndrome, senile trembles, metrorrhagia and metrostaxis, peptic ulcer, and so on.

13.2.5 Si-Ni-San (Shigyaku-San, Powder for Treating Cold Limbs)

Source: *Treatise on Febrile Diseases*
Ingredients: Radix Bupleuri, Radix Paeoniae Alba, Fructus Aurantii Immature Praeparata, Radix Glycyrrhizae Praeparata

Effects and Indications: The recipe has the functions of soothing the liver and allaying fever. It is always used in depressed fever due to internal stagnant heat and gastralgia and abdominal pain caused by disharmony between liver and stomach. Modern pharmacological research has proved that the recipe had the effect of relieving spasm, resisting ulcer and syphilis, potentiating interferon, tranquilizing the mind, decreasing the temperature, increasing blood pressure, resisting shock and arrhythmia, tonifying the heart, resisting oxygen deficit, improving cerebrovascular volume, promoting blood microcirculation, lowering cholesterol level, protecting the liver, resisting inflammation, alleviating pain, etc. At present, it is mainly used in liver and gallbladder diseases, gastric diseases, urinary diseases, epilepsy, neurosis, gynopathy, and other diseases.

13.2.5.1 Liver and Gallbladder Diseases

The prescription produced remarkable effects when treating chronic postponed hepatitis, chronic hepatitis, and acute icterohepatitis; the effective rates were 90, 96.3, 97.1%, respectively. It also had significant effects when treating acute or chronic cholecystitis, cholelithiasis, biliary ascariasis (Yang, 1978; Zhang, 1989).

13.2.5.2 Gastric Diseases

When using the recipe to treat 65 cases of gastric ulcer, the result was that 46 cases were significantly effective, 14 improved, and 5 showed no effect. The whole effective rate was 92.3%. When using the modified recipe to treat 54 cases of choler reflex gastritis, 34 had remarkable effect, 16 improved, 5 showed no effect; the whole effective rate was 90.2%. In addition, it also had a significant effect in treating acute and chronic gastritis (Zhang, 1986; He, 1988).

13.2.5.3 Intercostal Neuralgia

When using the modified recipe to treat 50 such cases, all the symptoms disappeared after taking 4 to 8 doses on average (Chen, 1964).

13.2.5.4 Diseases of Intestinal Tract

When using the modified recipe to treat 31 cases of chronic ulcerative colitis, the whole effective rate was 93.5%. It also proved effective when treating the diseases like allergic colitis, bacillary dysentery, and intestinal neurosis (Lv, 1995).

13.2.5.5 Epilepsy and Neurosis

Using the modified recipe to treat epilepsy had some degree of effect. Among 30 cases of neurasthenia, 83.3% of the patients showed improved symptoms after taking 4 doses of the recipe (Zhou et al., 1989).

13.2.5.6 Surgical Diseases

The recipe was also significantly effective when used to treat acute mastadenitis, costal cartilagitis, chronic suppurative otitis media, exudative pleuritis, and other diseases (Liang, 1978).

13.2.5.7 Gynopathy

When using the recipe to treat 50 cases of obstructive fallopian tube, the whole effective rate was 84.3%; in treating 30 cases of secondary sterility, half were completely cured. The recipe also had a remarkable effect when used to treat chronic adnexitis, climacteric syndrome, irregular menstruation, and other gynopathies (Li, 1985).

When using the recipe to treat hyperthyroidism, pediatric fever, abdominal pain, diarrhea, and impotency, it also had a significant effect.

13.2.6 CHAIHU-SHU-GAN-SAN (POWDER OF *BUPLEURUM* ROOT TO SOOTHE THE QI OF LIVER)

Source: *Complete Works of Zhang Jing Yue*

Ingredients: Radix Bupleuri, Pericarpium Citri Reticulatae, Rhizoma Ligustici Chuanxiong, Fructus Aurantii Immature Praeparata, Radix Paeoniae Alba, Rhizoma Cyperi, Radix Glycyrrhizae Praeparata

Effects and Indications: The recipe has the function of soothing the liver to graduate qi, relieving depression and dispersing stagnation. Its indications are liver depression and qi stagnation marked by hypochondriac pain, distention in the abdomen, anorexia, dysmenorrheal, and irregular menstruation. Modern research has proved that the recipe had the effect of increasing the blood flow volume of brain and liver, protecting the liver, and promoting the function of the gallbladder. At present, it is mainly used to treat the diseases such as hepatitis B, intestinal adhesion after operation, premenstrual tension syndrome, and inejaculation syndrome.

13.2.6.1 Hepatitis B

When using the recipe to treat the patients with positive HBsAg, 32 cases had remarkable effect, 5 had effect, and the whole effective rate was 46.25%. Treating 80 cases of hepatitis B resulted in 16 complete cures, 15 with significantly effective results, 26 effective results; the effective rate was 71%. It was proved that the recipe had the function of preventing the infection of hepatitis B virus (Ran, 1984).

13.2.6.2 Intestinal Adhesion after Operation

Using the recipe to treat intestinal adhesion after operation resulted in a quick positive response with no side effect. The symptom of abdominalgia was significantly alleviated after taking the medicine, and in some of the patients the symptoms were completely eliminated.

13.2.6.3 Premenstrual Tension Syndrome

When using the recipe to treat 70 cases of this syndrome, in the long run and in the short run, the effects were both significant. In addition, the recipe was also completely effective when used to treat gynopathy, such as female amenorrhea and menstrual distention of breast.

13.2.6.4 Male Inejaculation Syndrome

When using the recipe to treat 19 cases of male sterility due to inejaculation, the result was that 17 cases were completely cured (Zhao, 1990).

13.2.6.5 Orchitis

When using the modified recipe to treat 37 such cases, the result was that 32 were completely cured (Zhang and Wang, 1993).

If a patient has the side effect of a reddish tongue with scanty fur, dry mouth and throat, dysphoria, and insomnia while taking the recipe, stop the medication.

13.2.7 CHAIHU-JIA-LONGGU-MULI-TANG (SAIKO-KA-RYUKOTSU-BOREI-TO, *BUPLEURUM* PLUS DRAGON BONE AND OYSTER SHELL DECOCTION)

Source: Treatise on Febrile Diseases

Ingredients: Radix Bupleuri, Os Draconis, Radix Ginseng, Radix Scutellariae, Ramuslus Cinnamomi, Fresh ginger, Rhizoma Pinelliae, Poria, Oyster, Radix et Rhizoma Rhei, Fructus Ziziphi Fujubae, Plumbum Preparata

Effects and Indications: The recipe has the functions of harmonizing qi and blood, resolving phlegm to relieve depression, tranquilizing mind. Its indications are fullness in chest, vexation and anxiety, difficulty in urination, delirium, and dreaminess. Modern research has ascertained that the recipe had the activity of regulating the function of the central nervous system, protecting the cardiovascular system, lowering blood-fat, preventing atherosclerosis, promoting blood coagulation, arresting blood, and increasing the content of estrin. At present, it is mainly used to treat neurosis, epilepsy, depression, mania, hypertension, atherosclerosis, hyperthyroidism, climacteric syndrome.

13.2.7.1 Neurosis

When using the recipe to treat 32 cases of neurosis, several syndromes, such as dysphoria, insomnia, tension, susceptibility to fatigue, decline in judgment, and insecurity, were remarkably improved. When using it to treat 35 cases of neurosis due to neurasthenia and climacteric age, a significant effect was produced except in only 1 case (Yang, 1984).

13.2.7.2 Manic Psychosis and Schizophrenia

When using the recipe to treat 36 cases of manic psychosis, taking the medicine for 1 to 3 months, the result was that 21 cases were completely cured, and did not relapse within 1 year. There were 3 cases whose symptoms recurred because they did not persevere in taking the medicine, and 2 cases whose symptoms were controlled and continue to be treated. When using the recipe to treat 67 cases of schizophrenia, the effect was very satisfying (Liu and Liu, 1993).

13.2.7.3 Epilepsy

When using the recipe to treat 36 cases of epilepsy, the result was that 18 were completely cured, 11 improved, 7 showed no effect (Jin, 1992).

13.2.7.4 Hyperthyroidism

When using the modified recipe to treat 100 cases of hyperthyroidism, 1 to 3 months for a medical process, there were 50 cases whose symptoms completely disappeared; 9 cases showed no effect (Yu, 1986).

13.2.8 BUZHONG-YIQI-TANG (HOCHU-EKKI-TO, DECOCTION FOR REINFORCING MIDDLE-WARMER AND REPLENISHING)

Source: Treatise on the Spleen and Stomach

Ingredients: Radix Asbragali seu Hedysari, Radix Codonopsis, Radix Glycyrrhizac Praepareta, Radix Angelicac Sinensis, Rhizoma Atractylodis Macrocephalac, Rhizoma Cimicifugac, Radix Bupleuri

Effects and Indications: The recipe has the functions of invigorating the spleen, replenishing qi, and elevating the spleen-yang to treat qi collapse. It is indicated for a syndrome due to weakness of spleen and stomach, prolapse of gastrosplenic qi, manifested by fatigue and lack of strength, reduced appetite and abdominal distention, protracted diarrhea, splanchnoptosis. Modern studies confirmed that the recipe had the effects of regulating the movement of stomach and intestine, resisting gastric ulcer and traumatism of gastric mucosa, exciting uterus, strengthening the function of the heart, affecting secretion of digesting fluid, regulating the immune function, promoting metabolism, resisting rumor and mutation. At present, it is mainly used in diseases such as splanchnoptosis, metror-rhagia and metrostaxis, diarrhea, myasthenia gravis, chylous urine, lower fever, chronic hepatitis, hypotension, insomnia, leukocytopenia, chronic colitis, peptic ulcer.

13.2.8.1 Gastroptosis

When using the recipe to treat 103 such cases, the result was that 54 were completely cured, 25 had significant effect, 22 had effect, and 2 had no effect. Among the completely cured patients, after visiting them at any time for more than 2 years, we found that their symptoms did not reappear (Zhou, 1976).

13.2.8.2 Prolapse of the Gastric Mucosa

When using the modified recipe to treat 35 such cases, taking the medicine for 2 weeks, the result was that 12 cases were completely cured, 8 improved, and in 5 it had no effect (Li et al., 1991).

13.2.8.3 Hysteroptosis

When using the recipe to treat 218 such cases, the result was that 172 cases were completely cured, 45 improved, and only 1 had no effect.

13.2.8.4 Prolapse of the Rectum

When using the recipe to treat 134 such cases, 119 cases were completely cured, 12 had effective results, and 3 experienced no effect (Zhang and Li, 1995).

13.2.8.5 Metrorrhagia and Metrostaxis

When using the recipe to treat 56 cases of metrorrhagia and metrostaxis, 22 cases were completely cured, 13 had remarkable effect, 9 had some effect, and 5 cases had no effect (Wu, 1989).

13.2.8.6 Chylous Urine

When using the modified recipe to treat 44 cases of chylous urine, the result was that 38 cases were completely cured, 4 had effective results, and 2 experienced no effect (Li, 1984).

13.3 OTHER PREPARATIONS

Other preparations containing *Bupleurum* used in TCM are listed in Table 13.1.

APPENDIX

Chaihu Oral Liquid

> **Ingredient:** Chaihu Oral Liquid is prepared from the root of *Bupleurum chinense* DC. or *B. scorzonerifolium* Willd.
>
> **Procedure:** To Radix Bupleuri, pulverized to coarse powder, add 4 portions of water, macerate at 80°C for half an hour, heat under reflux for 1 hour, and then perform water

steam distillation (add 4 portions of water during distillation), collect a quantity of initial distillate, add sodium chloride to a content of 12%, salt out for 12 hours, redistill, collect a quantity of redistillate, add propylene glycol, shake, and allow to stand. Continue to collect a quantity of redistillate. Filter and concentrate the above decoction to a quantity, refrigerate for 24 hours, filter, to the filtrate add sucrose, warmly heat to dissolve, cool, combine with redistillate, filter, add flavoring essence and successive distillate to a fixed volume, filter with G3 sintered glass filter, pack, seal, and sterilize at 100°C for 30 minutes.

Description: A brownish-red liquid; taste, slightly sweet and bitter.

Identification:

1. Distill 10 ml of the oral liquid with 50 ml of water in a 250-ml flask, collect 10 ml of the distillate. To 2 ml of the distillate, add 2 drops of fuchsin-sulfurous acid TS, mix well, and let stand for 5 minutes; a rose color is produced.

2. Evaporate 5 ml of the oral liquid to dryness on a water bath, dissolve the residue in 10 ml of methanol. To 0.5 ml of the supernatant, add 0.5 ml of *p*-dimethylaminoben-zaldehyde solution in methanol (1→30), mix well, and then add 2 ml of phosphoric acid, mix well, and allow to stand in a hot water bath; a pale reddish-purple color is produced.

3. Measure 30 ml of the oral liquid in separator, extract with three 15-ml quantities of ether, discard ether solutions, extract with three 15-ml quantities of *n*-butanol saturated with water again. Combine *n*-butanol extracts and add a same quantity of ammonia TS, mix well, allow to stand. Separate the supernatant, recover *n*-butanol to dryness in vacuum, dissolve the residue in 1 ml of methanol as test solution. Heat under reflux 3 g of Radix Bupleuri reference drug, in 30 ml of ether for 30 minutes; discard ether solution. To the residue, expel ether, add 30 ml of methanol and heat under reflux for 30 minutes, filter, and recover methanol to dryness in vacuum. Dissolve the residue in 15 ml of water, carry out the same manner as described under the preparation of the test solution, beginning at the words "extract with three 15-ml quantities of *n*-butanol saturated with water," to prepare the reference drug solution. Dissolve saiko-saponin-a CRS and saikosaponin-d CRS in methanol to produce a mixture solution containing 0.5 ml of each/ml as the reference solution. Carry out the method for thin layer chromatography, using silica gel G containing sodium carboxymethylcellulose as the coating substance and the lower layer of chloroform–methanol–water (13:7:2, stand below 10°C) as the mobile phase. Apply separately to the plate 5 μl each of the above three solutions. After developing and removal of the plate, dry it in air. Spray with a 1% solution of *p*-dimethylaminobenzaldehyde in sulfuric acid-ethanol (110), heat at 70°C until the spots clear. Three main spots in the chromatogram obtained with the test solution correspond in position and color to the spots in the chromatogram obtained with the reference drug solution. The spots in the chromatogram obtained with the solution correspond in position and color the spots in the chromatogram obtained with the reference solution. Examine under ultraviolet light (365 nm), showing the same yellow fluorescent spots.

Relative density: Not less than 1.01

PH value: 3.0 to 5.0

Specific absorbance: Measure accurately 25 ml of the oral liquid in a 250 ml flask, add 50 ml of water, heat to distill (the speed of distillation is adjusted by distillating the fixed volume in 20 to 30 minutes). Collect the distillate in a 50-ml volumetric flask, stop distillating while the distillate is almost to 50 ml, dilute with water to volume, and mix well. Transfer accurately 3 ml in 10-ml volumetric flask, add water to volume, mix well. Transfer accurately another 3 ml in a evaporating dish, evaporate to dryness on a water bath, dissolve the residue in water, and transfer to a 10-ml volumetric flask, dilute with

TABLE 13.1
Other Useful Preparations Containing *Bupleurum* Used in Traditional Chinese Medicine

Preparation	Source	Ingredients	Clinical Applications
Xuefu-Zhuyu-Tang (Decoction for Removing Blood Stasis in the Chest)	Some Correction of Chinese Traditional Medicine	Semen Persicae, Flos Carthami, Radix Angelicae Sinensis, Radix Remanniae, Rhizoma Chuanxiong, Radix Achyranthis Bidentayae, Radix Platycodi, Radix Bupleuri, Fructus Aurantii, Radix Paeoniae Rubra, Radix Glycyrrhizae	Oxidative stress state of angina pectoris (Ning, 2004); hepatocirrhosis (Wang, 2004); oral ulcer (Yan, 2004); hyperviscosity syndrome (Wang, 2004)
Chai-Ling-Tang (Sairein-To) (Decoction of *Bupleurum* and Poria)	ZhuDanxi's Thoughtway and Methods in Traditional Chinese Medicine	Radix Bupleuri, Radix Scutellariae, Rhizoma Pinelliae, Rhizoma Zingiberis Recens, Radix Ginseng, Fructus Ziziphi Fujubae, Radix Glycyrrhizae Praeparata, Poria, Ramulus Cinnamoni, Rhizoma Alismatis, Rhizoma Atractylodis Macrocephalae	Nephrotic syndrome (Chi et al., 2004; Xu et al., 2004); hepatocirrhosis ascites (He et al., 2000); catarrhal tympanitis (Xu, 1996); acute nephritis (Hu et al., 1994)
Chaiping-Tang (Decoction of *Bupleurum* for Stomach)	Complete Works of Zhang Jing Yue	Radix Bupleuri, Radix Scutellariae, Rhizoma Pinelliae, Rhizoma Atractylodis, Pericarpium Citri Reticulatae, Cortex Magnoliae	Chronic gastritis (He et al., 2004); choler reflex gastritis (Huang, 2004); cholecystitis (Sun, 2001); intestinal constipation (He, 1998)
Longdan-Xiegan Tang	Golden Mirror for Orthodox Medicine	Radix Gentianae, Radix Scutellariae, Fructus Gardeniae, Rhizoma Alismatis, Caulis Aristolochiae Manshuriensis, Semen Plantago, Radix Angelicae Sinensis, Radix Bupleuri, Radix Glycyrrhizae, Radix Remanniae	Herpes zoster (Zhang, 2003); gout (Xu, 2002); tympanitis with effusion (Ye et al., 1995); male infertility (Chen, 1997)
Diankuang-Mengxing-Tang	Some Correction of Chinese Traditional Medicine	Semen Persicae, Radix Bupleuri, Rhizoma Cyperi, Caulis Aristolochiae Manshuriensis, Radix Paeoniae Rubra, Rhizoma Pinelliae, Pericarpium Arecae Catechu, Pericarpium Citri Reticulatae Viride, Pericarpium Citri Reticulatae, Cortex Mori, Fructus Perillae, Radix Glycyrrhizae	Chronic schizophrenia (Wang et al., 1995); manic psychosis (Ding et al., 2001); epilepsy (Ye, 2001)
Xuanyu-Tongjing Tang	Gynaecology of Fu Qing Zhu	Radix Bupleuri, Rhizoma Cyperi Radix Angelicae Sinensis, Radix Paeoniae Alba, Rhizoma Curcumae, Semen Sinapii, Radix Scutellariae, Fructus Gardeniae, Radix Glycyrrhizae, Cortex Moutan	Adolescent dysmenorrhea (Zhuang et al., 2003); infertility (Lin et al., 2001)
Chaihu-Guizhi–Ganjiang-Tang (Saiko-Keishi-Kankyo-To) (Decoction of *Bupleurum*, Cinnamon Twig and Dried Zingiberis)	Treatise on Febrile Disease	Radix Bupleuri, Ramulus Cinnamoni, Radix Scutellariae, Pollen, Ostrea, Rhizoma Zingiberis Recens, Radix Glycyrrhizae	Peptic ulcer (Ye, 2001); chronic hepatitis B (Zhang et al., 1999); irritable bowel syndrome (Pang and Liu, 2002)

TABLE 13.1 (CONTINUED)
Other Useful Preparations Containing *Bupleurum* Used in Traditional Chinese Medicine

Preparation	Source	Ingredients	Clinical Applications
Chaihu-Xianxiong Tang (Chaihu Decoction for Dropping Chest)	Exoteric Treatise on Febrile Disease	Radix Scutellariae, Rhizoma Pinelliae, Semen Trichosanthis. Radix Bupleuri, Radix Coptidis, Radix Platycodi, Fructus Aurantii Immature Praeparata Rhizoma zingiberis Recens	Chronic hepatitis B (Zhang and An, 2004); stable angina pectoris (Xie and Chen, 2002); choler reflex gastritis (Tao, 1997)
Shengyang-Yiwei Tang (Decoction for elevating yangqi and nourishing the stomach)	Treatise on the Spleen and Stomach	Radix Astragali, Radix Genseng, Rhizoma Atractylodis Macrocephalae, Radix Glycyrrhizae, Radix Paeoniae Alba, Rhizoma Pinelliae, Radix Bupleuri, Radix Saposhnikoviae, Poria, Rhizoma Alismatis, Radix et Rhizoma Notopterygii, Radix Angelicae Pubescentis, Radix Coptidis, Cortex Citri Reticulatae, Rhizoma Zingiberis Recens, Fuctus Ziziphi Jujubae	Chronic fatigue syndrome (Shen, 2003); irritable bowel syndrome (Zhang and Liang, 2002); chronic diarrhea (Shi, 1999); senile chronic bronchitis (Gao, 1995)
Wandai-Tang (Decoction for Regulating Leukorrhea)	Gynaecology of Fu Qing Zhu	Rhizoma Atractylodis Macrocephalae, Rhizoma Dioscorerae, Radix Genseng, Radix Paeoniae Alba, Semen Plantago, Rhizoma Atractylodis, Pericarpium Citri Reticulatae, Fructus Brassicae nigrae, Rhizoma Cyperi, Radix Bupleuri, Radix Glycyrrhizae	Chronic diarrhea (Ma et al., 2002); chronic endometritis (Yang et al., 2001); protraction of menses (Li, 2001); leukorrhagia (Guo et al., 1997); chronic colonitis (Chen, 1995)
Shengxian-Tang (Decoction for Decline in Vigor)	Practical Records of Traditional Chinese Medicine with Reference to Western Medicine	Radix Astragali, Rhizoma Anemarrhenae, Radix Bupleuri, Radix Platycodi, Rhizoma Cimicifugae	Chronic fatigue syndrome (Xie, 1998); splanchnoptosis (Wu, 1998); chronic diarrhea (Yu et al., 2002)
Chaihu-Xixin-Tang (Saiko-SaiShin-To) (Decoction of *Bupleurum* and Asarum)	*Trauma Science* (Guangzhou, TCM College, Ed.)	Radix Bupleuri, Radix Angelicae Sinensis, Radix Salviae Miltiorrhizae, Rhizoma Pinelliae, Folium Lycopus, Herba Asari, Eupolyphaga sinensis, Rhizoma Chuanxiong, Radix Coptidis, Herbal Menthae	Hemicrania (Zhuang, 2001); cerebral concussion (Lin et al., 1997); cerebral trauma syndrome (Li et al., 2000)
Chai-Pu-Tang (Saiboku-To) (Decoction of *Bupleurum* and Magnolia Bark)		Radix Bupleuri, Rhizoma Pinelliae, Poria, Radix Scutellariae, Cortex Magnoliae, Fuctus Ziziphi Jujubae, Radix Ginseng, Radix Glycyrrhizae, Folium Perillae, Rhizoma Zingiberis Recens	Asthma (Kanehiro, 1996); mental diseases during aftertreatment (Matsuhashi, 1990)

water to volume, mix well as a blank. Carry out the method for spectrophotometry, measure the absorbance at 277 nm; the value of absorbance is not less than 0.50.

Other requirements: Complies with the general requirements for mixtures

Action: To remove *heat*, expel superficial evils

Indications: Fever caused by superficial evils

Usage and dosage: 10 to 20 ml, 3 times a day; appropriate reduction of the dosage for children

Specification: 10 ml per ampule (equivalent to 10 g of the crude drug)

Storage: Preserve in tightly closed containers, stored in a cool place

BUZHONG-YIQI-WAN

Ingredients: Radix Astragali Preparata 200 g; Radix Codonopsis 60 g; Radix Glycyrrhizae Preparata 100 g; Rhizoma Atractyloidis Macrocephalae (stir-baked) 60 g; Radix Angelicae Sinensis 60 g; Rhizoma Cimicifugae 60 g; Radix Bupleuri 60 g; Pericarpium Citri Reticulatae 60 g

Procedure: Pulverize the above eight ingredients to fine powder, sift, and mix well. Decoct 20 g of Rhizoma Zingiberis recens and 40 g of Fructus Jujubae with water twice and filter. Make watered pill with the decoction and dry; alternatively, concentrate the decoction, to each 100 g of powder add 100 to 120 g of refined honey and concentrated decoction, make small honeyed pills, or to each 100 g of the powder add 100 to 120 g of refined honey, make honeyed pills.

Description: Brown watered pills; or brown to blackish-brown small or big honeyed pills; taste, slightly sweet, slightly bitter and pungent.

Identification:

1. Microscopical: Fibers in bundles or scattered, walls thickened, with longitudinal fissures on the surface, both ends broken to broom-like or slightly truncate. Fiber bundles surrounded by parenchymatous cells containing prisms of calcium oxalate, forming crystal fibers, walls slightly lignified. Needles of calcium oxalate minute, 10 to 32 μm long, irregularly filled in parenchymatous cells. Prisms of calcium oxalate abundant in parenchyma. Anastomosing laticiferous tuber 12 to 15 μm in diameter, containing fine granules. Parenchymatous cells fusiform, walls slightly thickened, with very minute oblique crisscross striations. Wood fibers in bundles, mostly broken, pale yellowish green, with narrowly acute or obtuse-rounded ends, some branched, 14 to 41 μm in diameter, walls slightly thickened, with cross-shaped pit-pairs, sometimes containing yellowish brown contents. Vittae containing pale yellow or yellowish-brown stripped secretion, 8 to 25 μm in diameter.

2. Triturate well 5 g of the watered pills and 10 ml of *n*-hexane, or triturate 9 g of small honeyed pills or big honeyed pills, mix well with 5 g of kieselguhr, add 20 ml of *n*-hexane, ultrasonicate for 15 minutes, and filter. Evaporate the filtrate to dryness at a low temperature. Dissolve the residue in 1 ml of *n*-hexane as the test solution. Prepare a solution with 0.2 g of Rhizoma Atractylodis Macrocephalae reference drug and 5 ml of *n*-hexane as the reference drug solution in the same manner. Carry out the method for thin layer chromatography, using silica gel G as the coating substance and a mixture of petroleum ether (60 to 90°C)-ethyl acetate (20:0.1) as the mobile phase. Apply separately to the plate 10 μl each of the above two solutions. After developing and removal of the plate, dry it in air. Spray with a 5% solution of vanillin in sulfuric acid and heat until the spots clear. The pink spot in the chromatogram obtained with the test solution corresponds in position and color to the spot in the chromatogram obtained with the reference drug solution.

3. Triturate well 5 g of the watered pills, add 20 ml of water; or cut 9 g of small honeyed pills or big honeyed pills into pieces, add 30 ml of water, decoct for 30 minutes, and filter. To the filtrate add 5 ml of dilute hydrochloric acid, ultrasonicate for 5 minutes, allow to stand, and centrifuge. Separate the precipitate and dissolve in 1 ml of dilute ethanol, neutralize with 10% solution bicarbonate solution, and heat for a while as the test solution. Dissolve ammonium glycyrrhizinate CRS in dilute ethanol to produce a solution containing 1 mg/ml as the reference solution. Carry out the method for thin layer chromatography, using silica gel GF254 as the coating substance and a mixture of *n*-butanol–glacial acetic acid–water (6:1:3) as the mobile phase. Apply separately to the plate 5 μl each of the above two solutions. After developing and removal of the plate, dry it in air and examine under ultraviolet light (254 nm). The fluorescent spot in the chromatogram obtained with the test solution corresponds in position and color to the spot in the chromatogram obtained with the reference solution.

Other requirements: Comply with the general requirements for pills
Action: To reinforce the function of the *spleen* and the *stomach*, and to relieve prolapse
Indications: Weakness of the *spleen* and *stomach,* collapse of *qi* in the *middle-jiao* marked by lassitude, anorexia, abdominal distension, chronic diarrhea, or accompanied with pro-lapse of the rectum or the uterus
Usage and dosage: 6 g of watered pills, or 9 g of small honeyed pills or 1 big honeyed pill, 2 to 3 times a day
Specification: 9 g per big honeyed pill
Storage: Preserve watered pills in well closed containers, protected from moisture; preserve small honeyed pills and big honeyed pills in tightly closed containers

Chaihu-shugan-Wan

Ingredients: Poria 100 g; Fructus Aurantii (stir-baked) 50 g; Fructus Amomi Rotundus 40 g; Radix Paeoniae Alba (stir-baked with wine) 50 g; Radix Glycyrrhizae 50 g; Rhizoma Cyperi (processed with vinegar) 75 g; Pericarpium Citri Reticulatae 50 g; Radix Platycodi 50 g; Cortex Magnoliae Officinalis (processed with ginger) 50 g; Fructus Crataegi (stir-baked) 50 g; Radix Saposhnikoviae 50 g; Massa Medicata Fermentata (stir-baked) 50 g; Radix Bupleuri 75 g; Radix Scutellariae 50 g; Herba Menthae 50 g; Caulis Perillae 75 g; Radix Aucklandiae 25 g; Semen Arecae (stir-baked) 75 g; Rhizoma Sparganii (processed with vinegar) 50 g; Radix et Rhizoma Rhei (stir-baked with wine) 50 g; Pericarpium Ciri Reticulatae Virde (stir-baked) 50 g; Radix Angelicae Sinensis 50 g; Rhizoma Pinelliae (processed with ginger) 75 g; Radix Linderae 50 g; Rhizoma Curcumae (processed) 50 g.
Procedure: Pulverize the above 25 ingredients to fine powder, sift, and mix well. To each 100 g of the powder add 180 to 190 g of refined honey to make big honeyed pills.
Description: Blackish-brown big honeyed pills; taste, sweet and bitter
Identification:
1. Microscopical: Clusters of calcium oxalate large, 60 to 140 μm in diameter. Irregular branched masses colorless, dissolved in choral hydrate solution; hyphae colorless or pale brown, 4 to 6 μm in diameter. Fiber bundles surrounded by parenchymatous cells containing prisms of calcium oxalate, forming crystal fibers. Fibers pale yellow, fusiform, with thickened walls and fine pit-canals. Fragments of endosperm colorless, with relatively thickened walls and many large subrounded pits.
2. Heat under reflux 2 pills, ground well with 8 g of kieselguhr, in 50 ml of ether on a water bath at a lower temperature for 1 hour. Filter and evaporate the filtrate to dryness, dissolve the residue in 1 ml of ethyl acetate as the test solution. To 0.5 g of Radix Aucklandiae reference drug, add 10 ml of ether, prepare a solution as the reference

drug solution in the same manner. Carry out the method for thin layer chromatography, using silica gel G as the coating substance and a mixture of cyclohexane-acetone (10:3) as the mobile phase. Apply separately to the plate 5 to 10 µl of the test solution and 1 µl of the reference drug solution. After developing and removal of the plate, dry it in air. Spray with a 5% solution of vanillin in sulfuric acid, heat until the spots clear. The blue spots in the chromatogram obtained with the test solution correspond in position and color to the spots in the chromatogram obtained with the reference drug solution.

3. Grind well 3 pills with 10 g of kieselguhr to fine powder, add 90 ml of chloroform, and heat under reflux for 1 hour. Filter and extract the filtrate with three 20-ml quantities of 2% solution hydroxide solution. Combine the alkaline solution, adjust the pH value to 1 to 2 with dilute hydrochloric acid. Extract with three 20-ml quantities of chloroform. Combine the chloroform extracts and wash with water, evaporate to dryness after dehydrating with anhydrous sodium sulfate. Dissolve the residue in 1 ml of dehydrated ethanol as the test solution. Dissolve magnolol CRS and honokiol CRS in dehydrated ethanol to prepare a mixture containing 1 mg of each/ml as the reference solution. Carry out the method for thin layer chromatography, using silica gel GF254 prepared with 1% sodium hydroxide solution as the coating substance and mixture of benzene-ethyl acetate (6:1) as the mobile phase. Apply separately to the plate 5 µl each of the above two solutions, allow to stand in a condition of relative humidity >80% for 15 minutes, and then develop immediately. After developing and removal of the plate, dry it in air, examine under ultraviolet light (254 nm). The spots in the chromatogram obtained with the test solution correspond in position and color to the spots in the chromatogram obtained with the reference solution. Spray with a 5% solution of vanillin in sulfuric acid, heat at 105°C until the spots clear. The spots show reddish-brow or purplish-brown under sunlight.

Other requirements: Comply with the requirements for pills
Action: To disperse the stagnated *liver-qi*, to active the flow of *qi*, to relieve distension and pain
Indications: Stagnation of *liver-qi*, distension of chest and hypochondria, indigestion, acid eructation
Usage and dosage: 1 pill, 2 times a day
Specification: 10 g per pill
Storage: Preserve in tightly closed containers

Xiaoyao-Wan

Ingredients: Radix Bupleuri 100 g; Radix Angelicae Sinensis 100 g; Radix Paeoniae Alba 100g; Rhizoma Atractylodis Macrocephalae (stir-baked) 100 g; Pria 100 g; Radix Glycyr-rhizae Preparate 80 g; Herba Minthae 20 g
Procedure: Pulverize the above seven ingredients to fine powder, sift, mix well. To each 100 g of the powder add 135 to 145 g of refined honey to make big honeyed pills.
Description: Dark brown big honeyed pills; taste, sweet
Identification:

1. Microscopical: Irregularly branched masses colorless, dissolved in chloral hydrate solution; hyphae colorless or pale brown, 4 to 6 µm in diameter. Parenchymatous cells fusiform, with slightly thickened walls and very fine and oblique crisscross striations. Clusters of calcium oxalate occurring in parenchymatous cells, usually in rows, or several clusters in one cell. Needle crystals of calcium oxalate fine, irregularly filling in parenchymatous cells. Fiber bundles surrounded by parenchymatous cells

containing prisms of calcium oxalate, forming crystal fibers. Vittae contain yellow or brownish-yellow secretion.

2. Cut 2 g of the pills into pieces, add 15 ml of ethanol, allow to stand for 1 hour while shaking, filter, and evaporate the filtrate to dryness. Dissolve the residue in 1 ml of acetone to produce a solution as the test solution. Prepare a solution with 0.1 g of Radix Angelicae Sinensis reference drug and 10 ml of ethanol as the reference drug solution in the same manner. Carry out the method for thin layer chromatography, using silica gel G as the coating substance and a mixture of *n*-hexane–ethyl acetate (9:1) as the mobile phase. Apply separately 5 μl each of the two solutions to the plate. After developing and removal of the plate, dry it in air and examine under ultraviolet light (365 nm). The fluorescent spots in the chromatogram obtained with the test solution correspond in position and color to the spots in the chromatogram obtained with the reference drug solution.

3. Triturate well 18 g of the pills, cut into pieces, with 10 g of kieselguhr; add 60 ml of ethanol, ultrasonicate for 30 minutes, filter, and evaporate the filtrate to dryness. Dissolve the residue in 30 ml of water, extract with two 10-ml quantities of ether, discard the ether solution, extract the aqueous solution with three 30-ml quantities of *n*-butanol saturated with water, wash the combined *n*-butanol solution with three 20-ml quantities of water saturated with *n*-butanol. Discard the washing and evaporate the *n*-butanol solution to dryness. Dissolve the residue in 1 ml of methanol to produce a solution as the test solution. Prepare a solution with 1 g of Radix Glycyrrhizae reference drug and 20 ml of ethanol as the reference drug solution in the same manner. Carry out the method for thin layer chromatography, using silica gel G as the coating substance prepared with a 10% solution of sodium hydroxide and a mixture of ethyl acetate-formic acid–glacial acetic acid–water (15:1:1:2) as the mobile phase. Apply separately to the plate 3 μl each of the two solutions. After developing and removal of the plate, dry it in air, spray with a 10% solution of sulfuric acid in ethanol, heat at 105°C until the spots appear and examine under ultraviolet light (365 nm). The fluorescent spots in the chromatogram obtained with the test solution correspond in position and color to the spots in the chromatogram obtained with the reference drug solution.

4. Mix the test solution obtained in the test for Identification 3 with a small quantity of neutral aluminum oxide, dry on a water bath, apply to a column packed with neutral aluminum oxide (200 mesh, 2 g , 8 to 10 mm in internal diameter), elute with 40 ml of a mixture of ethyl acetate–methanol (1:1), collect the eluate, and evaporate to dryness. Dissolve the residue in 1 ml of ethanol to produce a solution as the test solution. Dissolve paeoniflorin CRS in ethanol to produce a solution containing 2 mg/ml as the reference solution. Carry out the method for thin layer chromatography, using silica gel G as the coating substance and a mixture of chloroform–ethyl acetate–methanol–formic acid (40:5:10:0.2) as the mobile phase. Apply separately to the plate 15 μl of the test solution and 3 μl of the reference solution. After developing and removal of the plate, dry it in air, spray with a 5% solution of vanillin in sulfuric acid, and heat until the spots appear. The spot due to paeoniflorin in the chromatogram obtained with the test solution corresponds in position and color to the spot in the chromatogram obtained with the reference solution.

Other requirements: Comply with the general requirements for pills

Assay: Carry out the method for high-performance liquid chromatography:

Chromatographic system and system suitability: Use octadecylsilane bonded silica gel as the stationary phase and a mixture of acetonitrile–1% solution of phosphoric acid (15:85) as the mobile phase. The wavelength of the detector is 230 nm. The number of theoretical plates of the column is not less than 2000, calculated with the reference to the peak of paeoniflorin.

Preparation of reference solution: Dissolve 10 mg of paeoniflorin CRS, weighted accurately, in dilute ethanol TS in a 100-ml volumetric flask, dilute to volume with the same solvent, and mix well. Transfer 5 ml, measured accurately, to a 10-ml volumetric flask, dilute to volume with dilute ethanol TS, and mix well (containing 0.05 mg of paeoniflorin per ml).

Preparation of test solution: To 1 g of the pills obtained in the test of weight variation, cut into pieces and weighed accurately, add accurately 25 ml of dilute ethanol TS in a stoppered conical flask, stopper tightly, and weigh. Ultrasonicate for 30 minutes, cool to ambient temperature, and weigh again. Replenish the lost weight with dilute ethanol TS, mix well, filter, and use the successive filtrate.

Procedure: Accurately inject 10 μl each of the reference solution and the test solution, respectively, into the column and determine. Each pill may not contain less than 6.3 mg paeoniflorin ($C_{23}H_{28}O_{11}$), referred to as Radix Paeoniae Alba.

Action: To soothe the *liver*, invigorate the function of the *spleen*, nourish blood. and to regulate menstruation

Indication: Depression of the *liver qi* marked by distending pain in the chest and hypochondriac regions, dizziness, impaired appetite, and menstrual disorders

Usage and dosage: 1 pill, 2 times a day.

Specification: 9 g per pill

Storage: Preserve in tightly closed containers

REFERENCES

Beijing An'ding Hospital. (1982) The Study Group of Integrated Traditional and Western Medicine: a clinical analysis of effects on 150 cases of schizophrenia treated by combining Chinese-Western medical means, *Chin. J. Modern Dev. Trad. Med.*, 2(3), 170–171.

Cai, J.W. (1986) Da-Chaihu-Tang treatment of acute pancreatitis-experiences of 132 cases, *Liaoning J. Trad. Chin. Med.*, 10(2), 21.

Chen, L.B. (1997) 27 cases of male infertility treated by Longdan-Xiegan-Tang, *J. Anhui TCM Coll.*, 116(6), 28.

Chen, W.C. (1995) Wandai Decoction for 49 cases of chronic colonitis, *Hubei J. Trad. Chin. Med.*, 17(2), 18.

Chen, X.Q. (1964) Clinical observation of 50 cases of intercostal neuralgia treated with Si-Ni-San and Decoction of Trichosanthes and Macrostem with liquor, *Zhejiang J. Trad. Chin. Med.*, 6, 15.

Chi, R.P., Kimber, L.W.J., and Guo, T.L. (2004) Immunomodulation by Chai-Ling-Tang, a formula consisting of twelve Chinese herbs, *Chin. J. Pharmacol. Toxicol.*, 18(2), 146–151.

Ding, G.A. and Yu, G.H. (2001) A treatment of 36 manic patients by combining traditional and Western medicine, *Chin. J. Civil Admin. Med.*, 13, 229.

Fang, D. (1988) Treatment of acute infectious diseases of liver, gallbladder and pancreas with Modified Da-Chaihu-Tang, *J. Trad. Chin. Med. Chin. Mater. Med. Jilin*, (1), 25, 30.

Fu, C.G. (1992) Observation on the short-term effect of "Xiao-Chaihu-Tang" with additives on reflex esophagitis, *Chin. J. Integrated Trad. West. Med.*, 12(11), 686.

Gao, J. (1995) Shengyang Yiwei Decoction for 50 cases of senile chronic bronchitis, *Liaoning J. Trad. Chin. Med.*, 229, 19–20.

Gong, C. (1984) Clinical effectives of urinary infection in children treated with minor decoction of *Bupleurum*, *J. Mod. East. Med.*, 5(3), 82.

Gong, L.L. et al. (1985) Clinical observation of primary dysmenorrheal treated with reinforced Xiao-Yao-San-Analysis of 52 cases, *J. Guiyang Coll. Trad. Chin. Med.*, 3, 42.

Guo, Q.P. and Wang, S.L. (1997) Wandai Decoction for 117 cases of leukorrhagia, *Gansu J. Trad. Chin. Med.*, 10(4), 35.

He, F. and Wang, M.J. (2000) Combination of Chai-Ling-Tang and phentolamine for 60 cases of hepatocirrhosis ascites, *Guiding J. Med.*, 19, 157.

He, J.C., and Li, C.Y. (2004) Clinical observation of therapeutic effect of modified Chai-Ping-Tang for 80 cases of chronic gastritis, *Yunnan J. Trad. Chin. Med.*, 25, 22.

He, L.X. (1988) 49 Cases of epigastric pain treated with Si-Ni-San, *Shanxi J. Trad. Chin. Med.*, 9(10), 441.

He, Q.Q. (1998) Clinical observation of therapeutic effect of Modified Chai-Ping-Tang for 36 cases of chronic intestinal constipation, *J. N. Trad. Chin. Med.*, 30(9), 18–19.

He, S.A. (1985) Application of Ease Powder in ophthalmiatrics, *J. Sichuan Trad. Chin. Med.*, 3(8), 25–26.

Hu, W.K. and Hui, Y.J. (1994) Modified Chai-Ling-Tang for 60 cases of acute nephritis, *For. Trad. Chin. Med.*, 9, 30.

Huang, J. (2004) Clinical observation on treating choler reflex gastritis by Chai-Ping-Tang, *Hubei J. Trad. Chin. Med.*, 26(4), 29.

Jin, G.R. (1992) Observation on the effect of *Bupleurum*, Dragon's Bone and Oyster Decoction on epilepsy, *Chin. Trad. Patent Med.*, 9, 49.

Kanehiro, A. (1996) Clinical effect of Chaipu Decoction on treating stubborn asthma, *Jpn. J. Toyo Med.*, 46(6), 61.

Li, B.M. (1984) Treatment of 44 cases of chylous urine with Buzhong-Yiqi-Tang *Shandong J. Trad. Chin. Med.*, 5, 26.

Li, D.G. (1985) Application of Si-Ni-San in gyniatrics, *Hubei J. Trad. Chin. Med.*, 5, 40.

Li, K. et al. (1983) Observation on the short-term effect of "Xiao-Chaihu-Tang" with additives on regurgitated cholerrhagic gastritis, *J. Trad. Chin. Med.*, 24(5), 41–42.

Li, S.H., Sun, Z.L., Yuan, S.C., Wang, X.E., Wang, F.L., Chen, S.Y., and Jin, X.M. (1991) Treatment of prolapse of the gastric mucosa with bolus of Buzhong-Yiqi-Tang and gentamicin, *Acta Chin. Med. Pharmacol.*, 1, 30.

Li, S.L. and Zhou, J.L. (2000) Clinical observation on treating 60 cases of cerebral trauma syndrome by Chaihu-Xixin Decoction, *Sci. TCM*, 7, 290.

Li, W.Y. (2001) Wandai Decoction for 56 cases of protraction of menses, *Sichuan J. Trad. Chin. Med.*, 19(3), 55–56.

Li, X.H. (1982) 50 cases of acute pancreatitis treated with Modified Xiao-Chaihu-Tang, *J. Trad. Chin. Med.*, 23(9), 40.

Li, X.Z. et al. (1991) Treatment of hypergalatonemia with Reinforced Ease Powder: analysis of 54 cases, *Chin. J. Mod. Dev. Trad. Med.*, 11(7), 439–440.

Liang, R.R. (1978) Treatment of mastocarbunculosis with reinforced Si-Ni-San: analysis of 15 cases, *Guangxi J. Trad. Chin. Med.*, 4, 34.

Liang, Y.J. and Dong, R.L. (1994) Treatment of fever with Modified Minor Decoction of *Bupleurum*, *Chin. J. Trad. Chin. Med. Pharm.*, 9(2), 32–33.

Lin, J.Z. and Qiu, Y.M. (1997) Chaihu-Xixin Decoction for 40 cases of cerebral concussion, *Fujian J. Trad. Chin. Med.*, 28, 7.

Lin, Y. and Miao, Y.P. (2001) Xuanyu Tongjing Decoction 51 case of infertility induced by endometriosis, *Res. Trad. Chin. Med.*, 17(4), 23–24.

Lin, Y.K. (1998) *The Chinese Materia Medica*. Shanghai Science and Technology Press, Shanghai.

Liu, D.L. (1993) 60 Cases of treating diabetes mellitus with modified powder Xiao-Yao-San, *Shizhen J. Trad. Chin. Med. Res.*, 4(4), 8–9.

Liu, Q. and Wang Z.M. (1991) Treatment of symptoms after hepatitis with "Chaihu-Guizhi-Tang": analysis of 116 cases, *Hunan J. Trad. Chin. Med.*, 7(4), 42.

Liu, X.W and Liu, F.Q. (1993) Treatment of manic psychosis with *Bupleurum*, Dragon's Bone and Oyster Decoction, *J. Sichuan Trad. Chin. Med.*, 11(10), 27.

Lv, W.J. (1995) Application of Ease Powder in gastrointestinal diseases, *J. Nanjing Univ. Trad. Chin. Med.*, 11(6), 26.

Ma, G.J. and Sun, T.S. (2002) Clinical observation on treating 60 cases of chronic diarrhoea by Wandai Decoction, *Shanxi J. TCM*, 18(4), 16–17.

Matsuhashi, M. (1990) Clinical effect of Chaipu Decoction on treating mental diseases during aftertreatment, *Jpn. J. New Drugs Clin.*, 39(7), 98–99.

Ning, B.G. (2004) Xuefuzhuyu Decoction for 130 cases of oxidative stress state of angina pectoris, *Shanxi J. Trad. Chin. Med.*, 250, 150.

Pang, Z.R. and Liu, B.S. (2002) Clinical observation on treating 86 cases of irritable bowel syndrome by Chaihu Guizhi Ganjiang Decoction, *J. Hebei TCM*, 24(2), 32.

Qu, Z.Q. and Han, B. (1991) Observation on treatment of chronic pancreatitis with "Chaihu-Guizhi-Tang," *Zhejiang J. Trad. Chin. Med.*, 26(12), 535.

Ran, Y.R. (1984) Analysis of therapeutic effect of treatment of hepatitis B in 80 cases using "Chaihu-Shugan-San" (Powder of *Bupleurum* Root to Soothe the Qi of Liver), *Yunnan J. Trad. Chin. Med.*, 5(5), 19–20.

Shen, L.Y. (2003) Clinical observation on treating 41 cases of chronic fatigue syndrome by Shengyang Yiwei Decoction, *Inf. Trad. Chin. Med.*, 20, 49.

Shi, Y.F. (1999) Shengyang Yiwei Decoction for 46 cases of chronic diarrhoea, *Hebei J. Integrated Trad. West. Med.*, 8, 940.

Sun, Q.W. (2001) Chai-Ping-Tang for 27 cases of chronic cholecystitis, *Anhui J. Prev. Med.*, 25, 22.

Sun, W.J. (1986) Viral myocarditis treated with "Xiao-Chaihu-Tang," *Chin. J. Integrated Trad. West. Med.*, 6(5), 282.

Tao, H.C. (1997) Clinical observation on treating 35 cases of choler reflex gastritis by Chaihu Xianxiong Decoction, *Practical J. Combination Chin. West. Med.*, 1455–1456.

Wan, Z.C. (1999) Modified Chaihu-Guizhi-Ganjiang Decoction for 120 cases of peptic ulcer, *Guangxi J. Trad. Chin. Med.*, 22, 236.

Wang, A.N. (2004) Treatment of Xuefuzhuyu Decoction for 68 cases of hyperviscosity syndrome, *J. Practical Trad. Chin. Intern. Med.*, 18, 236.

Wang, C.C. (1986) Major Decoction of *Bupleurum* treatment of biliary colic: analysis of 324 cases, *J. Trad. Chin. Med.*, 27(10), 44.

Wang, C.S. (1986) Treatment of pernicious vomiting with Xiao-Chaihu-Tang, *J. Trad. Chin. Med.*, 27(5), 27.

Wang, D.J. (2004) Clinical observation on treating hepatocirrhosis by Decoction for removing blood stasis in the chest, *Chin. J. Practical Chin. Mod. Med.*, 4, 2396.

Wang, D.L. (1960) Primary conclusion of 253 cases of icterohepatitis treated with Xiao-Yao-San, *Guangdong J. Trad. Chin. Med.*, 8, 389.

Wang, J.X. (1984) 182 cases of udder adenoidism treated with Modified Powder Xiao-Yao-San, *J. Trad. Chin. Med. Chin. Mater. Med. Jilin*, 2, 25.

Wang, W. (1988) Treatment of epilepsy with Modified Minor Decoction of *Bupleurum*, *Sichuan J. Trad. Chin. Med.*, 6(10), 26.

Wang, X.F., Yang, S.L., and Wang, J.F. (1999) Modified Wandai Decoction for 113 cases of chronic prostatitis, *For. Trad. Chin. Med.*, 14, 70.

Wang, X.X. (1986) Treatment of cough due to accumulated fire with Xiao-Chaihu-Tang: analysis of 50 cases, *J. Trad. Chin. Med.*, 27 (4), 43–44.

Wang, Y.X., Zhao, L.M., and Li, H.P. (1995) A contradistinctive clinical observation on treating chronic schizophrenia by Diankuang Mengxing Decoction, *J. Binzhou Med. Coll.*, 18, 100–101.

Wang, Z.R. and Liu, C.M. (1991) 24 cases of arrhythmia treated with modified "Chaihu-Guizhi-Tang," *Henan Trad. Chin. Med.*, 11(4), 11.

Wu, J.L. (1998) Clinical observation on treating 26 cases of splanchnoptosis by Modified Shengxian Decoction, *Beijing J. Trad. Chin. Med.*, 4, 26.

Wu, M.H. (1989) Large dose of Buzhong-Yiqi-Tang for uterine bleeding, *Shanxi J. Trad. Chin. Med.*, 10(8), 340–341.

Xiao, G.W.Z. (1986) Study on the effect of "Xiao-Chaihu-Tang" with a large long dose on chronic hepatitis, *Diagn. Treat.*, 74, 2247.

Xie, H.L. and Liu, F.L. (2003) Observation on clinical effectives on treatment of 57 cases of primary dysmenorrheal by Modified Minor Decoction of *Bupleurum*, *Jiangxi J. Trad. Chin. Med.*, 34(7), 36.

Xie, H.N. (1998) Modified Shengxian Decoction for 23 cases of chronic fatigue syndrome, *Jiangsu J. Trad. Chin. Med.*, 19, 20.

Xie, Y.F. and Cheng, C.F. (2002) Treating 45 cases of stable angina pectoris with Chaihuxianxiongtang as main prescription, *Hunan Guiding J. TCM*, 8, 330–331.

Xu, C.H. and Ye, Y.L. (1996) Modified Chai-Ling-Tang for 60 cases of catarrhal tympanitis, *Practical J. Integrated Trad. Chin. West. Med.*, 9, 606.

Xu, D.L. and Liu, C.X. (2004) Study of Chai-Ling-Tang and Tao-Hong Siwu Decoction on hyperlipermia in nephritic syndrome, *Mod. J. Integrated Trad. Chin. West. Med.*, 13, 722–723.

Xu, G. (2002) Clinical observation on treating 78 cases of gout by Longdan Xiegan Decoction, *Bonesetting Trad. Chin. Med.*, 14(4), 29.

Yan, X. (2004) Xuefuzhuyu Decoction for 44 cases of oral ulcer, *Liaoning J. Trad. Chin. Med.*, 31, 501.

Yang, D.N., Yang, D.Y., and Zhang, H.Q. (1995) 84 cases of hyperlipidemia treated with Xiao-Yao-Wan, *Shanxi J. Trad. Chin. Med.*, 16(3), 109–120.

Yang, P.Q. (1984) Treatment of 35 cases of melancholia with *Bupleurum*, Dragon's Bone and Oyster Decoction, *J. Sichuan Trad. Chin. Med.*, 3, 24.

Yang, X.X., Cui, W.P., and Wu, G.Y. (2001) Wandai Decoction for 60 cases of chronic endometritis, *Chin. J. Commun. Phys.*, 12, 37.

Yang, Y.F. (1978) Clinical analysis of 75 cases of chronic postponed hepatitis treated with Si-Ni-San, *J. Guangxi Bare Footed Doctor*, 11, 15.

Ye, D.L. (2001) A treatment of 23 epilepsy patients with Diankuang Mengxing Decoction, *Beijing J. Trad. Chin. Med.*, 1, 24.

Ye, S.P. and Han, H.B. (1995) 44 cases of tympanitis with effusion treated by Longdan-Xiegan-Tang, *J. Zhejiang Coll. TCM*, 19, 30.

Yu, J.G. (1986) Treatment of 100 cases of hyperthyroidism with Decoction of Buzhong-Yiqi-Tang and gentamicin, *Hunan J. Trad. Chin. Med.*, 2, 29.

Yu, Y.H., Liang, Y., and Wang, A.P. (2002) Clinical observation on treating chronic diarrhoea by Modified Shengxian Decoction, *Chin. J. Spaceflight Med.*, 4(5), 60.

Zeng, W.C. (1990) Clinical observation of 84 cases of epilepsy treated with decoction of *Bupleurum* and cinnamon twig, *Liaoning J. Trad. Chin. Med.*, 14(6), 23–24.

Zhang, H.J. and Wang, D.J. (1993) Modified Chaihu-Shugan-San Decoction for 37 cases of orchitis, *Shanxi J. Trad. Chin. Med.*, 14(2), 54.

Zhang, J. (2003) Observation of therapeutic effect of Traditional Chinese Medicine in treating 58 cases herpes zoster, *Tianjin J. Trad. Chin. Med.*, 20(2), 79.

Zhang, J.C. and An, D.M. (2004) Chaihu Xianxiong Decoction for 62 cases of chronic hepatitis B, *Chin. J. Integrated Trad. West. Med.*, 14, 105.

Zhang, J.J. (1990) Treatment of higher fever in children with Da-Chaihu-Tang, *Chin. J. Integrated Trad. West. Med.*, 10(3), 167.

Zhang, L.J., Zhang, A.J., and Zheng, B. (1999) Clinical observation on treating 49 cases of chronic hepatitis B by Chaihu-Guizhi-Ganjiang Decoction, *J. Hebei Med. Univ.*, 20, 310.

Zhang, S.F. and Li, H.Y. (1995) Report of prolapse of the rectum treated with Reinforced Decoction for Reinforcing Buzhong-Yiqi-Tang and gentamicin, *Acta Chin. Med. Pharmacol.*, 3, 42.

Zhang, S.J. and Liang, G.S. (2002) Shengyang Yiwei Decoction for 150 cases of irritable bowel syndrome, *Henan Trad. Chin. Med.*, 22(6), 42–43.

Zhang, W.Y. (1986) Treatment of abnormal proliferation of gastric mucous membrane with Reinforced Si-Ni-San: analysis of 30 cases, *J. Trad. Chin. Med.*, 27(12), 35–36.

Zhang, Y.W. (1989) Treatment of chronic cholecystitis with Modified Si-Ni-San: analysis of 103 cases, *Hubei J. Trad. Chin. Med.*, 4, 39.

Zhao, G.R. (1990) Treating infertility with Modified Powder of *Bupleurum* Root to Soothe the Qi of Liver, *Zhejiang J. Trad. Chin. Med.*, 25(6), 253.

Zhou, D.H. (1994) Treatment of gynecomastism with Powder Xiao-Yao-San, *Gansu J. Trad. Chin. Med.*, 7(6), 35–36.

Zhou, H.Z. et al. (1989) Electroencephalogram observation of 30 cases of neurasthenia treated with Si-Ni-San, *Shenyang J. Army Med. Pharm.*, 2, 82.

Zhou, Z.S. (1976) Observation on the effect of Modified Decoction of Buzhong-Yiqi-Tang and gentamicin on gastroptosis, *J. N. Med.*, 6, 276.

Zhuang, C.S., Zhu, J.Y., and Chen, N.M. (2003) Gan-Draining and Yu-Dispelling therapy for 48 cases of adolescent dysmenorrhea, *Shanxi J. Trad. Chin. Med.*, 24, 400.

Zhuang, W.M. (2001) Chaihu-Xixin Decoction for 47 cases of Hemicrania, *Fujian J. Trad. Chin. Med.*, 32(3), 29.

14 Anti-Hepatofibrotic Effect of Xiao-Chaihu-Tang (Sho-Saiko-To)

Ichiro Shimizu

CONTENTS

14.1 INTRODUCTION

Chinese herbal medicines have now attracted the attention of practitioners of Western medicine, and are being manufactured in uniform quality and in sufficient quantities for utilization as hospital drugs in Japan. Among these herbal medicines, Xiao-Chaihu-Tang (Sho-saiko-to), which has been used in the treatment of pyretic diseases in China, is an officially approved prescription drug in Japan. As the most commonly administered herbal medicine, Sho-saiko-to is used for the treatment of patients with chronic liver disease, especially those with chronic hepatitis C virus (HCV) infection, chronic hepatitis C (Hirayama et al., 1989; Tajiri et al., 1991), and cirrhosis (Oka et al., 1995). The root of *Bupleurum falactum* is one of the chief components of Japanese Sho-saiko-to. The usual daily dose of Sho-saiko-to is 7.5 g,, which is administered orally in three equal doses. The 7.5 g of Sho-saiko-to contains 4.5 g of dried Sho-saiko-to extract, which is prepared from boiling water extracts of seven herbs: 7.0 g of *Bupleurum* root, 5.0 g of *Pinellia* tuber, 3.0 g of *Scutellaria* root, 3.0 g of jujube fruit, 3.0 g of ginseng root, 2.0 g of glycyrrhiza root, and 1.0 g of ginger rhizome.

HCV infections are widespread throughout the world, and are recognized as a major causative factor in chronic hepatitis, cirrhosis, and hepatocellular carcinoma (HCC) (Takano et al., 1995; Shiratori et al., 1995). In fact, the World Health Organization reported that up to 3% of the world's population is infected with HCV, suggesting that more than 170 million chronic carriers are currently at risk of developing cirrhosis and HCC (WHO, 1997). Although Sho-saiko-to is widely used in the treatment of chronic hepatitis C and cirrhosis, little is known about the mechanism by which it protects against hepatic fibrosis. This chapter summarizes our current knowledge of the biological functions of Sho-saiko-to as it relates to fibrogenesis in the liver.

14.2 CLINICAL SIGNIFICANCE OF SHO-SAIKO-TO IN CHRONIC LIVER DISEASE

Sho-saiko-to has been shown to improve liver function (Hirayama et al., 1989; Tajiri et al., 1991), as well as to alleviate the subjective symptoms associated with chronic liver disease, such as nausea, vomiting, and digestive discomfort. In a double-blind multicenter clinical trial, Sho-saiko-to was shown to lower the serum levels of aspartate aminotransferase (AST), alanine aminotransferase (ALT), and γ-glutamyl transpeptidase (γ-GTP) (Hirayama et al., 1989), in patients with chronic liver disease. As shown in Figure 14.1, in addition to serum ALT levels, serum concentrations of hepatic fibrogenesis markers of the 7S domain of type IV collagen (7S-IV), and the amino terminal propeptide of type III procollagen (P-III-P) were significantly attenuated by Sho-saiko-to in patients with chronic hepatitis C with fibrosis of stages 1 to 3 (Shimizu, 2002). Hepatic fibrosis, or the deposition of extracellular matrix (ECM), is classified on a scale of 0 to 4: 0, no fibrosis; 1, portal fibrosis without septa; 2, few septa; 3, numerous septa without cirrhosis; 4, cirrhosis. The proteins and metabolites of hepatic connective tissue, including 7S-IV and P-III-P, have been used for monitoring hepatic fibrosis, and changes in these parameters might reflect accelerated synthesis or degradation of collagen in the liver (Biagini and Ballardini, 1989; Risteli and Risteli, 1995).

Hepatic fibrosis is often associated with inflammation and cell death, which accompanies the repair processes, and is a consequence of severe liver damage that occurs in many patients with chronic liver disease, including chronic HCV infection. The main origin of the abnormal ECM proteins is a cell known as the hepatic stellate cell (HSC) (also known as the fat-storing cell, lipocyte, or the Ito cell). HSCs are located in the space of Disse in close contact with hepatocytes and sinusoidal endothelial cells. Their three-dimensional structure consists of the cell body and several long and branching cytoplasmic processes (Wake, 1999) (Figure 14.2). It is now evident that HSCs undergo proliferation and transformation under inflammatory and peroxidative stimuli into myofibroblast-like cells, which serve as the origin of much of the collagen hypersecretion and nodule formation that occurs during hepatic fibrosis and cirrhosis (Shimizu, 2001).

14.3 PROTECTIVE EFFECT OF SHO-SAIKO-TO ON HEPATOCYTE INJURY INDUCED BY HCV INFECTION

During the course of a chronic HCV infection, hepatocytes are continuously damaged and replicated, and hepatic fibrosis appears to progress. In 80 to 85% of those infected with the virus,

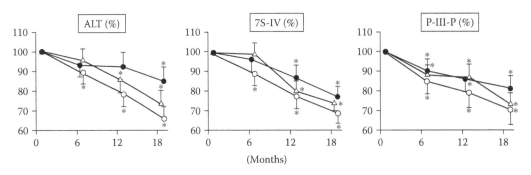

FIGURE 14.1 Changes in individual percentages of the initial values for serum levels of ALT and hepatofibrogenesis markers of 7S domain of type IV collagen (7S-IV) and amino terminal propeptide of type II procollagen (P-III-P) after administration of Sho-saiko-to to patients with chronic hepatitis C with fibrosis of stages 1 (○, n = 6), 2 (△, n = 8), and 3 (●, n = 8). Values are expressed as mean percentages (± SD) of each initial value before treatment. *P < 0.05.

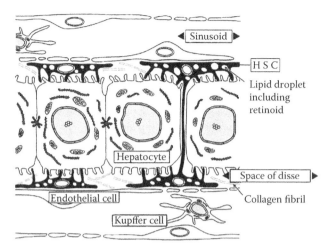

FIGURE 14.2 Schema of the sinusoidal wall of the liver. Mononuclear cells including Kupffer cells rest on fenestrated endothelial cells. Hepatic stellate cells (HSCs) contact both endothelial cells and hepatocytes. Collagen fibrils course through the space of Disse. HSCs are the main storage sites for retinoids.

chronic hepatitis C eventually develops, which can lead to cirrhosis. However, the mechanisms by which HCV induces liver injury and hepatocyte death remain mostly ambiguous.

Cytotoxic T lymphocytes (CTLs) are not only thought to be a major host defense against viral infection, but also have been implicated in immunopathogenesis. Two pathways, the perforin and Fas/Fas ligand pathways, have been proposed to account for all cytolytic activity of CTLs (Kagi et al., 1994), although tumor necrosis factor-α (TNF-α), a proinflammatory cytokine, is released by all HCV-specific CTL clones studied to date (Koziel et al., 1995) and may also contribute to the cytotoxicity of CTLs (Braun et al., 1996). The core protein of HCV has been recognized as a target for CTLs (Shimizu et al., 1997; Kato et al., 2000). Viral proteins possess various accessory functions that target host proteins and thus alter normal cellular growth properties, affecting many signaling molecules, such as the nuclear factor κB (NF-κB) and activator protein 1 (AP-1), have been reported to be activated by HCV proteins. The NF-κB pathway plays an important role in the cellular response to a variety of extracellular stimuli, including TNF-α and interleukin-1 (IL-1). Because the HCV core protein binds both the TNF receptor and p53 (Zhu et al., 1998; Lu et al., 1999), the induction of NF-κB by HCV proteins may either cause or suppress hepatocyte death and, on other occasions, may promote cellular proliferation, thus contributing to liver injury or tumorigenesis induced by HCV. Likewise, the activation of AP-1, a transcription factor that regulates a number of genes involved in the control of cellular growth, by viral proteins presumably would promote oncogenesis and a myriad of other effects. Our preliminary study demonstrated that prooxidants induce the activation both of AP-1 and NF-κB with degradation of IκB-α, an inhibitory subunit of NF-κB, in cultured rat hepatocytes, and that Sho-saiko-to inhibited the oxidative stress-induced activation of NF-κB and AP-1 in a dose-dependent manner (Shimizu, 2003). In addition, oxidative stress was observed to induce early apoptosis, by decreasing the expression of antiapoptotic proteins Bcl-2 and Bcl-X_L, and by increasing the expression of proapoptotic protein Bad in cultured rat hepatocytes, whereas Sho-saiko-to was found to suppress the oxidative stress-induced early apoptosis by modulating the Bcl-2 family protein expression (Shimizu, unpublished data, 2002).

Sho-saiko-to has also been reported to modulate *in vitro* cytokine production in peripheral blood mononuclear cells, downregulating the synthesis of IL-4 and IL-5 in favor of IL-10 in patients with chronic hepatitis C. IL-10 production in mononuclear cells of patients with hepatitis C was reported to be lower than that of healthy subjects (Yamashiki et al., 1997b). IL-10 would be expected to have an effective activity for inflammatory bowel disease (Kuhn et al., 1993) and endotoxin shock (Howard et al., 1993). These findings suggest that Sho-saiko-to may play a role in the repair of abnormalities in the cytokine production system in patients with chronic HCV infection.

Parenchymal cell membrane damage could result in the release of oxygen-derived free radicals and other reactive oxygen species (ROS) derived from lipid peroxidative processes, which represent a general feature of sustained inflammatory response and liver injury, once the antioxidant mechanisms have been depleted (Houglum et al., 1990). Many cells have their own unique enzymatic defense systems against oxidative stress, including the production of superoxide dismutase (SOD) and glutathione peroxidase (GPx). In addition, histopathological studies associated with chronic HCV infection showed fatty changes in 31 to 72% of patients (Scheuer et al., 1992; Bach et al., 1992; Lefkowitch et al., 1993), indicating that hepatic steatosis is a characteristic feature of chronic HCV infection. It has been suggested that hepatic steatosis may reflect a direct cytopathic effect of HCV and may play a role in the progression of the disease. In support of these proposals, a transgenic mouse model, which expresses the HCV core gene, was observed to develop progressive hepatic steatosis (Moriya et al., 1997). It is conceivable that following hepatocyte injury, hepatic steatosis leads to an increase in lipid peroxidation, which might contribute to HSC proliferation and transformation by releasing soluble mediators (Gressner et al., 1992; Lee et al., 1995), and, thus, induce hepatic fibrosis.

We previously reported that, in two rat models of hepatic fibrosis, hepatic concentrations of malondialdehyde (MDA), an end product of lipid peroxidation, in Sho-saiko-to-fed animals were significantly lower than in those fed a basal diet, and that Sho-saiko-to inhibited the prooxidant-enhanced lipid peroxidation in cultured rat hepatocytes, and inhibited lipid peroxidation induced in rat liver mitochondria by Fe^{2+}/adenosine 5′-diphosphate (Shimizu et al., 1999). In addition, we observed that Sho-saiko-to scavenges the free radical 1,1-diphenyl-2-picrylhydrazyl (DPPH) (Shimizu et al., 1999). Free radicals, generated mainly by Kupffer cells, are thought to cause tissue injury by initiating lipid peroxidation and inducing irreversible modifications of cell membrane structure and function (Sevanian et al., 1988). In an animal model of endotoxemia, the preadministration of Sho-saiko-to was found to significantly increase the activity of SOD and GPx, suggesting that Sho-saiko-to acts by protecting against plasma membrane damage by ROS such as free radicals (Sakaguchi et al., 1983).

14.4 INHIBITORY EFFECT OF SHO-SAIKO-TO ON HEPATIC FIBROSIS

In the injured liver, HSCs are regarded as the primary target cells for inflammatory and peroxidative stimuli, and are transformed into myofibroblast-like cells. These HSCs are referred to as activated cells, and this activation is accompanied by a loss of cellular retinoid, and the synthesis of α-smooth muscle actin (α-SMA) and large quantities of the major components of the ECM, including collagen types I, III, and IV, fibronectin, laminin, and proteoglycans. α-SMA is an activation marker of HSCs. It has been shown that, *in vivo*, HSCs express the genes that encode for enzymes such as matrix metalloproteinase (MMP)-1 and MMP-2, as well as a tissue inhibitor of metalloproteinase (TIMP)-1. The net effect of the production of proteins involved in matrix synthesis and degradation could be reduced matrix degradation, which could account for the marked increases in matrix deposition and nodule formation observed during hepatic fibrosis and cirrhosis (Shimizu, 2001).

Several reports concerning the role of Sho-saiko-to with respect to the prevention and treatment of experimental liver damage induced in rats by D-galactosamine (Ymamoto et al., 1985), carbon tetrachloride (Amagaya et al., 1988a), dimethylnitrosamine (DMN) (Amagaya et al., 1988b), and pig serum (PS) (Amagaya et al., 1988b) have appeared. Although the mechanism by which Sho-saiko-to prevents hepatic fibrosis is not at present clear, it has been reported that the preadministration of this herbal medicine protects the liver plasma membrane and HSCs against injury (Sakaguchi et al., 1983). Moreover, Sho-saiko-to was reported to prevent the development of hepatic fibrosis by the inhibition of HSC activation in a different animal model, the choline-deficient rat (Sakaida et al., 1998a). We confirmed the preventive and therapeutic effects of Sho-saiko-to on rat experimental hepatic fibrosis induced by DMN and PS (Shimizu et al., 1999). The rats were fed a basic diet that contained Sho-saiko-to for 2 weeks prior to the induction of hepatic fibrosis, or during the last 2 weeks of treatment. Sho-saiko-to suppressed the induction of hepatic fibrosis, maintained hepatic retinoid stores, and reduced hepatic collagen levels and the hepatic expression of α-SMA and type I collagen. In addition, when incubated with cultured rat HSCs, the presence of Sho-saiko-to led to an increase in lipid droplets, which include retinoid and occupy the cytoplasmic space, and inhibit type I collagen production, α-SMA expression, cell spreading, and DNA synthesis. Furthermore, Sho-saiko-to was also reported to induce the arrest at the G_0/G_1 phase in the cell cycle of HSCs (Kayano et al., 1998). These findings suggest that the antifibrogenic activities of Sho-saiko-to are associated with the regulation of ECM proteins including type I collagen and α-SMA expression, retinoid disappearance, as well as HSC proliferation.

In investigating the mechanism by which Sho-saiko-to inactivates HSCs, Kakumu et al. (1991) showed that Sho-saiko-to enhanced the *in vitro* production of interferon (IFN)-γ and antibodies to the hepatitis B core and e antigens, produced by peripheral blood mononuclear cells from patients with chronic hepatitis (Kakumu et al., 1991). IFN-γ is a potent cytokine with immunomodulatory and anti-proliferative properties, which inhibits HSC activation and ECM production in *in vivo* models of hepatic schistosomiasis and carbon tetrachloride-, DMN-, and PS-induced hepatic fibrosis (Czaja et al., 1989; Rockey et al., 1992; Rockey and Chung, 1994; Baroni et al., 1996; Sakaida et al., 1998b). Oxidative stress, including the generation of ROS, has also been implicated as a cause of hepatic fibrosis. There is evidence to show that the products of lipid peroxidation modulate collagen gene expression (Houglum et al., 1991; Iredale et al., 1992), suggesting that lipid peroxidation is a link between liver tissue injury and fibrosis (Houglum et al., 1990; Bedossa et al., 1994). It has been reported that paracrine stimuli derived from hepatocytes undergoing oxidative stress induce HSC proliferation and collagen synthesis (Baroni et al., 1998). HSCs have also been shown to be activated by the generation of free radicals with Fe^{2+}/ascorbate (Lee et al., 1995) and by MDA and 4-hydroxynonenal (Parola et al., 1993; Baraona et al., 1993), aldehydic products of lipid peroxidation, and antioxidants such as α-tocopherol were observed to inhibit HSC activation (Lee et al., 1995). We also reported that Sho-saiko-to supplementation led to a dose-dependent suppression in oxidative stress in cultured rat HSCs in parallel with the inhibition of the type I collagen production (Shimizu et al., 1999). In hepatic fibrosis, Sho-saiko-to may exert its suppressive effects, at least in part, by acting as an antioxidant, and/or by stimulating IFN-γ.

Inflammatory cells, such as Kupffer cells and invading mononuclear cells, which release cytokines, transforming growth factor-β1 (TGF-β1), and platelet-derived growth factor (PDGF), may also contribute to the fibrogenic response to liver injury. It has been shown that TGF-β1 and PDGF activate cultured HSCs (Pinzani et al., 1989; Matsuoka and Tsukamoto, 1990). HSCs also produce and respond to TGF-β1 in an autocrine manner with increased collagen expression. These findings suggest that these growth factors may act as paracrine and autocrine (i.e., from HSCs) mediators that trigger the transformation of HSCs *in vivo* . PDGF is a major mitogen that drives HSC proliferation (Friedman and Arthur, 1989). Importantly, TGF-β1 is a key fibrogenic mediator that is capable of enhancing ECM deposition and inhibiting MMP activity (Casini et al., 1993). TGF-β is also an inhibitor of the proliferation of hepatocytes (Sanchez et al., 1996), and that, at higher concentrations, TGF-β induces oxidative stress leading to hepatocyte apoptosis (Sanchez et al., 1996). A preliminary report concluded that Sho-saiko-to inhibited the PDGF-induced proliferation of HSCs (Kayano et al., 1998).

Because of their anatomical location, their ultrastructural features, and similarities with pericytes that regulate blood flow in other organs, it has been proposed that HSCs function as liver-specific pericytes (Pinzani et al., 1992). Previous studies have shown that the contraction and relaxation of HSCs regulate hepatic sinusoidal blood flow (Pinzani et al., 1992; Bataller et al., 2000). Two vasoregulatory compounds with obvious effects on HSCs include endothelin (ET)-1 and nitric oxide (NO) (Rockey et al., 1993; Sakamoto et al., 1993; Rockey, 1997). Experimental evidence suggests that ET-1 is a potent vasoconstrictor in the liver microcirculation *in vivo* (Bauer et al., 1994), and that exogenous NO prevents ET-induced contraction as well as causing pre-contracted cells to relax (Rockey and Chung, 1995). HSCs and sinusoidal endothelial cells produce NO in response to various stimuli in the presence and absence of endotoxins (Helyar et al., 1994; Shah et al., 1997). It should be pointed out that Sho-saiko-to upregulates the inducible NO synthase in hepatocytes, when cultured in the presence of IFN-γ (Hattori et al., 1995).

14.5 CONCLUSION

Although herbal medicines are thought to be safe drugs, a complicating factor, which has caused physicians and patients to lose confidence in the safety of Sho-saiko-to, is the development of severe interstitial pneumonia associated with its use, particularly when it is used in combination with interferon (IFN) in treating some Japanese patients with chronic hepatitis C. Interstitial pneumonia is also induced by granulocyte colony-stimulating factor (G-CSF), whereas Sho-saiko-to induced G-CSF production in peripheral blood mononuclear cells in patients with chronic hepatitis C (Yamashiki et al., 1997a). These findings suggest that Sho-saiko-to, when used in combination with IFN, may be a cause of interstitial pneumonia.

Because Sho-saiko-to has been shown to have a stronger anti-proliferative effect than any one of its active ingredients, these effects are difficult to explain, based on a single ingredient, and the combination of several ingredients may possess synergistic or additive effects (Shimizu, 2000). In any case, it should be noted that Sho-saiko-to may have some beneficial effects on hepatic fibrosis in patients with chronic liver disease.

REFERENCES

Amagaya, S., Hayakawa, M., Ogihara, Y., and Fujiwara, K. (1988a) Effects of Sho-saiko-to and Dai-saiko-to on carbon tetrachloride-induced hepatic injury in rats, *J. Med. Pharm. Soc. Wakan-Yaku,* 5, 129–136.

Amagaya, S., Hayakawa, M., Ogihara, Y., and Fujiwara, K. (1988b) Effects of Sho-saiko-to and Dai-saiko-to on experimental hepatic fibrosis in rats, *J. Med. Pharm. Soc. Wakan-Yaku,* 5, 137–145.

Bach, N., Thung, S.N., and Schaffner, F. (1992) The histological features of chronic hepatitis C and autoimmune chronic hepatitis: a comparative analysis, *Hepatology,* 15, 572–577.

Baraona, E., Liu, W., Ma, X.L., Svegliati, B.G., and Lieber, C.S. (1993) Acetaldehyde-collagen adducts in *N*-nitrosodimethylamine-induced liver cirrhosis in rats, *Life Sci.,* 52, 1249–1255.

Baroni, G.S., D'Ambrosio, L., Curto, P., Casini, A., Mancini, R., Jezequel, A.M. et al. (1996) Interferon gamma decreases hepatic stellate cell activation and extracellular matrix deposition in rat liver fibrosis, *Hepatology,* 23, 1189–1199.

Baroni, G.S., D'Ambrosio, L., Ferretti, G., Casini, A., Sario, A.D., Salzano, R., et al. (1998) Fibrogenic effect of oxidative stress on rat hepatic stellate cells, *Hepatology,* 27, 720–726.

Bataller, R., Gines, P., Nicolas, J.M., Gorbig, M.N., Garcia-Ramallo, E., Gasull, X. et al. (2000) Angiotensin II induces contraction and proliferation of human hepatic stellate cells, *Gastroenterology,* 118, 1149–1156.

Bauer, M., Zhang, J.X., Bauer, I., and Clemens, M.G. (1994) ET-1 induced alterations of hepatic microcirculation: sinusoidal and extrasinusoidal sites of action, *Am. J. Physiol.,* 267, G143–G149.

Bedossa, P., Houglum, K., Trautwein, C., Holstege, A., and Chojkier, M. (1994) Stimulation of collagen α1(I) gene expression is associated with lipid peroxidation in hepatocellular injury: a link to tissue fibrosis? *Hepatology,* 19, 1262–1271.

Biagini, G. and Ballardini, G. (1989) Liver fibrosis and extracellular matrix,. *J. Hepatol.,* 8, 115–124.

Braun, M.Y., Lowin, B., French, L., Acha-Orbea, H., and Tschopp, J. (1996) Cytotoxic T cells deficient in both functional fas ligand and perforin show residual cytolytic activity yet lose their capacity to induce lethal acute graft-versus-host disease, *J. Exp. Med.,* 183, 657–661.

Casini, A., Pinzani, M., Milani, S., Grappone, C., Galli, G., Jezequel, A.M. et al. (1993) Regulation of extracellular matrix synthesis by transforming growth factor β1 in human fat-storing cells, *Gastroenterology*, 105, 245–253.

Czaja, M.J., Weiner, F.R., Takahashi, S., Giambrone, M.A., van der Meide, P.H., Schellekens, H. et al. (1989) Gamma-interferon treatment inhibits collagen deposition in murine schistosomiasis, *Hepatology*, 10, 795–800.

Friedman, S.L. and Arthur, M.J. (1989) Activation of cultured rat hepatic lipocytes by Kupffer cell conditioned medium. Direct enhancement of matrix synthesis and stimulation of cell proliferation via induction of platelet-derived growth factor receptors, *J. Clin. Invest.*, 84, 1780–1785.

Gressner, A.M., Lotfi, S., Gressner, G., and Lahme, B. (1992) Identification and partial characterization of a hepatocyte-derived factor promoting proliferation of cultured fat-storing cells (parasinusoidal lipocytes), *Hepatology*, 16, 1250–1266.

Hattori, Y., Kasai, K., Sekiguchi, Y., Hattori, S., Banba, N., and Shimoda, S. (1995) The herbal medicine Shosaiko-to induces nitric oxide synthase in rat hepatocytes, *Life Sci.*, 56, L143–L148.

Helyar, L., Bundschuh, D.S., Laskin, J.D., and Laskin, D.L. (1994) Induction of hepatic Ito cell nitric oxide production after acute endotoxemia, *Hepatology*, 20, 1509–1515.

Hirayama, C., Okumura, M., Tanikawa, K., Yano, M., Mizuta, M., and Ogawa, N. (1989) A multicenter randomized controlled clinical trial of Shosaiko-to in chronic active hepatitis, *Gastroenterol. Jpn.*, 24, 715–719.

Houglum, K., Filip, M., Witztum, J.L., and Chojkier, M. (1990) Malondialdehyde and 4-hydroxynonenal protein adducts in plasma and liver of rats with iron overload, *J. Clin. Invest.*, 86, 1991–1998.

Houglum, K., Brenner, D.A., and Chojkier, M. (1991) d-alpha-Tocopherol inhibits collagen alpha 1(I) gene expression in cultured human fibroblasts. Modulation of constitutive collagen gene expression by lipid peroxidation, *J. Clin. Invest.*, 87, 2230–2235.

Howard, M., Muchamuel, T., Andrade, S., and Menon, S. (1993) Interleukin 10 protects mice from lethal endotoxemia, *J. Exp. Med.*, 177, 1205–1208.

Iredale, J.P., Murphy, G., Hembry, R.M., Friedman, S.L., and Arthur, M.J. (1992) Human hepatic lipocytes synthesize tissue inhibitor of metalloproteinases-1. Implications for regulation of matrix degradation in liver, *J. Clin. Invest.*, 90, 282–287.

Kagi, D., Vignaux, F., Ledermann, B., Burki, K., Depraetere, V., Nagata, S. et al. (1994) Fas and perforin pathways as major mechanisms of T cell-mediated cytotoxicity, *Science*, 265, 528–530.

Kakumu, S., Yoshioka, K., Wakita, T., and Ishikawa, T. (1991) Effects of TJ-9 Sho-saiko-to (Kampo medicine) on interferon gamma and antibody production specific for hepatitis B virus antigen in patients with type B chronic hepatitis, *Int. J. Immunopharmacol.*, 13, 141–146.

Kato, N., Yoshida, H., Kioko Ono-Nita, S., Kato, J., Goto, T., Otsuka, M. et al. (2000) Activation of intracellular signaling by hepatitis B and C viruses: C- viral core is the most potent signal inducer, *Hepatology*, 32, 405–412.

Kayano, K., Sakaida, I., Uchida, K., and Okita, K. (1998) Inhibitory effects of the herbal medicine Sho-saiko-to (TJ-9) on cell proliferation and procollagen gene expressions in cultured rat hepatic stellate cells, *J. Hepatol.*, 29, 642–649.

Koziel, M.J., Dudley, D., Afdhal, N., Grakoui, A., Rice, C.M., Choo, Q.L. et al. (1995) HLA class I-restricted cytotoxic T lymphocytes specific for hepatitis C virus. Identification of multiple epitopes and characterization of patterns of cytokine release, *J. Clin. Invest.*, 96, 2311–2321.

Kuhn, R., Lohler, J., Rennick, D., Rajewsky, K., and Muller, W. (1993) Interleukin-10-deficient mice develop chronic enterocolitis, *Cell*, 75, 263–274.

Lee, K.S., Buck, M., Houglum, K., and Chojkier, M. (1995) Activation of hepatic stellate cells by TGF alpha and collagen type I is mediated by oxidative stress through c-myb expression, *J. Clin. Invest.*, 96, 2461–2468.

Lefkowitch, J.H., Schiff, E.R., Davis, G.L., Perrillo, R.P., Lindsay, K., Bodenheimer, H.C., Jr. et al. (1993) Pathological diagnosis of chronic hepatitis C: a multicenter comparative study with chronic hepatitis B. The Hepatitis Interventional Therapy Group. *Gastroenterology*, 104, 595–603.

Lu, W., Lo, S.Y., Chen, M., Wu, K., Fung, Y.K., and Ou, J.H. (1999) Activation of p53 tumor suppressor by hepatitis C virus core protein., *Virology*, 264, 134–141.

Matsuoka, M. and Tsukamoto, H. (1990) Stimulation of hepatic lipocyte collagen production by Kupffer cell-derived transforming growth factor beta: implication for a pathogenetic role in alcoholic liver fibrogenesis, *Hepatology*, 11, 599–605.

Moriya, K., Yotsuyanagi, H., Shintani, Y., Fujie, H., Ishibashi, K., Matsuura, Y. et al. (1997) Hepatitis C virus core protein induces hepatic steatosis in transgenic mice, *J. Gen. Virol.*, 78(7), 1527–1531.

Oka, H., Yamamoto, S., Kuroki, T., Harihara, S., Marumo, T., Kim, S.R. et al. (1995) Prospective study of chemoprevention of hepatocellular carcinoma with Sho-saiko-to (TJ-9), *Cancer*, 76, 743–749.

Parola, M., Pinzani, M., Casini, A., Albano, E., Poli, G., Gentilini, P. et al. (1993) Stimulation of lipid peroxidation or 4-hydroxynonenal treatment increases procollagen (I) gene expression in human liver fat-storing cells, *Biochem. Biophys. Res. Commun.*, 194, 1044–1050.

Pinzani, M., Gesualdo, L., Sabbah, G.M., and Abboud, H.E. (1989) Effects of platelet-derived growth factor and other polypeptide mitogens on DNA synthesis and growth of cultured rat liver fat-storing cells, *J. Clin. Invest.*, 84, 1786–1793.

Pinzani, M., Failli, P., Ruocco, C., Casini, A., Milani, S., Baldi, E. et al. (1992) Fat-storing cells as liver-specific pericytes. Spatial dynamics of agonist-stimulated intracellular calcium transients, *J. Clin. Invest.*, 90, 642–646.

Risteli, J. and Risteli, L. (1995) Analysing connective tissue metabolites in human serum. Biochemical, physiological and methodological aspects, *J. Hepatol.*, 22, 77–81.

Rockey, D. (1997) The cellular pathogenesis of portal hypertension: stellate cell contractility, endothelin, and nitric oxide, *Hepatology*, 25, 2–5.

Rockey, D.C. and Chung, J.J. (1994) Interferon gamma inhibits lipocyte activation and extracellular matrix mRNA expression during experimental liver injury: implications for treatment of hepatic fibrosis, *J. Invest. Med.*, 42, 660–670.

Rockey, D.C. and Chung, J.J. (1995) Inducible nitric oxide synthase in rat hepatic lipocytes and the effect of nitric oxide on lipocyte contractility, *J. Clin. Invest.*, 95, 1199–1206.

Rockey, D.C., Maher, J.J., Jarnagin, W.R., Gabbiani, G., and Friedman, S.L. (1992) Inhibition of rat hepatic lipocyte activation in culture by interferon-gamma, *Hepatology*, 16, 776–784.

Rockey, D.C., Housset, C.N., and Friedman, S.L. (1993) Activation-dependent contractility of rat hepatic lipocytes in culture and *in vivo*, *J. Clin. Invest.*, 92, 1795–1804.

Sakaguchi, S., Tsutsumi, E., and Yokota, K. (1983) Preventive effects of a traditional Chinese medicine (Sho-saiko-to) against oxygen toxicity and membrane damage during endotoxemia., *Biol. Pharm. Bull.*, 16, 782–786.

Sakaida, I., Matsumura, Y., Akiyama, S., Hayashi, K., Ishige, A., and Okita, K. (1998a) Herbal medicine Sho-saiko-to (TJ-9) prevents liver fibrosis and enzyme-altered lesions in rat liver cirrhosis induced by a choline-deficient L-amino acid-defined diet, *J. Hepatol.*, 28, 298–306.

Sakaida, I., Uchida, K., Matsumura, Y., and Okita, K. (1998b) Interferon gamma treatment prevents procollagen gene expression without affecting transforming growth factor-beta1 expression in pig serum- induced rat liver fibrosis *in vivo*, *J. Hepatol.*, 28, 471–479.

Sakamoto, M., Ueno, T., Kin, M., Ohira, H., Torimura, T., Inuzuka, S. et al. (1993) Ito cell contraction in response to endothelin-1 and substance P, *Hepatology*, 18, 978–983.

Sanchez, A., Alvarez, A.M., Benito, M., and Fabregat, I. (1996) Apoptosis induced by transforming growth factor-beta in fetal hepatocyte primary cultures: involvement of reactive oxygen intermediates, *J. Biol. Chem.*, 271, 7416–7422.

Scheuer, P.J., Ashrafzadeh, P., Sherlock, S., Brown, D., and Dusheiko, G.M. (1992) The pathology of hepatitis C, *Hepatology*, 15, 567–571.

Sevanian, A., Wratten, M.L., McLeod, L.L., and Kim, E. (1988) Lipid peroxidation and phospholipase A2 activity in liposomes composed of unsaturated phospholipids: a structural basis for enzyme activation, *Biochim. Biophys. Acta*, 961, 316–327.

Shah, V., Haddad, F.G., Garcia-Cardena, G., Frangos, J.A., Mennone, A., Groszmann, R.J. et al. (1997) Liver sinusoidal endothelial cells are responsible for nitric oxide modulation of resistance in the hepatic sinusoids, *J. Clin. Invest.*, 100, 2923–2930.

Shimizu, I. (2000) Sho-saiko-to: Japanese herbal medicine for protection against hepatic fibrosis and carcinoma., *J. Gastroenterol. Hepatol.*, 15, D84–D90.

Shimizu, I. (2001) Antifibrogenic therapies in chronic HCV infection, *Curr. Drug Targets Infectious Disord.*, 1, 227–240.

Shimizu, I. (2004) Sho-saiko-to. In *Herbal Medicines: Molecular Basis of Biological Activity and Health,* L. Packer, Ed. Marcel Dekker, New York, pp. 573–594.

Shimizu, I., Yao, D.-F., Horie, C., Yasuda, M., Shiba, M., Horie, T. et al. (1997) Mutations in a hydrophilic part of the core gene of hepatitis C virus in patients with hepatocellular carcinoma in China., *J. Gastroenterol.,* 32, 47–55.

Shimizu, I., Ma, Y.-R., Mizobuchi, Y., Liu, F., Miura, T., Nakai, Y. et al. (1999) Effects of Sho-saiko-to, a Japanese herbal medicine, on hepatic fibrosis in rats [see comments], *Hepatology,* 29, 149–160.

Shiratori, Y., Shiina, S., Imamura, M., Kato, N., Kanai, F., Okudaira, T. et al. (1995) Characteristic difference of hepatocellular carcinoma between hepatitis B- and C-viral infection in Japan, *Hepatology,* 22, 1027–1033.

Tajiri, H., Kozaiwa, K., Ozaki, Y., Miki, K., Shimuzu, K., and Okada, S. (1991) Effect of Sho-saiko-to (Xiao-Chai-Hu-Tang) on HBeAg clearance in children with chronic hepatitis B virus infection and with sustained liver disease, *Am. J. Chin. Med.,* 19, 121–129.

Takano, S., Yokosuka, O., Imazeki, F., Tagawa, M., and Omata, M. (1995) Incidence of hepatocellular carcinoma in chronic hepatitis B and C: a prospective study of 251 patients. *Hepatology,* 21, 650–655.

Wake, K. (1999) Cell–cell organization and functions of "sinusoids" in liver microcirculation system., *J. Electron. Microsc.,* 48, 89–98.

WHO (1997) Hepatitis C: global prevalence, *Wkly. Epidemiol. Rec.,* 72, 341–344.

Yamashiki, M., Nishimura, A., Nobori, T., Nakabayashi, S., Takagi, T., Inoue, K. et al. (1997a) *In vitro* effects of Sho-saiko-to on production of granulocyte colony-stimulating factor by mononuclear cells from patients with chronic hepatitis C, *Int. J. Immunopharmacol.,* 19, 381–385.

Yamashiki, M., Nishimura, A., Suzuki, H., Sakaguchi, S., and Kosaka, Y. (1997b) Effects of the Japanese herbal medicine "Sho-saiko-to" (TJ-9) on *in vitro* interleukin-10 production by peripheral blood mononuclear cells of patients with chronic hepatitis C, *Hepatology,* 25, 1390–1397.

Ymamoto, K., Araki, N., and Ogawa, K. (1985) Ultrastructural and utlaracytochemical examination of the effects of preadministration of Xiao-Chai-Hu-Tang on hepatic disorders induced by D-galactosamine HCl., *Acta Histochem. Cytochem.,* 18, 403–418.

Zhu, N., Khoshnan, A., Schneider, R., Matsumoto, M., Dennert, G., Ware, C. et al. (1998) Hepatitis C virus core protein binds to the cytoplasmic domain of tumor necrosis factor (TNF) receptor 1 and enhances TNF-induced apoptosis. *J. Virol.,* 72, 3691–3697.

15 Preventive Effects of Sho-Saiko-To against Septic Shock Symptoms

Shuhei Sakaguchi

CONTENTS

15.1 INTRODUCTION

Endotoxin from Gram-negative bacteria induce shock symptoms in humans and animals, a state characterized by fever, hypotension, intravascular coagulation, and finally multi-organ failure. Therefore, investigators have recently turned their attention to the metabolic alterations that develop during Gram-negative sepsis or endotoxic shock. Most endotoxin administered is localized within cells of the reticuloendothelial system (RES) in animals, particularly in Kupffer cells and splenic macrophages. Macrophages stimulated with endotoxin also release lysosomal enzymes and cytokines. Tumor necrosis factor-α (TNF-α), a macrophage-derived cytokine inducible by endotoxin, has frequently been reported to cause a shock syndrome similar to that caused by endotoxins, and TNF-α is considered to be a major early mediator in the systemic inflammatory response syndrome (SIRS) observed during Gram-negative sepsis (Vassalli, 1992). This mediator is responsible, at least in part, for a number of pathophysiological responses in the liver including the acute phase response, inflammatory cell infiltration, hepatocyte proliferation, hyperlipidemia, free oxygen radical formation, fibrogenesis, and cholestasis (Camussi et al., 1991; Fiers, 1991).

In Japan, many herbal medicines that originated and have been used for several thousands of years in China are manufactured with uniform quality and quantity of components as ready-for-use prescriptions for hospital use. These medicines have received official approval, have been used by Japan's Occidental-medicine practitioners for 20 years, and their clinical efficacy has been well recognized. Among them, Sho-saiko-to, which has been used in the treatment of pyretic diseases in China, is well known for gradually improving subjective symptoms and abnormal liver functions of patients with chronic viral liver disease. Sho-saiko-to is associated with low side effects and can be administered long term. Despite the remarkable progress in clinical medicine, sepsis and shock continue to be major clinical problems in intensive care units. We reported previously that "Sho-saiko-to" (used as Tsumura's granules TJ-9) improved endotoxin shock, in a series of studies on metabolic pharmacological effects (Sakaguchi et al., 1991, 1993a, 1994, 1995, 1996a). We therefore suggested that Sho-saiko-to may protect animals from the severe shock syndrome induced by endotoxin.

15.2 PREVENTIVE EFFECT OF SHO-SAIKO-TO ON FREE RADICAL GENERATION DURING ENDOTOXEMIA

The liver is one of the main target organs of endotoxin attack. Detoxification of endotoxin is considered to be mediated mainly by the RES, particularly Kupffer cells, in the liver (Cook et al., 1980; Sakaguchi et al., 1982). Ischemia causes functional and structural damage to tissues or organs by generation of active oxygen species. The modification induced in the apolar side residues of the membrane phosphoglycerides by active oxygen generation are considered to bring about structural alterations in the membrane. Therefore, biomembranes and subcellular organelles are the major sites of lipid peroxide damage. In previous studies (Sakaguchi et al., 1981a, 1981b), endotoxin injection was shown to result in lipid peroxide formation and membrane damage in experimental animals, causing decreased levels of scavengers or quenchers of free radicals. Therefore, we investigated whether or not Sho-saiko-to can defend mice from damage by free radicals generated in the ischemic state of tissues during endotoxemia (Sakaguchi et al., 1993a).

Despite marked high levels of lipid peroxide in the liver of endotoxemic (6 mg/kg, i.p.) mice, it was noted here that lipid peroxide formation was markedly lower in the liver of endotoxemic mice given Sho-saiko-to (500 mg/kg/day, p.o). However, xanthine oxidase activity notably increased in the liver of these mice, while, superoxide dismutase (SOD) and glutathione peroxidase (GSH-Px) activities showed a significant recovery in endotoxin/Sho-saiko-to-treated mice (Figure 15.1A). SOD dismutates from O_2^- to H_2O_2 formation, and the ensuing molecular interaction generates a more toxic hydroxyl radical and perhaps singlet oxygen, while GSH-Px is the enzyme responsible for the destruction of H_2O_2 and organic hydroperoxide compounds inducing cellular membrane damage. It follows, therefore, that the upkeep of these enzymic activities by Sho-saiko-to pretreatment may play a key role in providing a defense against endotoxin-induced O_2^- toxicity by catalytically scavenging O_2^-. Moreover, the nonprotein SH (NpSH) and α-tocopherol levels showed a significant increase in the liver of endotoxemic mice given Sho-saiko-to than in endotoxemic mice (Figure 15.1B). Previously, we observed that α-tocopherol can be helpful in preventing membrane instability in endotoxin-poisoned mice (Sakaguchi et al., 1981b). Furthermore, GSH plays an important role in tissues, especially in the oxidation-reduction system, which is responsible for the inner tissue metabolism, and also protects SH-enzymes and membrane SH from free radical attack. Interestingly, Sho-saiko-to shows a preventive effect on endotoxin-induced hypoferremia (Sakaguchi et al., unpublished data). Iron not only participates in numerous biological processes but also plays a central role in oxidative stress as the major catalyst for hydroxyl radical formation via Fenton reaction. Miyahara and Tatsumi (1990) suggested that Sho-saiko-to markedly inhibited iron-induced lipid peroxidation in microsomes and mitochondria in the rat liver, and also identified active components as ginsenoside Rf and baicalein.

The administration of Sho-saiko-to clearly prevented the membrane protein damage arising from endotoxin challenge (Figure 15.2). Thus, it may be inferred that the administration of Sho-saiko-to prevented the peroxidation of membrane lipid by superoxide free radicals generated in endotoxicosis as described above. The role of lysosome as an intracellular target for endotoxin has been proposed on the basis that endotoxin induces lysosomal instability and causes the release of lysosomal enzymes into tissues. In our experiment, endotoxin/Sho-saiko-to-treated mice exhibited less leakage of lactate dehydrogenase and acid phosphatase in the serum, suggesting that the liver

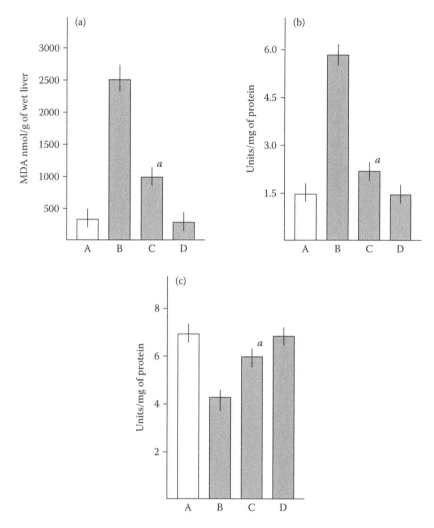

FIGURE 15.1 (A) Effects of Sho-saiko-to preadministration on lipid peroxide level (a), xanthine oxidase (b), and SOD activities (c) in mouse liver 18 h after endotoxin challenge. A, saline; B, endotoxin (6 mg/kg, i.p.); C, endotoxin and Sho-saiko-to (500 mg/kg/day, p.o); D, Sho-saiko-to. Each bar represents the mean ± S.E. of 10 mice. *(a)* Significant difference from the value of endotoxin-poisoned mice at $p < 0.05$.

tissue membrane was stabilized by the administration of Sho-saiko-to. Our series of studies (Sakaguchi et al., 1981a, 1981b, 1989, 1996b, 2000; Sakaguchi and Yokota, 1995) demonstrated that oxidative stress caused by endotoxin can decrease the levels of scavengers or quenchers of free radicals, and Ca^{2+} or selenium may participate in free radical formation during endotoxemia. Kampo prescription Sho-saiko-to thus appears to protect the liver plasma membrane from injury by free radicals, which occur in a tissue ischemic state during endotoxemia. Sho-saiko-to may, therefore, prove to be important for shock induced by Gram-negative bacteria.

15.3 APPROACHED FROM THE BEHAVIOR OF CALCIUM ION ON PREVENTIVE EFFECT OF SHO-SAIKO-TO DURING ENDOTOXEMIA

Ca^{2+} plays important roles in many cellular functions. Several of our studies over the past years have implicated endotoxin-mediated alterations in transmembrane Ca^{2+} movement and cellular Ca^{2+}

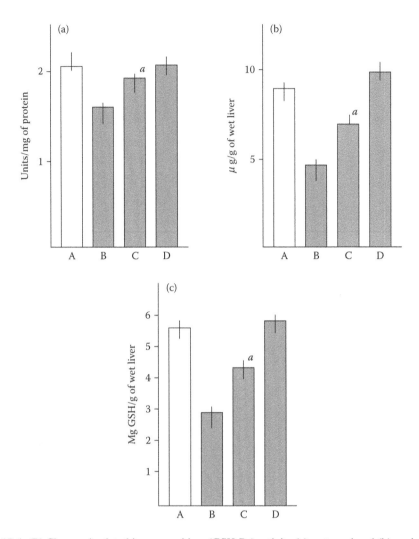

FIGURE 15.1 (B) Changes in glutathione peroxidase (GSH-Px) activity (a), α-tocopherol (b), and nonprotein SH (NpSH) (c) levels in liver of Sho-saiko-to-pretreated mice at 18 h after endotoxin administration. A, saline; B, endotoxin (6 mg/kg, i.p.); C, endotoxin and Sho-saiko-to (500 mg/kg/day, p.o.); D, Sho-saiko-to. Each bar represents the mean ± S.E. of 10 mice. *(a)* Significant difference from the value of endotoxin-poisoned mice at $p < 0.05$.

homeostasis (Sakaguchi et al., 1984, 1989, 1993b; Sakaguchi and Yokota, 1995). For example, we suggested that the increase of cytosolic-free Ca^{2+} concentration ($[Ca^{2+}]i$) in liver cytoplasm may partially explain various endotoxin-induced metabolic disorders. In addition, in support of our findings previous studies showed that intracellular Ca^{2+} may mediate glycogenesis, rather than glycogenolysis, in the depletion mechanism of liver glycogen during endotoxemia. On the other hand, it was found that endotoxin-induced lipid peroxide formation in mouse liver was markedly inhibited by administration of the Ca^{2+}-channel blocker verapamil or by feeding a Ca^{2+}-deficient diet. It seems that intracellular Ca^{2+} may play an important role in free radical formation during endotoxemia. We have already shown that administration of Sho-saiko-to can protect mice against the toxicity of free radical generated during endotoxemia (Sakaguchi et al., 1993a). Therefore, the present study was conducted to discuss the role of intracellular Ca^{2+} in its preventive effects against some of the various metabolic disorders during endotoxemia (Sakaguchi et al., 1994).

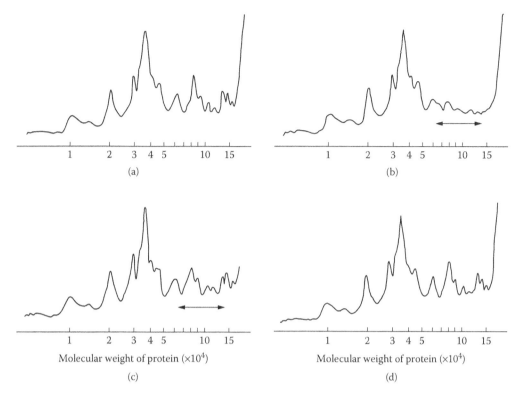

FIGURE 15.2 Sonograms of SDS-polyacrylamide gel electropherograms of liver plasma membrane protein. (A), control; (B), endotoxin; (C), endotoxin + Sho-saiko-to; (D), Sho-saiko-to. Endotoxin (6 mg/kg) was administered i.p. into Sho-saiko-to (500 mg/kg/day, p.o.)-pretreated mice. After treatment, the mice were sacrificed at 18 h postintoxication. Each sample (10 to 20 μg of protein) was subjected to SDS-gel electrophoresis. Gels were stained for protein with 0.1% Coomassie blue and decolored. Each plasma membrane preparation was from 10 mice. ↔, edotoxin-induced membrane protein damage.

In this experiment, we estimated the $[Ca^{2+}]i$ in liver single cells using a photonic microscope system. As observed in Figure 15.3, when the mice already given Sho-saiko-to (500 mg/kg/day, p.o.) were injected with endotoxin (6 mg/kg, i.p.), the $[Ca^{2+}]i$ levels in single cells were shown to be markedly lower in comparison to the levels in the cells of mice treated with endotoxin alone. We also observed that the administration of Sho-saiko-to greatly prevented the depression of Ca^{2+}-ATPase activity in the liver plasma membrane caused by endotoxin. Thus, it is suggested that increased Ca^{2+} pumping of the liver plasma membrane in endotoxin/Sho-saiko-to-treated mice is responsible for pumping Ca^{2+} from liver cytoplasm. Furthermore, as described above, we also reported (Sakaguchi et al., 1993a) that the administration of Sho-saiko-to clearly prevented the membrane protein damage that arose from an endotoxin challenge. It was of interest that the molecular weight (140 kDa) of Ca^{2+}-ATPase (Kessler et al., 1990) fell within the region of molecular weight (60000 to 150000) of liver plasma membrane protein injured by free radicals that generate in a tissue ischemic state during endotoxemia (Sakaguchi et al., 1981a), and that the membrane damage was prevented by the administration of Sho-saiko-to.

The mitochondria of animal cells carry out active intracellular transport of Ca^{2+}, and Ca^+ can accumulate against a steep gradient and with high affinity, with the energy provided by electron transport. Intracellular Ca^{2+} may be sequestered in liver mitochondria as the result of an increase in mitochondrial Ca^{2+}-ATPase activity 18 h after endotoxin injection. An increase in mitochondrial Ca^{2+} may be considered to damage mitochondrial function. In this study, the mitochondrial Ca^{2+}-ATPase activity showed a significant decrease in the liver of endotoxemic mice given Sho-saiko-to,

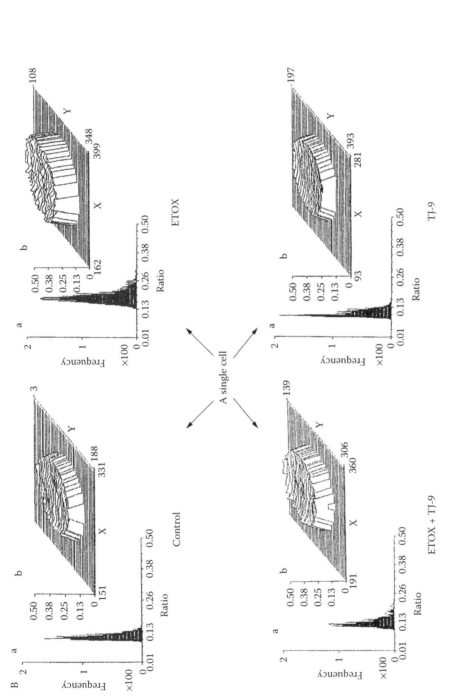

FIGURE 15.3 Changes in cytosolic-free Ca^{2+} concentration ([Ca^{2+}]i) in a single liver cell in Sho-saiko-to pretreated mouse 18 h after endotoxin administration. [Ca^{2+}]i in a single liver cell was measured by microfluorometric analysis using a Hamamatsu Photonics ARGUS-100CA image processor fitted with computer apparatus and a video camera. Changes of [Ca^{2+}]i in a single cell were shown by histogram (A) and digital (B) using the ARGUS-100CA system. Control: saline, ETOX: endotoxin (6 mg/kg, i.p), TJ-9: Sho-saiko-to (500 mg/kg/day, p.o.).

TABLE 15.1
Effect of TJ-9 Administration on
Respiratory Function in Liver
Mitochondria of Mice 18 h after
Endotoxin Challenge

Treatment	Mitochondrial Fraction (nmol O_2/min/mg of protein)	
	State 3	RCI[a]
Control	96.06 ± 6.57[b]	4.96 ± 0.06
ETOX	56.59 ± 2.78	3.23 ± 0.11
ETOX + TJ-9	81.97 ± 6.56[c]	4.31 ± 0.16[c]
TJ-9	112.65 ± 1.50	5.66 ± 0.36

Note: Control saline, ETOX: endotoxin (6 mg/kg, i.p.), TJ-9: Shosaiko-to (500 mg/kg/day, p.o.).

[a] RCI: respiratory control index.
[b] Mean value ± S.E. of 10 mice.
[c] $p < 0.05$ for difference from endotoxin-injected mice.

in comparison to purely endotoxemic mice. The finding indicates that Sho-saiko-to interferes with Ca^{2+} accumulation in the liver mitochondria of endotoxin-poisoned mice. The elevated levels of Ca^{2+} overload have been proved to cause the uncoupling of oxidative phosphorylation in the mitochondria. It is well known that the parameters of state 3 and respiratory control index (RCI) are often emphasized as indicators of damaged mitochondrial function. Thus, it was noted that the mitochondrial respiratory activity (state 3 and RCI) in liver of endotoxin/Sho-saiko-to–treated mice was markedly higher than that in mice treated with endotoxin alone (Table 15.1). Judging from these results, we conjectured that Sho-saiko-to might block the obstacle of ATP production caused by Ca^{2+} overload in cytoplasm and mitochondria.

These findings suggest the protective role of Sho-saiko-to in the damage of liver mitochondrial function in endotoxin-poisoned mice. This prescription may protect some of the various metabolic disorders caused by the change in Ca^{2+}-mobility in the ischemic state of tissues during endotoxemia.

15.4 DEPRESSIVE EFFECT OF SHO-SAIKO-TO ON ENDOTOXIN-INDUCED NITRIC OXIDE FORMATION IN ACTIVATED MURINE MACROPHAGE J774A.1 CELLS

Nitric oxide (NO) may play a role as an important regulator in many cellular functions in endotoxemic animals, and the NO radical functions efficiently as a mediator, a messenger, or a regulator of cell function in various physiological systems and pathophysiological states. NO also contributes to the cytotoxic or cytostatic actions of macrophages activated by various immunological stimuli. In addition, NO has been implicated in the pathogenesis of vascular injury, hypotension, and shock induced by endotoxin or TNF-α (Moncada et al., 1991; Titheradge, 1999). Sho-saiko-to improved endotoxin shock on metabolic pharmacological effects as described above. Therefore, we investigated whether Sho-saiko-to can suppress NO production caused by endotoxin challenge. In this report, using activated murine macrophage J774A.1 cells, we described the role of NO in the preventive effects of Sho-saiko-to against endotoxemia (Sakaguchi et al., 1995).

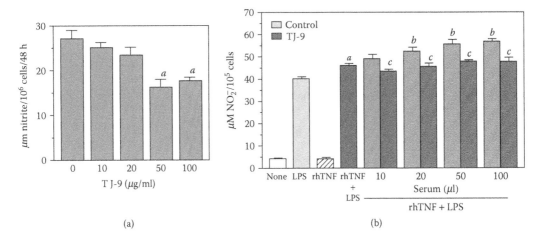

(a)   (b)

FIGURE 15.4 (A) Effect of Sho-saiko-to (TJ-9) on generation of nitric oxide by J774A.1 cells stimulated with endotoxin. Cells were incubated with combinations of endotoxin (0.1 μg/ml) and TJ-9 (10 to 100 μg/ml) for 48 h. Each bar represents the mean ± S.E. of three experiments. Significant difference from the value of cells treated with endotoxin alone at $p < 0.05$. (B) Effect of Sho-saiko-to-(TJ-9)-pretreated serum on production on nitric oxide in J774A.1 cells stimulated with endotoxin/rhTNF. Mice were pretreated with TJ-9 (500 mg/kg/day, p.o.). The pooled serum was obtained from 10 mice pretreated with TJ-9. Control serum was obtained from TJ-9-nontreated 10 mice. Cells (1×10^6 cells/well) were incubated with combinations of endotoxin/rhTNF and TJ-9-pretreated serum (10 to 100 μl). Each bar represents the mean ± S.E. of three experiments. None, unstimulated J774A.1 cells: LPS, endotoxin (1 μg/ml); rhTNF, recombinant human tumor necrosis factor (1×10^4 units/ml); Control, TJ-9-nontreated serum; TJ-9, Sho-saiko-to (500 mg/kg/day, p.o.)-pretreated serum. (a) $p < 0.05$, compared with LPS alone-treated group. (b) $p < 0.05$, compared with rhTNF/LPS-treated group. (c) $p < 0.05$, compared with group treated with rhTNF/LPS plus control serum.

In this study, our results clearly demonstrate that endotoxin (0.1 to 10 μg/ml) can effectively produce NO from activated J774A.1 cells, and NO production by endotoxin-activated J774A.1 cells showed an increase in a dose-dependent manner. NO produced by activated macrophages has been shown to be involved in TNF-α-induced shock, hypotension, and vasodilatation, and in addition NO, a highly reactive free radical produced by activated macrophages, has emerged as another important mediator of inflammatory responses (Moncada et al., 1991; Beckman and Koppenol, 1996). Moreover, NO may react with superoxides resulting in the formation of peroxynitrite, which can lead to the iron-independent generation of hydroxyl radicals (Radi et al., 1991). Our present result demonstrated that Sho-saiko-to (50 to 100 μg/ml) showed clear inhibition in the production of NO from endotoxin-activated J774A.1 cells (Figure 15.4A). On the other hand, we employed a seropharmacological method to investigate the suppressive effect of Sho-saiko-to (500 mg/kg/day, p.o.)-pretreated serum on NO production by endotoxin/TNF-α activated J774A.1 cells (Sakaguchi et al., 1996a). As shown in Figure 15.4B, since the serum contained a variety of cytokines, the effect of normal serum on NO production in J774A.1 cells was seen to be increased in dose-dependent fashion. In contrast, we noted that Sho-saiko-to showed a significant inhibition on the NO production in J774A.1 cells stimulated by endotoxin/TNF-α in the normal serum. Endothelium-derived NO plays (Moncada et al., 1991) a role in the physiological regulation of vascular tone and blood pressure. It has also been implicated in the pathogenesis of vascular injury, hypotension, and shock induced by endotoxin and TNF-α. Previously, we observed that the administration of Sho-saiko-to prevented the peroxidation of membrane lipid by superoxide-free radicals generated in endotoxicosis (Sakaguchi et al., 1993a). It is possible that the preventive effects of Sho-saiko-to in endotoxemia are caused, in part at least, by the inhibition of NO production. Sho-saiko-to may, therefore, prove to be important in Gram-negative bacteria-induced shock. Moreover, Sho-saiko-to is known to show a glucocorticoid-like action (Inoue et al., 1990). Glucocorticoids have been used in the treatment of endotoxin shock. Induction of NO synthase in macrophages is strongly inhibited by glucocorticoids such as dexamethasone and hydrocortisone (Di Rosa et al., 1990). It is, therefore, of interest that endotoxin-induced NO is inhibited by Sho-saiko-to, having a gluco-corticoid-like action. From the findings described above, the suppression of NO generation from endotoxin-activated macrophages by Sho-saiko-to may also prove useful in improving these endo-toxin-induced shock symptoms.

15.5 EFFECT OF ANTITUMOR ACTIVITY AND PROTECTION OF TNF-α-INDUCED SHOCK SYMPTOMS BY SHO-SAIKO-TO

Septic shock may be associated with a toxic state initiated by stimulation of monocytes by a bacterial toxin, such as endotoxin, which is released into the bloodstream. It seems that endotoxin exhibits its toxic effects by stimulating host cells, especially macrophages, to release various proinflamma-tory mediators which act as secondary messengers. Beulter and Cerami (1986) reported that TNF-α may be identical to cachectin. TNF-α/cachectin is a factor that has been found to play a pivotal role in the development of shock and tissue injury activity for some cancer cells. We reported (Sakaguchi et al., 1991, 1993a, 1994, 1995) that Sho-saiko-to improves endotoxin shock based on our series of studies on metabolic pharmacological effects. Therefore, we investigated whether or not Sho-saiko-to can protect from the severe shock symptoms induced by TNF-α, and can exhibit an enhancing effect of TNF-α on antitumor activity by Sho-saiko-to administration (Sakaguchi et al., 1996a).

In this study, we found that fibrinogen was at a markedly lower level in plasma of mice 4 h after TNF-α (5×10^4 units/ mouse, i.v.) injection than that in the control. It was noted that the level showed a significant increase in plasma of mice treated with TNF-α plus Sho-saiko-to (500 mg/kg/day, p.o.). TNF-α is known to have an enhancing effect on procoagulant activity and concomitant suppression of the protein C pathway. Thus, endothelial-directed actions of TNF-α may be relevant to intravascular coagulation and hemorrhagic tumor necrosis (Fiers, 1991). Kubo et al. (1985) suggested that the compounds bicalein and baicalin can prevent the decrease of blood platelets and fibrinogen in disseminated intravascular coagulation in rats, which is induced by endotoxin. We reported previously that Sho-saiko-to decreases the TNF-α-induced lethality in galactosamine-hypersensitized mice, and also that Sho-saiko-to-pretreated mice are protected against falling rectal temperature after TNF-α administration (Sakaguchi et al., 1991). On the other hand, as shown in Figure 15.5a, when cells were treated with endotoxin (1 μg/ml), TNF-α pro-duction was markedly increased, while Sho-saiko-to (20 μg/ml) treatment significantly decreased endototoxin-induced TNF-α production in J774A.1 cells (unpublished data). In addition, treatment with Sho-saiko-to (10 to 50 μg/ml) clearly prevented the endotoxin (10 μg/ml)-induced cytotoxicity in J774A.1 cells (unpublished data). It is, therefore, possible that the protective effect of Sho-saiko-to on endotoxin-induced shock syndrome caused by TNF-α is due to inhibition of TNF-α production in macrophages by the cell stability induced by this prescription.

The Meth-A sarcoma cell is immunogenic and the system is so sensitive that not only hemor-rhagic necrosis, but also the tumor can completely vanish with a single injection of a low, nontoxic concentration of TNF-α. It was originally a surprise, however, to find that Meth-A sarcoma cells in tissue culture were completely resistant to the action of TNF-α. Despite the *in vitro* findings in Figure 15.5B, it was noted in this study that TNF-α-induced cytotoxicity of Meth-A sarcoma cells was enhanced *in vitro* in a dose-dependent fashion by added Sho-saiko-to (1 and 10 μg/ml). We also observed *in vitro* the increase of antitumor activity of TNF-α by Sho-saiko-to pretreatment. It is of interest to note that TNF-α (1×10^4 units/mouse, i.v.) as a single injection had little effect on antitumor activity to Meth-A sarcoma cells, while the activity in TNF-α/Sho-saiko-to-treated

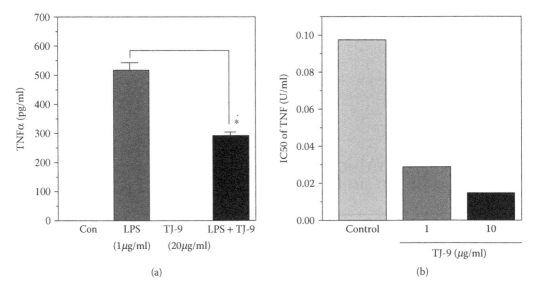

FIGURE 15.5 (A) Suppression of endotoxin-induced TNF-α production in J774A.1 cells by Sho-saiko-to. J774A.1 cells were incubated with endotoxin (1 μg/ml) for 2 h. Sho-saiko-to (20 μg/ml) was added to cells (1×10^5 cells/ml) 18 h before treatment with endotoxin. TNF-α concentration in the culture supernatant was measured by ELISA. Data represent the mean ± S.E. from three independent experiments performed in triplicate. *Significant difference from the value of cells treated with endotoxin alone ($p < 0.05$). (B) rhTNF cytotoxicity in Meth-A sarcoma cells by Sho-saiko-to. Meth-A sarcoma cells (1×10^5 cells) were incubated for 48 h with various concentrations of recombinant human TNF(rhTNF) in the presence of absence of TJ-9 (1 and 10 μg/ml). Then, drug effects on cell proliferation were determined using MTT assay. rhTNF cytotoxicity is expressed as IC_{50}, i.e. rhTNF concentration providing a 50% reduction in cell numbers as compared to controls cultured in parallel without drug. Each value represents the mean of quadruplicate determinations varying less than 10%.

TABLE 15.2
Enhanced Antitumor Activity of rhTNF by TJ-9 Injection

Treatment	Tumor Weight (g) ± S.E.	Inhibition (%)
Control	7.44 ± 0.59	—
TJ-9 500 mg/kg (p.o.)	7.03 ± 0.91	5.6
rhTNF 1×10^4 units/mouse (i.v.)	6.44 ± 0.72	13.4
TJ-9 + rhTNF	4.26 ± 0.56*	52.8

Note: Male BALB/C mice were inoculated i.m. with 1×10^5 Meth-A sarcoma on day 0. On days 11, 12, 13, 14, and 15, they were given p.o. injection of TJ-9 (500 mg/kg) and on day 15 an i.v. injection of rhTNF (1×10^4 units/mouse). Each group consisted of 10 mice. The antitumor activity was evaluated by weighing the solid tumor on day 30 after Meth-A sarcoma inoculation.

$* p < 0.05$, significantly different from the group treated with rhTNF alone.

(500 mg/kg/day, p.o.) mice was significantly increased compared with that in mice treated with TNF-α or Sho-saiko-to alone (Table 15.2). Two active ingredients of Sho-saiko-to, i.e., glycyrrhizin and baicalein, have been reported to suppress proliferation of human hepatocellular carcinoma cell line (HuH-7) *in vitro,* interfering with the cell cycle at the G_0/G_1 phase and with DNA synthesis.

Thus, the present *in vitro* or *in vivo* investigation clearly demonstrated a synergistic effect on cytotoxicity or antitumor activity in Meth-A sarcoma cells by TNF-α and Sho-saiko-to, since Sho-saiko-to alone did not effectively show cytotoxicity *in vitro*. It is, therefore, of interest that TNF-α-induced shock symptoms are prevented by Sho-saiko-to, which has an antitumor activity.

The systemic administration of TNF-α can mediate the regression of a number of established experimental murine tumors, but has no therapeutic effect when administered to humans, probably because humans can tolerate only 2% of the dose required for regression in mice (Feinberg et al., 1988). TNF-α has been delivered via isolation perfusion of the limbs or by direct intralesional injection. Although it has been effective in mediating tumor regression in patients with cancer, our findings suggest that antitumor effects after administration of Sho-saiko-to are more probable if high TNF-α concentration can be used at a local site (Lienard et al., 1992). From the findings described above, the preventive effect of Sho-saiko-to from shock symptoms by TNF-α might be made use of in tumor therapy.

REFERENCES

Beckman, J.S. and Koppenol, W.H. (1996) Nitric oxide, superoxide, and peroxynitrite: the good, the bad, and the ugly, *Am. J. Physiol.*, 271, C1424–C1437.

Beutler, B. and Cerami, A. (1986) Cachectin and tumour necrosis factor as two sides of the same biological coin, *Nature*, 320, 584–588.

Camussi, G., Albano, E., Tetta, C., and Bussolino, F. (1991) The molecular action of tumor necrosis factor-α, *Eur. J. Biochem.*, 202, 3–14.

Cook, J.A., Dougherty, W.J., and Holt, T.M. (1980) Enhanced sensitivity to endotoxin induced by the RES stimulant, glucan, *Circ. Shock*, 7, 225–238.

Di Rosa, M., Radomski, M., Carnuccio, R., and Moncada, S. (1990) Glucocorticoids inhibit the induction of nitric oxide synthase in macrophages, *Biochem. Biophys. Res. Commun.*, 172, 1246–1252.

Feinberg, B., Kurzrock, R., Talpaz, M., Blick, M., Saks, S., and Gutterman, J.U. (1988) A phase 1 trial of intravenously-administered recombinant tumor necrosis factor-alpha in cancer patients, *J. Clin. Oncol.*, 6, 1328–1334.

Fiers, W. (1991) Tumor necrosis factor: characterization at the molecular, cellular and *in vivo* level, *FEBS Lett.*, 285, 192–212.

Inoue, M., Kikuta, Y., Nagatsu, Y., and Ogihara, Y. (1990) Response of liver to glucocorticoid is altered by administration of Shosaikoto (Kampo medicine), *Chem. Pharm. Bull.*, 38, 418–421.

Kessler, F., Bennardini, F., Bachs, O., Serratosa, J., James, P., Caride, A.J., Gazzotti, P., Penniston, J.T., and Carafoli, E. (1990) Partial purification and characterization of the Ca^{2+}-pumping ATPase of the liver plasma membrane, *J. Biol. Chem.*, 265, 16012–16019.

Kubo, M., Matsuda, H., Tani, T., Arichi, S., and Kimura, Y. (1985) Studies on scutellariae radix. XII: anti-thrombic actions of various flavonoids from scutellariase radix, *Chem. Pharm. Bull.*, 33, 2411–2415.

Lienard, D., Ewalenko, P., Delmotte, J.J., Renard, N., and Lejeune, F.J. (1992) High-dose recombinant tumor necrosis factor alpha in combination with interferon gamma and melphalan in isolation perfusion of the limbs for melanoma and sarcoma, *J. Clin. Oncol.*, 10, 52–60.

Miyahara, M. and Tatsumi, Y. (1990) Suppression of lipid peroxidation by Sho-saiko-to and its components in rat liver subcellular membranes, *Yakugaku Zasshi*, 110, 407–413.

Moncada, S., Palmer, R.N.J., and Higgs, E.A. (1991) Nitric oxide: physiology. pathophysiology and pharmacology, *Pharmacol. Rev.*, 43, 109–142.

Radi, R., Beckman, J.S., Bush, K.M., and Freeman, B.A. (1991) Peroxynitrite-induced membrane lipid per-oxidation: the cytoxic potential of superoxide and nitric oxide, *Arch. Biochem. Biophys.*, 288, 481–487.

Sakaguchi, S. and Yokota, K. (1995) Role of Ca^{2+} on endotoxin-sensitive by galactosamine challenge: lipid peroxide formation and hepatotoxicity in zymosan-primed mice, *Pharmacol. Toxicol.*, 77, 81–86.

Sakaguchi, S., Kanda, N., Hsu, C.C., and Sakaguchi, O. (1981a) Lipid peroxide formation and membrane damage in endotoxin-poisoned mice, *Microbiol. Immunol.*, 25, 229–244.

Sakaguchi, O., Kanda, N., Sakaguchi, S., Hsu, C.C., and Abe, H. (1981b) Effect of α-tocopherol on endotox-icosis, *Microbiol. Immunol.*, 25, 787–799.

Sakaguchi, O., Abe H., Sakaguchi, S., and Hsu, C.C. (1982) Effect of lead acetate on superoxide anion generation and its scavengers in mice given endotoxin, *Microbiol. Immunol.*, 26, 767–778.

Sakaguchi, S., Abe, H., and Sakaguchi, O. (1984) Calcium behavior in endotoxin-poisoned mice: especially calcium accumulation in mitochondria, *Microbiol. Immunol.*, 28, 517–527.

Sakaguchi, S., Ibata, H., and Yokota, K. (1989) Effect of calcium ion on lipid peroxide formation in endotoxemic mice, *Microbiol. Immunol.*, 33, 99–110.

Sakaguchi, S., Tsutsumi, E., Yokota, K., Furusawa, S., Sasaki, K., and Takayanagi, Y. (1991) Preventive effects of a Chinese herb medicine (Sho-saiko-to) against lethality after recombinant human tumor necrosis factor administration in mice, *Microbiol. Immunol.*, 35, 389–394.

Sakaguchi, S., Tsutsumi, E., and Yokota, K. (1993a) Preventive effects of a traditional Chinese medicine (Sho-saiko-to) against oxygen toxicity and membrane damage during endotoxemia, *Biol. Pharm. Bull.*, 16, 782–786.

Sakaguchi, S. Tsutsumi, E., and Yokota, K. (1993b) Decline in plasma membrane Ca^{2+}-ATPase activity and increase in cytosolic-free Ca^{2+} concentration of endotoxin-injected mice livers, *Biol. Pharm. Bull.*, 16, 808–810.

Sakaguchi, S., Tsutsumi E., and Yokota, K. (1994) Defense effects of a traditional medicine (Sho-saiko-to) against metabolic disorders during endotoxemia: approached from the behavior of the calcium ion, *Biol. Pharm. Bull.*, 17, 232–236.

Sakaguchi, S., Furusawa, S., Yokota, K., Sasaki, K., and Takayanagi, Y. (1995) Depressive effect of a traditional Chinese medicine (Sho-saiko-to) on endotoxin-induced nitric oxide formation in activated murine macrophage J774 A.1 cells, *Biol. Pharm. Bull.*, 18, 621–623.

Sakaguchi, S., Furusawa, S., Yokota, K., Sasaki, K., Takayanagi, M., and Takayanagi, Y. (1996a) Effects of antitumor activity and protection of shock symptoms by a traditional Chinese medicine (Sho-saiko-to) in recombinant human tumor necrosis factor administered mice, *Biol. Pharm. Bull.*, 19, 1474–1478.

Sakaguchi, S., Furusawa, S., Yokota, K., Sasaki, K., Takayanagi, M., and Takayanagi, Y. (1996b) The enhancing effect of tumour necrosis factor-α on oxidative stress in endotoxemia, *Pharmacol. Toxicol.*, 79, 259–265.

Sakaguchi, S., Iizuka, Y., Furusawa, S., Tanaka, Y., Takayanagi, M., and Takayanagi, Y. (2000) Roles of selenium in endotoxin-induced lipid peroxidation in the rats liver and in nitric oxide production in J774A.1 cells, *Toxicol. Lett.*, 118, 69–77.

Titheradge, M.A. (1999) Nitric oxide in septic shock, *Biochim. Biophys. Acta,* 1411, 437–455.

Vassalli, P. (1992) The pathophysiology of tumor necrosis factors, *Annu. Rev. Immunol.*, 10, 411–452.

Section VI

Patents

16 Patents Containing *Bupleurum*

Patent No.	Title	Inventor*	Applicant
CN1593636	Orally disintegrating tablet of *Bupleurum* root and its preparation	Zhang Qinglong (CN)	Zhang Qinglong (CN)
CN1583158	Medicinal composition for wind-cold pathogen by exopathogen and its preparation	Wu Yifang (CN)	Wu Yifang (CN)
CN1586602	Medicinal composition for treating cholelithiasis and its preparation method	Mei Xi (CN)	Mei Xi (CN)
CN1586573	Pill for reducing transaminase and liver protection	Chaoying Zhang (HK)	Yangchuntang Chinese Medicine (HK)
CN1586572	Oral liquid for female sterility	Chaoying Zhang (HK)	Yangchuntang Chinese Medicine (HK)
CN1586541	External use medicine for preventing respiratory infectious disease and its preparation method	Wang Li (CN)	Wang Li (CN)
CN1586522	Chinese medicine capsule for treating hyperplasia of mammary glands and its production method	Geng Xinsheng (CN); Miao Mingsan (CN)	Geng Xinsheng (CN)
CN1586512	Medicine for treating liver disease	Yin Guisen (CN)	Yin Guisen (CN)
CN1583083	Natural medicine and its preparation of eliminating tumor internally	Zhang Longguang (CN); Zhang Guangyu	Zhang Longguang (CN)
CN1579531	Medicinal composition for treating anemopyretic cold and its preparation method	Zhang Hong (CN)	Zhang Hong (CN)
CN1579511	Ready-made traditional Chinese medicine for treating hyperplasia of mammary glans	Jiang Zhaojun (CN)	Gaohua Pharmaceutical Factory (CN)
CN1579507	Stomach-tonifying ulcer-healing effervescent tablets and preparation method	Li Yehua (CN); Jiang Yan (CN)	Yixiaotang Pharmaceutical Co L (CN)
CN1579485	Traditional Chinese medicinal composition for treating intestinal function disorder and its preparation method	Yang Xinghao (CN)	Univ Nanjing (CN)
CN1579467	Anti-virus medicine	Yang Rong (CN)	Yang Rong (CN)
CN1580043	Anti-malignant tumor southern radix bupleuri extract preparation method	Lin Xinrong (CN); Han Hongzhi (CN)	Buddhism Jici Comprehensive Ho (CN)
CN1575810	Chinese herbal medicine for treating intractable headache	Chen Wenhua (CN)	Chen Wenhua (CN)
CN1579446	Pill for treating liver disease	Hong Keqi (CN)	Hong Keqi (CN)
CN1575808	Medicine for treating hepatitis B and hepatic ascites and its preparation method and use	Jin Yu (CN)	Jin Yu (CN)
CN1579434	Chaihuang Tonic and its preparation method	Zhang Ling (CN); Wang Jing E (CN)	Fujiao Group Co Ltd Shandong (CN)
CN1579428	External ready-made preparation of traditional Chinese medicine to prevent lipsotrichia and promote hair growth	Qian Yong (CN)	Qian Yong (CN)
TW224005B	Pharmaceutical composition for nasal spray in treatment of cold and fever and method for producing the same	Shiu Wu-Ching (TW); Geng Shu-Shian (TW)	Shiu Wu-Ching (TW); Geng Shu-Shian (TW)

*AU: Austria; CN: China; FR: France; HK: Hong Kong; IT: Italy; JP: Japan; KR: Korea; LI: Liechtenstein; TW: Taiwan; US: United States.

Patent No.	Title	Inventor	Applicant
CN1562321	Chinese materia medica preparation for curing cholecystitis and preparation method	Gao Zhihong (CN); Wang Xiaoguang (CN)	Gao Zhihong (CN)
CN1562243	Rujiling effervescent tablet and preparation method	Li Yehua (CN); Jiang Yan (CN)	Yixiaotang Hunan Pharm Mfg Co (CN)
CN1562185	Chinese medica preparation for treating weaner exopathic diseases and fever heat, and preparation technique	Yu Wenyong (CN)	Qiyuanyide Medicines Inst Beij (CN)
CN1562183	Chinese medica preparation for curing hyperplasia of mammary glands and preparation method	Yu Wenyong (CN)	Qiyuanyide Medicines Inst Beij (CN)
CN1562178	Preparation of Chinese traditional medicine for curing gallstone and preparation method	Yu Wenyong (CN)	Qiyuanyide Medicines Inst Beij (CN)
CN1562175	Medicinal preparation for curing hepatitis and preparation method	Yu Wenyong (CN)	Qiyuanyide Medicines Inst Beij (CN)
CN1562160	Composite medicine for treating hepatitis B complication	Jin Haiqing (CN)	Jin Haiqing (CN)
CN1562140	Chinese–Western combined medicine for treating burn and scald and other external wounds	Li Xunfeng (CN)	Li Xunfeng (CN)
CN1562115	Antipyretic Chinese medicine preparation for child made of *Bupleurum* root and cinnamon twig	Wang Yongbin (CN); Yu Jiangbo (CN);	Aodong Yanbian Pharmaceutical (CN)
CN1572306	Chinese traditional medicine composition for treating cerebral infarction and hyperlipodemia	Zhang Jianeng (CN)	Zhang Jianeng (CN)
CN1559535	Chinese medicine oral preparation for treating urinary system infestation and its preparation method	Chen Lingling (CN)	Chen Lingling (CN)
CN1559521	Bag agent for treating gallstone disease and its preparation method	Zhang Jin (CN)	Zhang Jin (CN)
CN1559493	Medicine for treating hepatitis	Ju Hongfu (CN); Ju Ran (CN)	Tonghua Fangda Medicine Indust (CN)
CN1559467	Medicine for treating chronic nephritis, and its preparation method	Tian Naigeng (CN); Tian Jinghua (CN)	Li Guocheng (CN)
EP1527784	Method for extracting antineoplastic components from *Bupleurum scorzonerifolium*	Lin Shinn-Zong (TW); Harn Horng-Jyh (TW)	Buddhist Tzu Chi General Hospi (TW)
CN1554437	Medicinal composition for treating acne and chloasma	Chen Benshan (CN)	Benshan Pharmaceutical Co Ltd (CN)
CN1555878	Oral cavity convalescence liquid	Xu Haifei (CN)	Xu Haifei (CN)
CN1557428	Chinese traditional medicine for eliminating arteriosclerosis plaque	Yu Rui (CN)	Liaoning College Of Traditiona (CN)
CN1557385	Chinese medicine for treating catatonic type headache	Cao Wenbin (CN); Ni Jizhi (CN); (+1)	Cao Wenbin (CN)
CN1557380	Anticancer orally administered Chinese medicinal preparation	Que Feng (CN)	Que Feng (CN)
CN1557373	Chinese medicine preparation for treating climacteric syndrome of liver depression and qi stagnation	Liu Yinghui (CN)	Liu Yinghui (CN)
CN1546159	Hepatitis treating medicine and its preparation process	Liu Duzhou Wang (CN)	Beijing Runpu Medicine Dev Co (CN)
CN1546155	Anticancer Chinese traditional medicine	Liu Longguang (CN)	Liu Longguang (CN)
CN1546115	Jierening granule for abating fever and its preparation	Xi Xin (CN)	Xi Xin (CN)
CN1544035	Medicine for treating dyspepsia and fever of children	Wang Heng (CN); Xiong Bin (CN); (+1)	Xiong Bin (CN)
CN1537627	Capsule for treating hepatopathy	Ju Zhilun (CN)	Ju Zhilun (CN)

Patent No.	Title	Inventor	Applicant
CN1555816	Medicine for treating proliferation of mammary gland and its preparation process	Peng Jixiang (CN)	Peng Jixiang (CN)
CN1546084	Quick-acting hemorrhoid treating ointment	Hou Shuheng (CN)	Hou Shuheng (CN)
CN1546083	Animal used compound *Bupleurum* injection	Qi Kezong Zhu (CN)	Qi Kezong Zhu (CN)
CN1546078	Preparation of Chinese patent medicine for treating hyperplasia of mammary glands	Wang Tongsheng (CN)	Wang Tongsheng (CN)
CN1543993	Rhinitis-treating medicine and its preparation	Song Ge (CN); Wang Mingzhe (CN)	Song Ge (CN)
CN1537619	Traditional Chinese medicine for immunity and strengthening the body resistance	Zhang Chuanyin (CN); Lei Dapeng (CN)	Dong E Immunological Science R (CN)
CN1546074	Chinese herbal granule for treating viral myocarditis and its preparation process	Wang Xuefeng (CN)	Liaoning University of Traditi (CN)
CN1541678	Mastoplasia-treating medicine	Xu Ying Liu (CN)	Xu Ying (CN)
CN1537611	Medicine for treating cholecystitis, and its preparation method	Zhao Bingjun (CN)	Zhao Bingjun (CN)
CN1546066	Gastrointestinal ulcer-treating Chinese traditional medicine	Wang Dekui (CN)	Shi Zhong (CN)
CN1552408	Preparation method and quality control for Xiao Chaihu effervescent preparation	Lin Deliang (CN)	Handian Chinese Traditional An (CN)
CN1537568	Oral medicine for treating liver cancer	Deng Xinhe (CN)	Deng Xinhe (CN)
CN1548063	Hepatosis-treating Chinese medicine	Sun Shougui (CN)	Sun Shougui (CN)
CN1528438	External antipyretic medicinal liquor	Chen Huifu (CN); Chen Ke (CN)	Chen Huifu (CN)
CN1528182	Health care food and preparation method	Wang Tao (CN)	Wang Tao (CN)
CN1524567	Xuefu Zhuyu soft capsule and its preparation method	Xu Qun (CN)	Beijing Tong Ren Tang Medical (CN)
CN1531956	Chinese medicine compound composition and its preparation method and use	Xiao Youjuan (CN); Liu Zhongrong (CN); (+1)	Chengdu Diao Pharmaceutical Gr (CN)
CN1531943	Formula and production process of medicine for treating coronary heart disease and angina pectoris	Wang Xingkuan (CN); Huang Lijie (CN); (+1)	Yisheng Medicine Science and T (CN)
CN1524550	Traditional Chinese medicine for treating pancreatitis	Li Yanmei (CN)	Li Yanmei (CN)
CN1520854	Bone fracture therapeutic pharmaceuticals	Wang Jian (CN)	Wang Jian (CN)
CN1520833	Composition for alcohol type fatty liver	Wang Shuyue (CN)	Wang Shuyue (CN)
CN1520831	Health-preserving liver-protecting drug and preparation method	Wang Xiao (CN)	Wang Xiao (CN)
CN1491716	Fingered citron granule for stomach ailment and its preparation method	Zhu Honglong (CN)	Zhu Honglong (CN)
CN1491696	Composition for preventing and treating yellow dysentery of piglet	Zhang Wanfu (CN); Liu Fengxiang (CN); (+1)	Shannongda Pharmaceutical Co L (CN)
CN1491695	Composition for preventing and treating pig's epidemic diarrhea	Zhang Wanfu (CN); Liu Fengxiang (CN); (+1)	Shannongda Pharmaceutical Co L (CN)
CN1515304	Specific Chinese medicine preparation for curing pneumoconiosis and tuberculosis	Chen Chang An (CN)	Chen Chang An (CN)
CN1515302	Chinese medicine granule preparation for curing stomatocace	Wu Pingli (CN)	Wu Pingli (CN)
CN1515301	Medicine for curing upper respiratory tract infection and preparation method of its granules	Zhang Yi (CN); Zhang Mei (CN)	Weiao Sichuan Biolog Technolog (CN)

Patent No.	Title	Inventor	Applicant
CN1491691	Recipe composition of cold-resisting Chinese medicine sugar-less granular powder and tablets and preparation process	Wang Jianchun (CN)	Wang Jianchun (CN)
CN1524540	Chinese medicine preparation for treating fatty liver and its preparation method	Xie Fengying (CN); Su Jianjun (CN)	Tangshan Rongda Pharmaceutical (CN)
CN1511570	Method for producing brain heat-removing and blood pressure-reducing liquid	Guo Haoshan (CN)	Guo Haoshan (CN)
CN1511569	Method for producing stomach energy regulating medicine	Guo Haoshan (CN)	Guo Haoshan (CN)
CN1511563	Method for producing chromatic diarrhea-stopping capsule	Chang Wenqing (CN)	Chang Wenqing (CN)
CN1511562	Slow diarrhea-stopping capsule	Chang Wenqing (CN)	Chang Wenqing (CN)
CN1511553	Infantile antipyretic	Dai Long (CN)	Dai Long (CN)
CN1509745	Preparation of wutian liver-caring liquid	Bi Yedong (CN); Guo Fucheng (CN); (+1)	Hangu Traditional Chinese Medi (CN)
CN1500511	Cold proof medicine	Mei Zonghan (CN)	Mei Zonghan (CN)
CN1491677	Chinese medicine oral administration liquid for treating leukoderma	Wang Wei (CN)	Wang Wei (CN)
CN1504210	Prepared Chinese traditional medicine for alopecia	Han Yong (CN)	Han Yong (CN)
CN1507881	Oral preparation of Chinese medicine "kekeping" for treating cold	Li Xiangyang (CN)	Guangyang Traditional Chinese (CN)
CN1493308	Preparation technology of sugarless small radix bupleuri granular agent	Xiao Wei (CN); Dai Xiangling (CN); (+1)	Jiangsu Kangyuan Pharmaceutica (CN)
CN1486738	Medicine for treating upper respiratory tract infection type cold	Chang Licheng (CN)	Zhao Yixian (CN)
CN1486737	Hepatosis-treating Chinese medicine with four integrated functions	Li Wenxia (CN)	Li Wenxia (CN)
CN1470281	Spine osteopathy liquid	Nan Mingsen (CN)	Nan Mingsen (CN)
CN1471962	Oral liquid for biliary ascariasis	Xie Yuenan (CN)	Xie Yuenan (CN)
CN1473614	Chinese medicine for treading apoplexy, cancer, and other diseases	Wen Wenbin (CN)	Wen Wenbin (CN)
CN1486725	Chinese medicine preparation for treating epilepsy and its use	Jiang Hongying (CN); Liu Ping (CN); (+1)	Jiang Hongying (CN)
CN1473604	Capsule for treating epidemic parotitis	Ran Guangqi (CN)	Ran Guangqi (CN)
CN1486722	Spot-eliminating Chinese medicine with the functions of dispersing the stagnated liver energy and eliminating depressive syndrome	Yao Lianshu (CN)	Yao Lianshu (CN)
CN1475257	Medicinal plaster for treating chololithiasis	Jiang Mengxi (CN); Zhou Yichun (CN)	High & New Baicaohui Medical A (CN)
CN1473626	Chinese herbal medicine health sanitary incense	Wang Quanlin (CN)	Wang Quanlin (CN)
CN1468546	Liver strengthening agent for marine fishes	Tan Beiping (CN); Mai Kangsen (CN); (+1)	China Oceanology Univ (CN)
CN1490020	Oral Chinese patent drug for treating pelvis and nephritis and its preparation method	Wu Bingguang (CN)	Wu Bingguang (CN)
CN1468613	Chinese medicine composition and preparation for treating chronic cholecystitis	Shu Xin (CN); Wang Junyue (CN); (+1)	Shenzhen Tsinghua Modern Chine (CN)
CN1475240	Stone removing preparation	Chen Shengbin (CN); Chen Dayong (CN)	Chen Shengbin (CN)

Patent No.	Title	Inventor	Applicant
CN1466969	Chinese traditional medicine for treating purpuric disease and preparation method	Liu Guangyue (CN); Liu Guanghui (CN); (+1)	Liu Guangyue (CN)
CN1465378	Baicaoganfukang medicine for treating hepatopathy	Wu Yuquan (CN)	Wu Yuquan (CN)
CN1480161	Preparation of Chinese herbal medicine for treating lithiasis as well as its preparation method	Guo Derun (CN); Zhang Shunming (CN); (+1)	Guo Derun (CN)
CN1485060	Pungent and fragrant anti-rheum pillow	Liu Zengqi (CN)	Liu Zengqi (CN)
WO2005007127	Preparation to combat the unsightly skin effects of cellulite	Montanari Daniela (IT); Guglielmo Manuela (IT)	Gecomwert Anstalt (LI); Montanari Daniela (IT); (+1)
US2005013879	Method for extracting antineoplastic components from *Bupleurum scorzonerifolium*	Lin Shinn-Zong (TW); Harn Horng-Jyh (TW)	Buddhist Tzu Chi General Hospi (US)
WO2004091638	Herbal composition	Hilterman Karina Anna (AU)	Hilterman Karina Anna (AU)
CN1459314	Composition for preventing and treating milk cow from bacterial disease	Zhao Hongkun (CN); Wan Renzhong (CN); (+1)	Shandong Agricultural Univ (CN)
CN1457854	Health pill for liver	Yang Tao (CN)	Yang Tao (CN)
CN1457852	Chinese medicine composition for curing traumatic injury and pains in chest and hypochondrium and its preparation method	Ju Xiaoping (CN)	Ju Xiaoping (CN)
CN1449667	Chinese medicine preparation for killing virus and production process	Li Yuxin (CN); Zhang Duo (CN); (+1)	Inst of Genetics And Cytology (CN)
CN1449813	Medicine for treating SARS	Lan Jinchu (CN)	Lan Jinchu (CN)
CN1449794	Radix bupleuri soft capsule pharmaceutical and preparation process	Zhang Weidong (CN); Su Juan (CN); (+1)	Shanghai Botai Medicine Scienc (CN)
CN1442175	Chinese medicine for treating mammary gland lobular hyperplasia	Yang Xiuyun (CN)	Yang Xiuyun (CN)
CN1440799	Women's medicine and its preparation	Xu Chunxiang (CN)	Xu Chunxiang (CN)
CN1440802	Gastritis-treating Chinese medicine	Meng Lingyuan (CN); Chu Rongguang (CN)	Huiren Pharmaceutical Industry (CN)
CN1438027	Chinese medicine for treating breast disease	Li Xiuyun (CN); Lin Nianliang (CN)	Bailu Pharmaceutical Co Ltd Sh (CN)
CN1438017	Medicine for treating common cold and preparation method	Wu Meichun (CN)	Wu Meichun (CN)
CN1432399	Menstruation-regulating and pregnancy-promoting Chinese medicine and its preparation	Feng Guowei (CN)	Feng Guowei (CN)
CN1430999	Chinese herbal medicine combination for treating disease of disorder of bowel function and its production	Yang Xinghao (CN)	Univ Nanjing (CN)
CN1430996	Oral preparation of big *Bupleurum* root and its production methods	Zhou Yunzhong (CN); Ji Kesheng (CN)	Jinghua Pharmacy Co Ltd Nanton (CN)
CN1425449	Traditional Chinese medicine composition for curing wind-heat type cold and its preparation method	Li Guihai (CN)	Lunan Pharmaceutical Co Ltd (CN)
CN1425458	Medicine for curing endometriosis	Gao Yueping (CN)	Nanjing Univ of Traditional Ch (CN)
CN1424107	Medicinal composition for high examination syndromes	Liu Dianchi (CN)	Liu Dianchi (CN)
CN1453014	Chinese medicine preparation for preventing fibrillated liver and treating hepatocirrhosis	Zhang Lizhong (CN)	Zhang Lizhong (CN)

Patent No.	Title	Inventor	Applicant
CN1424106	Medicines for treating depression and its preparation method	Zhang Youzhi (CN)	Zhang Youzhi (CN)
CN1424079	Medicine for summer damp catch-cold and its preparation method	Zhang Qinglong (CN)	Zhang Qinglong (CN)
CN1424074	Capsule for constipation and its preparation method	Du Jialin (CN); Liang Maoxin (CN); (+1)	Liaoning Chinese Medical Acade (CN)
CN1425408	Pile internal treatment pill	Zhou Yijie (CN)	Zhou Yijie (CN)
CN1418475	Method for three-dimensional interplanting of Radix bupleuri together with chaenomeles fruit plants	Huang Lihai (CN)	Huang Lihai (CN)
CN1421140	Pesticidal matrine solution and its production process	Zhang Hengshan (CN); Xia Meiming (CN); (+1)	Zhang Hengshan (CN)
WO2004050106	A medicine for treating woman climacteric syndrome and its preparation method	Chan Hsiaochang (CN); Gou Yulin (CN); (+2)	Eu Yan Sang Hong Kong Ltd (CN); Chan Hsiaochang (CN); (+3)
CN1418683	Medicine composition for treating mammary gland proliferation, and its preparation method	Zhang Huifang (CN)	Zhang Huifang (CN)
CN1418682	Medicine composition for treating biliary calculus, and its preparation method	Zhang Huifang (CN)	Zhang Huifang (CN)
CN1429602	Medicine for treating throat disease and its preparation method	Kang Yongzheng (CN); Kang Xudong (CN)	Kang Xudong (CN)
CN1418679	Medicine compositions for treating hepatitis, and its preparation method	Zhang Huifang (CN)	Zhang Huifang (CN)
CN1416880	New use of powder for regulating liver and spleen and its active part	Shi Renbing (CN); Wang Qingguo (CN); (+1)	Beijing Traditional Chinese Me (CN)
CN1418664	Lireqing injecta (for clearing heat and diminishing inflammation)	Yu Jiansheng (CN)	Yu Jiansheng (CN)
CN1404865	Preparatory Chinese medicine for treating liver disease	Fang Yongsheng (CN)	Fang Yongsheng (CN)
CN1404864	Chinese medicine for treatment of depression	Zhao Lujun (CN); Xu Jiamin (CN); (+1)	Yumi Pharmaceutical Co Ltd Zhe (CN)
CN1415370	Medication for curing stomachache	Feng Xingbo (CN)	Feng Xingbo (CN)
CN1403144	Chinese medicine preparation with the functions of promoting blood circulation, dispersing blood clots, regulating vital energy, and stopping pain	Chen Keji (CN); Shi Dazhuo (CN)	Huiren Group Corp Ltd (CN)
CN1415358	Medication for curing lithiasis	Lai Guanhui (CN)	Lai Guanhui (CN)
CN1403114	Production process of cancer-eliminating pearl powder	Zhao Youlan (CN)	Zhao Youlan (CN)
CN1400008	Medicine for curing nasal sinusitis	Wang Ruzhi (CN)	Wang Ruzhi (CN)
CN1413663	Capsule for positive hepatitis B to negative	Liu Qingzhang (CN)	Liu Qingzhang (CN)
CN1398616	Medicine for treating upper respiratory tract infection and its preparation	Chen Jinghua (CN)	Zhuohai Science & Technology C (CN)
CN1389212	*Bupleurum* flavone composition for resisting influenza virus and its preparation	Yang Yong An (CN); Li Dongfang (CN); (+1)	Jiangsu Zhengda Tianqing Pharm (CN)
CN1395947	Medicine for treating wind-heat type common cold and its preparation process	Chen Jinghua (CN)	Zhuohai Science Technology Cul (CN)
CN1389213	Composite eye-moistening liquid and its application	Chen Qi (CN)	Shanghai Weikang Optics Co Ltd (CN)

Patent No.	Title	Inventor	Applicant
CN1389240	Gingko leaf powder for injection and its preparation	Zhang Ping (CN)	Zhang Ping (CN)
CN1385207	Desheng pellet	Shi Jingtian (CN); Shi Zhongnan (CN)	Shi Jingtian (CN)
CN1385191	Medicine for treating liver disease	Xu Lianhao (CN)	Xu Lianhao (CN)
CN1385190	Medicine for treating liver disease	Xu Lianhao (CN)	Xu Lianhao (CN)
CN1385203	Compound Chinese medicine preparation of damnacanthus	Mai Kaifeng (CN)	Mei Kaifeng (CN)
CN1383858	Medicine for treating diseases of liver, gallbladder, and spleen	Rong Xing (CN)	Rong Xing (CN)
CN1383874	External medicine for treating mastopathy and its preparation	Du Wei (CN)	Caihong Color Crt General Fact (CN)
CN1381265	Medicine for treating cholecystitis and its preparation	Sun Xiao (CN)	Sun Xiao (CN)
CN1381254	Medicine for treating fever by nasal application and its preparation process	Jiang Xinguo (CN); Lu Wei (CN); (+1)	Univ Fudan (CN)
CN1453006	Multifunctional treating and beautifying Chinese medicine acupoint plaster and its preparation	Sun Hualin (CN)	Sun Hualin (CN)
CN1380080	Medicine for curing fatty liver	Liu Guiying (CN); Wu Yongshun (CN); (+1)	Liu Guiying (CN)
CN1451414	Spot eliminating medicine and its preparation	Qi Honghui (CN)	Qi Honghui (CN)
CN1449777	Medicine for treating kidney disease	Han Yukun (CN)	Han Yukun (CN)
CN1448154	Medicine for treating exopathic disease and preparation process	Liu Jingjun (CN)	Liu Jingjun (CN)
CN1448163	Hepatosis-treating traditional Chinese medicine formula	Yang Guojun (CN)	Yang Guojun (CN)
CN1383867	Medicine for treating depression and its preparation	Wang Bingqi (CN)	Guilong Medicine Co Ltd Shanxi (CN)
CN1446559	Medicine for treating common cold and its preparation method	Zeng Kuansheng (CN)	Zeng Kuansheng (CN)
CN1375325	Composite medicine for treating hepatitis B	Wang Ziquan (CN)	Li Shaohua (CN)
CN1446554	Medicine for treating acute cholecystitis and chronic cholecystitis and its preparation method	Qiu Xueliang (CN)	Qiu Xueliang (CN)
CN1383855	Gastropathy-treating Chinese medicine	Zheng Guopeng (CN)	Zheng Guopeng (CN)
CN1444955	Chinese herbal medicine for treating hepatitis	Zhang Shufa (CN)	Zhang Shufa (CN)
CN1368380	Chinese medicine for treating hepatitis B and its preparation process	Liang Xinmeng (CN); Ren Yongxiang (CN)	Ren Yongxiang (CN)
CN1436554	*Bupleurum*-skullcap dripping pills	Huang Chenggang (CN); Zhu Qin (CN); (+1)	Shanghai Huatuo Medicine Sci T (CN)
CN1381250	Chinese medicine "lidandishi" for treating hepatobiliary calculus and cholecystitis	Li Bo (CN); Kou Shenyan (CN)	Li Bo (CN)
CN1365828	Medicine for treating diabetes	Liang Bangzhen (CN); Chen Yuzhou (CN)	Liang Bangzhen (CN)
CN1368379	Paishisan for treating cholecystolithiasis	Jian Yingkun (CN)	Jian Yingkun (CN)
CN1369262	Wrinkle-removing, skin-whitening cream	Wang Ling (CN)	Wang Ling (CN)
CN1367007	Medicine for curing common cold	Huang Ronghui (CN)	Huang Ronghui (CN)
CN1435208	Anticancer teabag and its production process	Wu Ge (CN)	Wu Ge (CN)
CN1367009	Medicine for curing hepatitis B	Feng Xiaomei (CN)	Feng Xiaomei (CN)
CN1413620	Shugan Zhitong soft extract for treating hepatitis	Hua Dejie (CN)	Hua Dejie (CN)
CN1430976	Medicine for treating liver disease	Sun Mingren (CN)	Sun Mingren (CN)
CN1429592	Liver-softening, spleen-reducing capsule	Li Donghai (CN); Li Junyi (CN); (+1)	Li Donghai (CN)

Patent No.	Title	Inventor	Applicant
CN1429574	Capsule for treating hepatitis B	Li Junyi (CN); Chen Liuxi (CN); (+1)	Li Donghai (CN)
CN1428158	Chinese medicine for curing gastropathy	Xu Zhongting (CN)	Xu Zhongting (CN)
CN1425304	Traditional Chinese medicine type sterilizer	Zhao Baorun (CN)	Zhao Baorun (CN)
CN1374106	Chinese medicine preparation for treating hepatitis B and its preparation process	Li Mingjiang (CN)	Li Mingjiang (CN)
CN1354010	Shuangjinlian oral liquid for curing cold and influenza, and its preparation method	Xing Zetian (CN)	He Nan Zhulin Zhongsheng Pharm (CN)
CN1356134	Capsule "Dankang" for treating cholecystitis	Zhang Guoguang (CN)	Zhang Guoguang (CN)
CN1419926	Medicine for treating bile backflow gastritis	Wang Shuiming (CN)	Wang Shuiming (CN)
CN1418647	Traditional Chinese medicine oral liquid for preventing and treating psychosis, and its preparation method	Chen Maoting (CN)	Chen Maoting (CN)
CN1416849	Externally applied medicine for treating mastopathy and its preparation	Zhang Gaojun (CN); Chen Juan (CN)	Zhang Gaojun (CN)
CN1356124	Medicine for treating hepatism	Liu Weidong (CN)	Liu Weidong (CN)
CN1341436	External-use Chinese medicine plaster for curing deafness and tinnitus	Qu Qiang (CN)	Qu Qiang (CN)
CN1408399	Medicine for curing hyperthermia and its preparation	Xu Yun (CN); Meng Fanlin (CN); (+1)	Liyuan Pharmaceutical Co Ltd J (CN)
CN1346654	Natural medicine material for interiorly eliminating cancer and its preparation	Zhang Longguang (CN); Zhang Guangyu (CN)	Zhang Longguang (CN)
CN1404844	Liver-tonifying stone-removing Chinese medicine	Huang Xinghai (CN)	Huang Xinghai (CN)
CN1399985	Medicine for curing rhinitis and its preparation method	Chen Junrui (CN); Lin Rongjin (CN)	Chen Junrui (CN)
CN1399914	Body-building face-nourishing nutrient liquor	Wu Duoqiang (CN); Pan Xianliang (CN); (+1)	Wu Duoqiang (CN)
CN1398610	*Bupleurum*-Puerariae granule and its preparation process	Zhang Zhonghai (CN)	No 1 Attached Hospital No 4 Mi (CN)
CN1389231	Composite Chinese medicine for treating venereal disease and dermatosis and its preparation	Chen Peiyun (CN)	Chen Peiyun (CN)
CN1337252	Chinese medicine for treating chronic bronchitis	Chen Hguaqin (CN); Wang Xingqin (CN); (+1)	Chen Huaqin (CN)
CN1394624	Chinese medicine prescription for curing eye disease and its preparation method	Shi Qiaozhi (CN)	Shi Qiaozhi (CN)
CN1394498	Chinese medicine composite health-care tea and its preparation method	Xu Qing (CN)	Xu Qing (CN)
CN1394578	Plant additive for shampoo	Chen Huinian (CN)	Chen Huinian (CN)
CN1394570	Plant additive for shampoo	Chen Huinian (CN)	Chen Huinian (CN)
CN1394569	Plant additive for shampoo	Chen Huinian (CN)	Chen Huinian (CN)
CN1328846	Chinese medicine preparation for curing headache	Gao Shuliang (CN); Zhang Ying (CN)	Gao Shuliang (CN)
CN1393255	Medicine for treating viral hepatitis C	Liu Yuzhang (CN)	Liu Yuzhang (CN)
CN1325740	Quick-acting defervescent wet tissue	Cui Danyang (CN)	Cui Danyang (CN)
CN1391919	Lifuji oral liquor	Liu Yuhui (CN)	Liu Yuhui (CN)
CN1390553	Liquid defervescent	Tang Yi (CN)	Tang Yi (CN)
CN1366982	Chinese medicine Tongshuyin for curing cardiopathy, biliary disease, and kidney disease	Yang Guoshuai (CN)	Yang Guoshuai (CN)

Patent No.	Title	Inventor	Applicant
CN1323621	Hypolycemic pellet made of ginseng and largehead atractylodes rhizome	Bu Deliang (CN)	Bu Deliang (CN)
CN1321499	Chinese patent medicine for curing deafness	Qu Qiang (CN)	Qu Qiang (CN)
CN1382460	Chinese medicinal capsule for treating hepatitis B and its preparation process	Bao Yuanxiang (CN)	Bao Yuanxiang (CN)
CN1378850	"Ganfukang" for treating hepatism	Pan Guiling (CN)	Pan Guiling (CN)
CN1377662	Stone-expelling pill	Su Liancun (CN)	Su Liancun (CN)
CN1377666	Medicine for curing cholecystitis and its preparation method	Sun Jinglu (CN)	Sun Jinglu (CN)
CN1377664	Pill for clearing away liver fire and reducing fat	Bai Jinlong (CN); Ru Yongxin (CN)	Bai Jinlong (CN)
CN1316263	Chinese medicine for treating hepatitis B	Xu Zhongting (CN)	Xu Zhongting (CN)
CN1374023	Bagged tea containing composite natural plant ingredients and its compounding process	Xu Qing (CN)	Xu Qing (CN)
CN1374012	Bagged tea containing composite natural plant ingredients and its compounding process	Xu Qing (CN)	Xu Qing (CN)
CN1374022	Bagged tea containing composite natural plant ingredients and its compounding process	Xu Qing (CN)	Xu Qing (CN)
CN1313125	Chinese patent medicine for treating tracheitis and whooping cough and its preparation process	Qian Sheng (CN)	Qian Sheng (CN)
CN1372884	Vegetative additive of hair protecting shampoo	Chen Huinian (CN)	Chen Huinian (CN)
CN1372882	Vegetative additive of hair protecting shampoo	Chen Huinian (CN)	Chen Huinian (CN)
CN1373186	Process for preparing health-care *Bupleurum* root-eucommia bark liquor	Chen Lie (CN)	Chen Lie (CN)
CN1372907	Process for preparing environment protection type health-care scent containing *Bupleurum* root	Jin Fengzhen (CN)	Jin Fengzhen (CN)
CN1368166	Nano medicine "Shuganzhitong" and its preparation process	Yang Mengjun (CN)	Yang Mengjun (CN)
CN1368161	Nano medicine "Jieyuhegan" and its preparation process	Yang Mengjun (CN)	Yang Mengjun (CN)
CN1368218	Nano compound medicine for treating hepatitis and its preparation process	Yang Mengjun (CN)	Yang Mengjun (CN)
CN1368118	Nano medicine "Rujiling" and its preparation process	Yang Mengjun (CN)	Yang Mengjun (CN)
CN1368060	Nano defervescent and digestion-promoting medicine and its preparation process	Yang Mengjun (CN)	Yang Mengjun (CN)
CN1366953	Nano midday tea preparation medicine and its preparation method	Yang Mengjun (CN)	Yang Mengjun (CN)
CN1366944	Nano common cold-fever-clearing preparation medicine and its preparation method	Yang Mengjun (CN)	Yang Mengjun (CN)
CN1366943	Nano *Bupleurum* preparation medicine and its preparation method	Yang Mengjun (CN)	Yang Mengjun (CN)
CN1365776	Nano medicine "Pinggan Shuluo" and its preparation process	Yang Mengjun (CN)	Yang Mengjun (CN)
CN1365814	Nano liver-protecting medicine and its preparation process	Yang Mengjun (CN)	Yang Mengjun (CN)
CN1365723	Nano compound medicine for treating hepatopathy and its preparation process	Yang Mengjun (CN)	Yang Mengjun (CN)
CN1308959	Medicine "Yishenjieyu" for treating mental diseases (psychosis)	Wang Dongqiao (CN)	Wang Dongqiao (CN)
CN1308958	Medicine "Huoxuexingshen" for treating mental diseases (psychosis)	Wang Dongqiao (CN)	Wang Dongqiao (CN)
CN1363347	Nano medicine "Nubao" and its preparation process	Yang Mengjun (CN)	Yang Mengjun (CN)

Patent No.	Title	Inventor	Applicant
CN1362246	Nano bupleuric medicine for regulating Shaoyang and its preparation	Yang Mengjun (CN)	Yang Mengjun (CN)
CN1362240	Nano medicine powder for treating cold limbs caused by Yang exhaustion and its preparation	Yang Mengjun (CN)	Yang Mengjun (CN)
CN1362217	Process for preparing liver-protecting liquor	Yang Mengjun (CN)	Yang Mengjun (CN)
CN1359697	Process for preparing liver-protecting liquor	Wang Yiyuan (CN)	Wang Yiyuan (CN)
CN1358512	Gallbladder normalizing soup	Liu Zhiguo (CN)	Liu Zhiguo (CN)
CN1352971	Eczema tablet	Xue Haichuan (CN)	Xue Haichuan (CN)
CN1328834	Capsule for curing cholecystitis	Zheng Guopeng (CN)	Zheng Guopeng (CN)
CN1352967	Medicine for treating chronic gastritis and gastric ulcer	Li Qingfu (CN)	Li Qingfu (CN)
CN1352959	Chinese medicine for treating heart disease	Qi Jiahe (CN)	Qi Jianhe (CN)
CN1308935	Medicinal patch for treating hepatism	Zhang Biyu (CN); Zhou Hua (CN)	Zhang Biyu (CN)
CN1299655	Hepatitis treating medicine	Yang Linghua (CN)	Yang Linghua (CN)
CN1349810	Kidney strengthening regenerating bolus	Yang Qingshan (CN)	Yang Qingshan (CN)
CN1291497	Mother liquid medicine for treating liver cancer and its preparation process	Li Guanqun (CN)	Li Guanqun (CN)
CN1345593	Gallbladder and appendix antiphlogistic	Zhou Xuetao (CN)	Zhou Xuetao (CN)
CN1345601	Chinese medicine composition for treating hepavirus disease its preparation and preparation process	Guoxiong Huang (HK)	Hongkong Res Ct of Traditional (HK)
CN1343505	Chinese medicine "Ruan capsule" for treating mastoplasia	Dong Shouyi (CN); Ma Xinpu (CN); (+1)	Dong Shouyi (CN)
CN1304730	Chinese medicine for treating cholecystitis	Liu Lanrong (CN)	Liu Lanrong (CN)
CN1281710	Chanyi compound preparation for curing cirrhosis	Li Jing E (CN)	Li Jing E (CN)
KR2002005343	Cosmetic composition containing extracts of *Bupleurum falcatum* L. and/or persicae semen	Bang Gi Man (KR); Chae Hui Nam (KR); (+4)	Rosee Cosmetics Co Ltd (KR)
CN1330943	Chinese medicinal honeyed pill for treating mastoplasia and its preparation process	Yang Suihuan (CN); He Jingkui (CN); (+1)	Yang Suihuan (CN)
CN1324644	Compound liver-protecting tea and its preparation	Chen Jianghui (CN)	Chen Jianghui (CN)
CN1324643	Compound Yeqing tea and its preparation	Chen Jianghui (CN)	Chen Jianghui (CN)
CN1323601	Diebestos treating medicine	Ma Yueqi (CN); Li Guirong (CN); (+1)	Ma Yueqi (CN)
CN1321474	Yigan Jiedu tea for curing hepatitis B and its preparation method	Chen Jianghui (CN)	Chen Jianghui (CN)
CN1280832	Chinese medicinal capsule for treating impotence	Zhang Yinwen (CN); Ma Xiu E (CN); (+1)	Zhang Yinwen (CN)
CN1269241	Chinese medicine for treating hepatitis B together with aweto-cephalosporin mycelium and its preparation	Li Xing (CN)	Li Xing (CN)
EP1038519	Use of a grafted silicone polymer as a tensioner	Toumi Beatrice (FR); Mougin Nathalie (FR); (+1)	Oreal (FR)
CN1265895	Specific medicine for treating common cold	Zhang Junfeng (CN)	Zhang Junfeng (CN)
CN1265893	Powder medicine for softening liver and eliminating ascites	Li Jinghai (CN); Zhang Xiaotao (CN); (+1)	Li Jinghai (CN)
CN1262936	Medicine for curing psoriasis	Yang Wenxi (CN)	Yang Wenxi (CN)
CN1262933	Soluble granules for curing vitreous opacity and vitreous hemorrhage, and their preparation method	Li Genlin (CN)	Li Genlin (CN)

Patent No.	Title	Inventor	Applicant
CN1262955	Chinese medicine powder preparation for curing leukemia	Dong Wuxin (CN); Liu Guoqi (Cn	Dong Wuxin (CN)
CN1263772	Hypolipemic capsule	Ju Kuixin (CN); Zhao Dezhu (CN); (+1)	Ju Kuixin (CN)
CN1299674	Preparation of cancer-treating medicine	Lu Haiqian (CN)	Lu Haiqian (CN)
CN129865	Process for preparing flavoring to prevent hepatitis B	Zuo Qicai (CN)	Zuo Qicai (CN)
CN1253830	Chinese medicine prescription for curing hepatitis, cholangitis, pancreatitis, and cirrhosis	Huang Peile (CN)	Huang Peile (CN)
CN1259380	Medicine for giving up drugs	Li Guoxin (CN); Qi Haiying (CN); (+1)	Li Guoxin (CN)
CN1257725	Chinese medicine for treating bone fracture	Wu Weidong (CN)	Wu Weidong (CN)
CA2389993	Herbal compositions for treating gastrointestinal disorders	Bensoussan Alan (AU); Yu Long Yu (AU)	Chinese Medicines Scient Consu (AU)
CN1294002	Chinese medicine for treating neuropathy	Zhang Anqiong (CN)	Zhang Anqiong (CN)
CN1253808	Chinese medicine abortifacient	Zhou Wenzhi (CN); Li Jianguo (CN)	Zhou Wenzhi (CN)
CN1289611	Quick-acting Chinese medicine for treating cirrhosis and its preparation process	Shen Huaizu (CN); Shen Guoshi (CN); (+1)	Shen Huaizu (CN)
CN1248469	Powder medicine for treating hepatitis B	Yuan Shuantian (CN)	Yuan Shuantian (CN)
CN1248465	Method for producing Anruneixiao medicinal liquid	Nie Cuixin (CN)	Nie Cuixin (CN)
CN1247079	Immersed-in-wine Chinese medicine for preventing and curing AIDS	Wen Binwu (CN)	Wen Binwu (CN)
CN1246356	Fetus-protecting instant particles for treating habitual or threatened abortion	Li Fu (CN)	Li Fu (CN)
CN1248462	Ganhuo mixture medicine for hepatosis	Liu Chunlan (CN)	Liu Chunlan (CN)
CN1247081	Chaiqi injection for treating viral hepatitis	Sun Chengzhai (CN); Sun Mengwen (CN); (+1)	Sun Chengzhai (CN)
CN1281722	Chinese medicine preparation for discharging toxic material and curing cold and its production method	Yao Jiming (CN); Li Guanxiang (CN); (+1)	Yao Jiming (CN)
RU2170519	Phytotea composition "otchischajuschy"	Malyshev RM; Tulupov AV	Chno Proizv Ts Vitius; Ooo Nau
CN1275396	Pill for radically treating male and female hemorrhoid	Zhu Xingming (CN); Zhu Baiman (CN)	Zhu Xingming (CN)
CN1271605	Process for preparing medicine to cure viral hepatitis	Quan Bingjie (CN)	Quan Bingjie (CN)
CN1254585	Chinese medicine for radically treating hepatitis A	Li Changzhong (CN)	Li Changzhong (CN)
CN1270054	Chinese patent medicine for treating prostatic diseases	Huang Tianrui (CN)	Huang Tianrui (CN)
CN1269237	Medicine for treating chronic cholecystitis	Zhang Renwei (CN)	Yunnan Prov Inst of Medicament (CN)
CN1231200	Traditional Chinese medicine composition for treating bleeding of blood disease	Niu Yuegui (CN)	Niu Yuegui (CN)
CN1268364	Medicine for curing prostatosis	Liang Ming (CN)	Liang Ming (CN)
CN1266703	Medicine for treating liver cancer and its preparation process	Lin Lushan (CN)	Lin Lushan (CN)
CN1228992	Antipyretic granular formulation containing ramulus cinnamomi, ephedra, and *Bupleurum* root	Gao Guiyu (CN)	Gao Guiyu (CN)

Patent No.	Title	Inventor	Applicant
CN1229644	Chinese herbs skin protective articles for eliminating women's facial stain	Wang Yuxi (CN); Wang Xiaoyan (CN)	Wang Yuxi (CN)
CN1260193	Medicinal composition for stasis of blood	Liu Lihua (CN)	Liu Lihua (CN)
CN1260189	Application of radix scutellariae stem and leaf to pharmaceutical industry	Zhao Tiehua (CN); Kang Shaowen (CN); (+1)	Traditional Chinese Medicine I (CN)
CN1223144	Weikang traditional Chinese medicine capsule	Xu Zhi (CN)	Xu Zhi (CN)
CN1255339	Chinese-medicinal instant particles for promoting milk secretion and recovery of puerperant	Wang Fuchen (CN); Zhang Dongsheng (CN)	Wang Fuchen (CN)
CN1223133	Medicine for curing hepatitis B	Lei Yuhong (CN)	Lei Yuhong (CN)
US6004560	Nasal spray (drop) for treating fever/cold, and its preparation	Hsu Wu-Ching (TW); Keng Su-Hsien (TW)	
CN1220163	Drug for curing premenstrual tension	Liang Feng (CN); Tian Fusheng (CN)	Yazhou Pharmaceutical Co Ltd D (CN)
CN1219422	Medicine for curing hepatic and gallbladder diseases	Wu Maocheng (CN)	Wu Maocheng (CN)
CN1213563	Chenxia medication for relieving asthma and its preparation method	Wu Weiping (CN); Li Yungu (CN); (+1)	Beijing Traditional Chinese Me (CN)
CN1214933	Medicine for curing hyperthyroidism	Zhang Jixu (CN)	Zhang Jixu (CN)
WO9917715	Extracellular matrix production promoter	Nakayama Yasukazu (JP); Akutu Nobuko (JP); (+2)	Shiseido Co Ltd (JP); Nakayama Yasukazu (JP); (+3)
CN1247073	Chinese medicine for treating acyesis	Zhang Qingrong (CN)	Zhang Qingrong (CN)
CN1245691	Chinese plaster for curing liver diseases and its preparation method	Zhao Xueyin (CN); Liu Dequan (CN); (+1)	Tai An City Hospital of Tradit (CN)
CN1245699	Fatigue-eliminating body-nourishing pill	Sun Baolin (CN)	Sun Baolin (CN)
CN1245695	Deodorant oral liquor	Ma Shukun (CN)	Ma Shukun (CN)
CN1242208	Special efficacy drug abstinence medicine	Zheng Yongjiang (CN)	Zheng Yongjiang (CN)
CN1240644	Face mask for eliminating maculae and wrinkles and whitening skin and its preparation process	Sun Shuqin (CN)	Sun Shuqin (CN)
CN1240142	Compound longshou soluble granules	Xu Hongsheng (CN)	Xu Hongsheng (CN)
CN1207311	Health drink for preventing and treating common cold	Li Yinliang (CN)	Li Yinliang (CN)
CN1238198	Chinese medicinal capsule for treating different kinds of epilepsy; Zhenxiankangnao capsule	Zhang Hewu (CN)	Dongfang Inst of Medicine And (CN)
CN1195554	Specific anti-cancer oral liquor	Si Zhaoqing (CN)	Si Zhaoqing (CN)
CN1235035	Medicine and prescription for toxoplasmic disease	Sun Baojiang (CN)	Sun Baojiang (CN)
CN1194855	Powder prescription for curing cholecystitis, gastritis, and pancreatitis and its preparation process	Guo Zhenwu (CN)	Hospital of Kailuan Mineral Bu (CN)
CN1207314	Chinese medicine for treating hepatitis B	Ye Tan (CN)	Ye Tan (CN)
CN1233477	Medicine for treating hepatitis and liver fibrosis, and its preparation method	Wang Xia (CN); Zhang Jianmin (CN); (+1)	Xindiya Medicine New Tech Dev (CN)
CN1233487	Medicine for treating hepatitis B	Wang Dongping (CN)	Wang Dongping (CN)
CN1192922	Preparatory Chinese medicine for treatment of hepatitis and hepatoascites	Zhang Juncai (CN)	Zhang Juncai (CN)
CN1231195	Capsule for treating prostate diseases and preparation process	You Wenxin (CN)	You Wenxin (CN)
CN1228326	Hypertension pill	Liao Qiu (CN)	Liao Qiu (CN)

Patent No.	Title	Inventor	Applicant
WO9843607	Slimming cosmetic compositions	Greff Daniel (FR)	Sederma SA (FR); Greff Daniel (FR)
WO9842306	Cosmetic or dermopharmaceutical slimming compositions	Greff Daniel (FR)	Sederma SA (FR); Greff Daniel (FR)
CN1223125	Injection for prevention and cure of AIDS and its preparation process	Li Pengfei (CN); Jiang Yan (CN); (+1)	Shi Hua (CN)
CN1225823	Chinese medicine for treating diabetes and its preparation method	Wang Gangzhu (CN)	Wang Gangzhu (CN)
CN1223872	"Ganduqing" antitoxic medicine for liver and its preparation process	Wang Jun (CN)	Wang Jun (CN)
CN1223868	Hepatitis B tablet and its preparation process	Wang Jun (CN)	Wang Jun (CN)
CN1223124	External-use medicine for curing hypertension	Wanyan Dejie (CN); Su Chaoli (CN)	Wanyan Dejie (CN)
CN1188667	Channel and collateral analgesic plaster for treating bone, joint, and nerve paralysis ache	Hou Shuheng (CN)	Hou Shuheng (CN)
CN1223119	Traditional Chinese medicinal preparation for curing gynecopathy	Cai Lishan (CN)	Cai Lishan (CN)
CN1217929	Chinese medicine for AIDS and its preparation process	Zhang Zhigang (CN)	Zhang Zhigang (CN)
CN1217210	Plaster for intensifying vigor of liver and its production process	Zheng Yulin (CN)	Zheng Yulin (CN)
CN1214921	Weikangning powder for gastric disease	Feng Genyuan (CN)	Feng Genyuan (CN)
CN1240147	Kunyuan glg oral liquor	Li Zongxian (CN)	Li Zongxian (CN)
CN1212155	Drug for curing hepatitis B	Zhang Fatian (CN)	Zhang Fatian (CN)
CN1173371	Chinese medicine for treating deafness	Wang Shuang (CN)	Wang Shuang (CN)
CN1209306	Shoe	Hong Yanxin (CN)	Hong Yanxin (CN)
CN1209296	Slice made mainly from sesame having blood-supplementing and spleen-tonifying functions	Huang Chengyao (CN)	Huang Chengyao (CN)
CN1209328	Liquor for giving up drug-taking	You Weifan (CN)	You Weifan (CN)
CN1179959	Chinese patent drug	Liu Fengsen (CN); Miao Cuiping (CN); (+1)	Liu Fengsen (CN)
CN1179319	Granular Chinese medicine composition for child's health	Liang Shengguo (CN); Meng Xiangzhu (CN); (+1)	Lude Co Ltd Beijing (CN)
CN1205217	Pure Chinese medicinal syrup preparation and its production method	Gan Ling (CN); Li Rongbin (CN); (+1)	Nat Hospital Dehong Dai Nation (CN)
CN1173362	Chinese compound medicine for treatment of hepatic calculus and cholecystitis	Lai Heng (CN); Li Xiaohong (CN)	Lai Heng (CN)
CN1200277	Compound oral liquid medicine for treating psychosis and nerve system disease	Yue Yunchun (CN)	Yue Yunchun (CN)
CN1196936	Medication for treating primary glomerular disease and its preparation method	Wang Chunru (CN)	Wang Chunru (CN)
CN1195544	Quick-acting traditional Chinese medicine for curing hepatitis B	Yi Yufa (CN)	Yi Yufa (CN)
CN1167629	Non-sugar	Liu Yifan (CN); He Chunhua (CN); (+1)	Liu Yifan (CN)
CN1192918	Medicinal powder for treatment of hepatitis B and its preparation method	Dai Fuhua (CN)	Dai Fuhua (CN)
CN1192917	Medicinal powder for treatment of hepatitis B	Xu Qixing (CN)	Xu Qixing (CN)
CN1191727	Medicine composite for digestive tract tumor	Zhang Xiaosu (CN)	Zhang Xiaosu (CN)
CN1189347	Nasal liquid for preventing cold	Xu Rui (CN)	Xu Rui (CN)

Patent No.	Title	Inventor	Applicant
US5804168	Pharmaceutical compositions and methods for protecting and treating sun-damaged skin	Murad Howard (US)	
CN1188012	Chinese herbal medicine composition for curing leukemia	Ren Yurang (CN)	Ren Yurang (CN)
CN1187995	Chinese patent drug for curing hepatitis	Shang Ershou (CN)	Shang Ershou (CN)
CN1159938	Eyesight-improving preparation for treatment of myopia and its preparation process	Guo Yinfeng (CN); Guo Shuqin (CN); (+1)	Guo Yinfeng (CN)
CN1188005	Chinese herbal medicine oral liquor for curing wind-heat common cold and its preparation method	Zhang Ling (CN); Wu Jibiao (CN); (+1)	Shandong Prov Inst of Traditio (CN)
CN1157736	Special medications ticking sheet dispensing for pneumonia therapeutic equipment and production technology	Zhao Jianli (CN); Huang Dongjie (CN); (+1)	Zhao Jianli (CN)
CN1157155	Chinese patent drug for curing monovesicle viral keratitis	Wang Shuang (CN)	Wang Shuang (CN)
CN1185960	Instant powder for hepatitis B by strengthening body resistance, removing dampness, and detoxicating	Cao Yousheng (CN)	Cao Yousheng (CN)
CN1185972	Decocted medicine for hepatitis B by strengthening body resistance, removing dampness, and detoxicating	Cao Yousheng (CN)	Cao Yousheng (CN)
CN1185327	Medicine for curing stagnation of circulation of vital energy about brestribs	Gong Junping (CN)	Gong Junping (CN)
CN1185339	Medicinal magnetic cap of plastering to acupuncture	Zuo Xinan (CN); Tu Jinwen (CN)	Zuo Xinan (CN)
CN1153060	Oral liquid for nephropathy and its preparation process	Wang Zheng (CN)	Wang Zheng (CN)
CN1149493	Traditional Chinese medicinal oral liquor for curing venereal disease	Chang Qing (CN)	Chang Qing (CN)
CN1178108	Weixiandan as medicine for gastropathy	Zheng Wenxue (CN)	Zheng Wenxue (CN)
CN1149489	Recovering powder for hepatitis B	Wu Yinfu (CN)	Wu Yinfu (CN)
CN1148977	Rescription of Yiganning capsule for hepatitis B and its processing method	Zhou Deming (CN); Qin Zhonghui (CN)	Xianghui Medical High and New (CN)
CN1172656	Medicine for treating asthenia-syndrome type viral myocarditis caused by enterovirus	He Zhong (CN)	He Zhong (CN)
CN1171242	Compound anticancer Chinese medicine	Song Shutian (CN); Zheng Shenling (CN); (+1)	Song Shutian (CN)
CN1156602	Compound Tibet capillary artemisia patent medicine	Guo Zhenchang (CN); Li Feng (CN)	Guo Zhenchang (CN)
CN1163771	Navel-treating-type medical bag for treating gastropathy	Hu Yuheng (CN)	Hu Yuheng (CN)
CN1149481	Capsule for enhancing eyesight	Guo Liangcai (CN)	Guo Liangcai (CN)
CN1157141	Mengxing quick-acting liquor for curing mad disease	Ma Li (CN)	Ma Li (CN)
CN1157145	Drug and its prescription for curing toxocariasis	Sun Baojiang (CN)	Sun Baojiang (CN)
CN1136943	"Mieyidan" pill for treating hepatitis and its production process	Yuzhen Liu (CN); Molin Liu (CN); (+1)	Liu Molin (CN)
CN1153044	Thyroid gland pill and its production process	Guan Chengjin (CN)	Guan Chengjin (CN)
CN1131035	Chinese herbal medicine composition	Liping Liao (CN)	Liao Liping (CN)
CN1132643	Medicine for diseases of liver and gall	Xuezhen Feng (CN); Huiqing Yao (CN)	Feng Xuezhen (CN)

Patent No.	Title	Inventor	Applicant
CN1129585	Fuming oral liquid for recovery of visual acuity	Zhenhua Liang (CN); Xiangyun Pan (CN); (+1)	Liang Zhenhua (CN)
CN1147943	Cancer-prevention and health-care medicine	Bai Weili (CN)	Bai Weili (CN)
CN1136939	Chinese drugs for curing hepatitis B	Ying Lu (CN)	Lu Ying (CN)
CN1144115	Gantai tablet for curing hepatic disease	Xuejun Xu (CN)	Hengyang City Traditional Chin (CN)
CN1145238	Wuling C-hepatitis powder	Yongguang Li (CN); Wenjuan Zhang (CN); (+1)	Li Yongguang (CN)
CN1144672	Preparation for treatment of gynecology disease	Jinqin Dou (CN)	Dou Jinqin (CN)
CN1123705	Belt for regulating qi, activating collateral, and protecting liver	Yulong Wan (CN); Yikun Yan (CN); (+1)	Lingling Health Care Products (CN)
CN1139564	Bupleurumone powder and injection made from *Bupleurum* root	Ming Wang (CN); Ye Lu (CN); (+1)	Hongjing Chinese Medicinal Her (CN)
CN1121827	"Jinshisan" powder for treatment of gallstones and lithangiuria	Jixiang Liu (CN)	Liu Jixiang (CN)
CN1144101	Antifebrile oral liquor	Jide Wang (CN)	Wang Jide (CN)
CN1137384	Changweiling medicine for curing enterogastritis	Guohua Zhou (CN)	Zhou Guohua (CN)
CN1144100	Medicine for curing bone tuberculosis and osteomyelitis	Changmao Huang (CN)	Huang Changmao (CN)
CN1132631	Health oral liquid for curing hepatitis B	Genxing Luo (CN)	Luo Genxing (CN)
CN1131019	Medical ointment for curing external hemorrhoids and anal fissure	Jingmin Li (CN)	Li Jingmin (CN)
CN1131018	Anti-inflammation debridement drug composition	Jianjun Lu (CN)	Lu Jianjun (CN)
CN1144662	Medicine composition for treatment of cold	Guojie Huang (CN)	Huang Guojie (CN)
CN1131030	Injection for curing edematous conjunctivitis of piglet	Shengming Shi (CN); Guishan Fu (CN)	Shi Shengming (CN)
CN1143503	Medicinal composition for curing eye injury	Jianping Gong (CN)	Gong Jianping (CN)
CN1109779	Once-granulating process of ginseng and *Bupleurum* root particles for curing hepatitis	Liankang Yu (CN); Ning Gao (CN); (+1)	Yu Liankang (CN)
CN1127664	External use medicinal bag for treating acute and chronic gastritis and cholecystitis, and its preparation method	Kai Wang (CN)	Wang Kai (CN)
CN1127650	External use medicine bag for treatment of dysmenorrhea and its production method	Kai Wang (CN)	Wang Kai (CN)
CN1125110	Drug for curing gastropathy	Yunsheng Zang (CN); Shuhua Fang (CN)	Zang Yunsheng (CN)
CN1124153	Medicine for recovery of and replenishing liver and its preparation method	Zhengwen Jiang (CN); Zhenghua Jiang (CN); (+1)	Jiang Zhengwen (CN)
CN1123159	Bag for curing dysmenorrhea and its preparation method	Kai Wang (CN)	Wang Kai (CN)
CN1123148	"Shencao" plaster for releasing ache resulting from cancer	Xiangqian Li (CN)	Li Xiangqian (CN)
CN1122721	Yin-Yang regulating liver function bag	Wan Jun (CN)	Wan Jun (CN)
CN1110592	Pill for treating hepatogastric vital energy stagnation type chronic superficial, atrophic gastritis	Lingyuan Meng (CN); Kecheng Gao (CN); (+1)	Meng Lingyuan (CN)
CN1117863	Chailian oral liquor	Haishui Shangguan (CN); Xinfeng Zhang (CN)	Sanyong Pharmaceutical Co Ltd (CN)

Patent No.	Title	Inventor	Applicant
CN1112834	Oral liquid for curing hepatitis B, and its production method	Yuehan Guo (CN)	Guo Yuehan (CN)
CN1117388	Compound bupleuri liniment	Lizhi Sui (CN)	Dongying City Flour Mill (CN)
CN1121820	Drug for external use for treating necrosis of femoral head	Keqin Huang (CN)	Huang Keqin (CN)
CN1121818	Drug for external use for treating necrosis of femoral head	Keqin Huang (CN)	Huang Keqin (CN)
CN1115245	Anti-cold inhalation and its preparation method	Qingchun Cao (CN)	Cao Qingchun (CN)
CN1109773	Healthful oral liquid for liver	Xudong Zhang (CN)	Zhang Xudong (CN)
CN1110919	Xugan oral liquor made of a plant material for curing deficiency cold	Zhongxin Li (CN); Jiye Li (CN)	Li Zhongxin (CN)
CN1110608	Natural medicine napkins for treating dysmenorrhea	Minyi Duan (CN)	Duan Minyi (CN)
CN1104108	Medicine for curing tuberculosis	Anguo Jiao (CN)	Jiao Anguo (CN)
CN1110168	Powder for curing wind-cold type of common cold and its preparation method	Qinglin Deng (CN); Yuzhen Li (CN); (+1)	Linqing Traditional Chinese Me (CN)
CN1108554	Series traditional Chinese medicines for curing cancer of the liver and its preparation method	Yongbo Yu (CN)	Yu Yongbo (CN)
CN1104523	Prescription of Jiumiduanyin pill and its preparation	Lei Du (CN)	Lei Du (CN)
CN1101862	Health band for gallbladder	Liqun Che (CN)	Che Liqun (CN)
CN1104097	"Yunquye," a medicine for delivery and abortion and its preparation method	Jingan Wang (CN)	Wang Jingan (CN)
CN1090778	"Qianzengshu" medical health bag	Haiming Huang (CN)	Huang Haiming (CN)
CN1112424	Toutongning medicine for headache	Mu Ding (CN); Yan Peng (CN)	Ding Mu (CN)
CN1102591	"Sanmiao" compound mixture and its prescription	Hongtao Xue (CN)	Xue Hongtao (CN)
CN1100594	Pesticide for fruit trees and its preparation method	Baichuan Li (CN)	Li Baichuan (CN)
CN1081906	Technology for producing granular preparation of *Bupleurum* root	Shouzhuo Li (CN)	Chengde Traditional Chinese Ph (CN)
CN1098926	Hepatitis capsule and its preparation technique	Baizhong Jiao (CN)	Jiao Baizhong (CN)
CN1098635	Medicine for treating gastric disease and its manufacturing method	Chengqi Zhao (CN)	Zhao Chengqi (CN)
CN1098294	Manganning medicine	Jisheng Gu (CN)	Tianjin No 1 Hospital (CN)
CN1080871	Effective thorowax-kudzu vine defervescent	Guangzhao Cheng (CN); Faxue Liu (CN); (+1)	Zichuan District Hospital of T (CN)
CN1095283	"Sancao" medicine powder for hepatitis B	Yongguang Li (CN); Wenjuan Zhang (CN); (+1)	Li Yongguang (CN)
CN1082913	Medical powder benefiting liver and gall	Shuquan Lin (CN); Guirong Gao (CN); (+1)	Lin Shuquan (CN)
CN1083375	Anshen san (sedative powder)	Shuquan Lin (CN); Liping Gao Guirong Lin (CN)	Lin Shuquan (CN)
CN1090193	Medicine for diabetes and its preparation	Zhiyuan Sun (CN)	Sun Zhiyuan (CN)
CN1078902	Traditional Chinese medicine for curing hepatitis B	Yu Zhou (CN)	Zhou Yu (CN)
EP0568001	Antiviral agent containing crude drug	Hozumi Toyoharu (JP); Matsumoto Takao (JP); (+6)	Namba Tsuneo (JP); Shiraki Kimiyasu (JP)

Patent No.	Title	Inventor	Applicant
CN1093532	Liver-strengthening, health care tea and its production method	Yongzhen Yang (CN)	Yang Yongzhen (CN)
CN1083712	Medicine for prevention and cure of hepatitis B	Fuhou Meng (CN)	Meng Fuhou (CN)
CN1093591	Capsule for strengthening sexual function of men	Jisheng Zou (CN); Dexiang Zou (CN)	Zou Jisheng (CN)
CN1087824	Chinese medicinal instant powder for treatment of B-hepatitis	Chengxing Li (CN)	Li Chengxing (CN)
CN1091630	Skin protective liquor	Jing Chen (CN)	Ex Pharmaceutical Factory Zhej (CN)
CN1091308	"Fukangling" for treating gynecologic common illnesses and its preparation method	Jingshu Gao (CN)	Gao Jingshu (CN)
CN1091026	Danshixiao medicine for treating cholelithiasis	Jingguo Su (CN)	Su Jingguo (CN)
CN1091026	Danshixiao medicine for treating cholelithiasis	Jingguo Su (CN)	Su Jingguo (CN)
CN1090183	*Artemisia scoparia* and ginseng pellet for nourishing liver and its preparation	Zhongyou Ao (CN)	Ao Zhongyou (CN)
CN1089853	Quick-acting antidiarrhea oral liquor for infant and its preparation method	Junying Ma (CN); Hanqing Dong (CN)	Ma Junying (CN)
CN1089851	Spray for preventing and curing common cold and its preparation method	Qingchun Cao (CN)	Cao Qingchun (CN)
CN1076626	Medicine that, after being mixed with boiling water, is taken for liver trouble	Xianwen Li (CN)	Li Xianwen (CN)
CN1086137	Anti-radiation medicine composite for enhancement of immune function	Biaochun Huang (CN)	Huang Biaochun (CN)
CN1088442	Medicine preparation process for curing nephritis	Wenxu Li (CN); Chunde Guo (CN)	Li Wenxu (CN)
CN1082907	Leukoderma pill	Cai Zhang (CN)	Zhang Cai (CN)
CN1072855	Preparation method of medication for climacteric syndrome	Jingzhu Yang (CN); Maoxin Liang (CN)	Yang Jingzhu (CN)
CN1086136	Preparation method for liver-protecting liquor	Mingyu Wang (CN); Zunlong Wang (CN); (+1)	Wuhan No 5 Pharmaceutical Fact (CN)
JP2004359732	Antioxidant	Daito Hajime; Murakami Akira; (+2)	Ryukyu Bio Resource Kaihatsu: Kk
JP2003299412	Method for improving germination rate and storage period of *Bupleurum falcatum* by using Chinese medicine	Matsui Masateru	Matsui Masateru
JP2003261457	Skin cosmetic, and beverage and food for beautifying	Shiyuu Enyou; Arao Daisuke; (+1)	Maruzen Pharmaceut Co Ltd
JP2003183123	Skin care preparation for beautifully whitening skin and its production method	Takita Masao	Takita Masao
JP2003089626	Agent for inhibiting hair growth	Wakizaka Etsuji; Kitahara Takashi; (+2)	Kao Corp
JP2003014739	Screening method of skin swell improvement agent, and skin swell improvement agent	Hosoi Junichi; Furuya Rikako; (+2)	Shiseido Co Ltd
JP2002284626	External skin preparation	Miki Tokutaro; Nishikawa Yoji	Nippon Hypox Lab Inc
JP2001335500	Refreshment promoter	Takenaga Takaaki; Morito Akihisa; (+1)	Taisho Pharmaceut Co Ltd
JP2001139487	Medicinal composition of nasal spray or nasal liquid medicine for pyrogenic common cold and method for producing the same	Kyo Bukei; Ko Shukuken	Kyo Bukei; Ko Shukuken

Patent No.	Title	Inventor	Applicant
JP2001039850	Agent for accelerating shrinkage of collagen gel	Sonehara Nobuko; Nishiyama Toshio; (+2)	Shiseido Co Ltd
JP2000319191	Cyclic GMP-specific phosphodiesterase inhibitor and sexual dysfunction-improving drug	Okuno Kenji; Tarui Naoki; (+1)	Takeda Chem Ind Ltd
JP2000178168	Elastase activity inhibitor and cosmetic composition	Nishibe Yukinaga	Ichimaru Pharcos Co Ltd
JP11335231	Skin lotion for slimming body	Nawamura Takeshi; Kawajiri Yasuharu	Shiseido Co Ltd
JP11236334	Cell adhesion inhibitor	Ito Kazunori; Shoji Fumiko; (+2)	Nissin Food Prod Co Ltd
JP11139980	Therapeutic agent for ulcerative colitis	Kawada Mitsuhiro; Hattori Kenichi; (+1)	Teikoku Seiyaku Co Ltd
JP10313856	Indolebutyrate 4-hydroxylase and production of rooting inducer using the same	Yokoyama Mineyuki; Yamaguchi Sachiko; (+1)	Shiseido Co Ltd
JP10077268	Indole derivative and rooting-inducing agent containing the same as active ingredient	Yokoyama Mineyuki; Yamaguchi Sachiko; (+3)	Shiseido Co Ltd
JP10045613	Interleukin 4 production inhibitor	Kondo Hidehiko; Tazaki Shinichi; (+2)	Kao Corp
JP9286736	Liquid drug for internal use	Okudaira Ichiro; Tsunoda Kenji	Taisho Pharmaceut Co Ltd
JP9252793	Production of organ culture product of plant belonging to genus *Bupleurum* and production of saikosaponin	Fukunishi Hirotada; Kusakari Takeshi; (+1)	Shiseido Co Ltd
JP9208479	Salicaceae plant mixture	Kato Tadashi	Kato Tadashi
JP9208431	Hair tonic that promotes action on growth of hair papilla cell	Miyauchi Yutaka; Hasegawa Shigeo	Miyauchi Yutaka
JP9087190	Renal dysfunction remedying agent	Kikuchi Kiyokimi; Shimizu Fujio	Kanebo Ltd; Taihoudou Yakuhin Kogyo Kk
JP8242878	Production of saikosaponin	Katagiri Chika; Inomata Shinji; (+2)	Shiseido Co Ltd
JP8208465	Therapeutic agent of cold	Nakano Masahiro; Tamashiro Hiroshi; (+4)	Kanebo Ltd
JP8140587	Pet food	Kanamaru Mutsumi	Lion Corp
JP8131183	Production of saikosaponin	Katagiri Kazuhana; Yokoyama Mineyuki	Shiseido Co Ltd
JP8051977	Method for introducing foreign gene into cell of genus *Bupleurum* plant	Morikawa Hiromichi; Others: 02	Shiseido Co Ltd
JP8038123	Production of herb beverage	Inoue Yoshio; Others: 03	Yoshio Inoue; Others: 03
JP7179354	Antiviral agent	Hozumi Toyoji; Others: 03	Showa Shell Sekiyu Kk
JP6321672	Organic fertilizer additive	Kobayashi Masayasu; Others: 01	Taiyo Nousan Kk; Others: 01
JP6293653	Antirheumatic agent	Sakane Takeshi; Others: 02	Tsumura & Co
JP6287144	Pharmaceutical preparation for common cold	Moriyama Ko; Others: 02	Takeda Chem Ind Ltd
JP6279305	Agent for treatment of dermatic disease such as atopic dermatitis	Kuga Masaaki	Takaaki Kuga; Others: 01

Patent No.	Title	Inventor	Applicant
JP6256204	Anti-glioma agent	Katakura Ryuichi; Others: 01	Tsumura & Co
JP6227995	Stabilized solid preparation	Imoto Soichiro; Others: 02	Takeda Chem Ind Ltd
JP6206891	Method for extracting saikosaponin	Fujii Akira; Others: 02	Takeda Chem Ind Ltd
JP5194248	External preparation for preventing and treating dermatitis	Aki Nobuchika; Others: 02	Takeda Chem Ind Ltd
JP5184379	Production of saikosaponin	Yokoyama Mineyuki; Others: 02	Shiseido Co Ltd
JP5139982	Ischemic encephalopathy improving agent	Nishizawa Koji; Others: 03	Kanebo Ltd
JP5103606	Honeybee product and its collection method	Hochido Yuko	Kojundo Chem Lab Co Ltd
JP5023069	Improved method for culturing *Bupleurum*	Kusakari Takeshi; Others: 02	Shiseido Co Ltd
JP4365476	Production of callus with high saikosaponin content	Sakurai Motoi; Others: 01	Mitsui Toatsu Chem Inc
JP4342535	Testosterone 5-alpha-reductase inhibitor	Kawaguchi Makoto; Others: 03	Rohto Pharmaceut Co Ltd
JP4159294	Na^+-K^+ ATPase inhibitor containing novel saikosaponin as active ingredient	Ehata Takafumi; Others: 03	Tsumura & Co
JP4159293	Novel saponin and Na^+-K^+ a ATPase inhibitor containing saikosaponin as active ingredient	Ehata Takafumi; Others: 03	Tsumura & Co
JP4059773	New chromone and use of the same chromone as medicine	Kobayashi Masaru; Others: 03	Tsumura & Co
JP4011875	Health tea	Watanabe Hitoshi; Others: 02	Takeda Chem Ind Ltd
JP3290124	Induction of adventitious embryo of plant of *Bupleurum* root	Ebe Yoji; Others: 01	Mitsui Toatsu Chem Inc
JP3232484	Preparation of protoplast of plant belonging to genus *Bupleurum*, culture of protoplast and regeneration methods	Kawasaki Wataru; Others: 02	Momoya:Kk
JP3232435	Plant belonging to genus *Bupleurum* and production of adventitious embryos	Kawasaki Wataru; Others: 02	Momoya:Kk
JP3151003	Method for refining *Bupleurum* root saponin	Oonaka Akane; Others: 02	Tosoh Corp
JP3099020	Stable crude drug-containing liquid preparation for internal use	Yamato Akihiro	Shiga Pref Gov Seiyaku Kk
JP2283247	Feed additive for pisciculture	Kajitani Shigeo	Sana Yakuhin Kogyo Kk
JP2273131	Production of *Bupleurum* plant	Komiya Takeya; Others: 02	Takeda Chem Ind Ltd
JP2268678	Production of callus containing cycosaponin	Ebe Yoji; Others: 02	Mitsui Toatsu Chem Inc
JP2255622	Carcinostatic assistant	Ikegawa Tetsuo; Others: 02	Tsumura & Co
JP2245180	Method for culturing protoplast of *Bupleurum falcatum* L.	Azuma Yoko; Others: 01	Shiseido Co Ltd
JP2171179	Callus cell containing high amount of useful component and production of such callus cell	Katakura Mitsuru; Others: 01	Tsumura & Co
JP2154684	Medium for producing callus-inducing cell containing large amount of useful plant component	Katakura Mitsuru; Others: 03	Tsumura & Co

Patent No.	Title	Inventor	Applicant
JP2111710	Cosmetic composition	Fujikawa Akio	Akio Fujikawa
JP1285116	Method for producing root of "saiko"	Yamamoto Osamu; Others: 02	Sekisui Plastics Co Ltd
JP1027465	Novel callus-inducing cell and its production	Tsunoda Mikio; Others: 02	Tsumura & Co
JP1026521	Improver for ischemic nervous cytotoxicity	Ishige Atsushi; Others: 02	Tsumura & Co
JP1019014	Skin-beautifying cosmetic	Mori Kenji; Others: 01	Kanebo Ltd
JP1233207	Hair tonic	Cho Akimitsu	Chiyuuwa Internatl: Kk
JP1160440	Culture of plant belonging to genus *Bupleurum*, anti-inflammatory agent containing said plant as active component and plant culture apparatus	Watanabe Hitoshi; Others: 02	Takeda Chem Ind Ltd
JP1071417	Culture of plant belonging to genus *Bupleurum*	Igari Naoki; Others: 03	Tsumura & Co
JP63276444	Bean jam blended with essence of crude drug	Shiina Shoji	Shoji Shiina
JP63255212	Skin cosmetic	Mori Kenji	Kanebo Ltd
JP63237784	Culture of root of plant belonging to *Bupleurum* genus	Katakura Mitsuru; Others: 02	Tsumura & Co
JP63090506	Novel polysaccharide	Yamada Akishiro; Others: 02	Tsumura Juntendo Inc; Others: 01
JP63090505	Novel polysaccharide	Yamada Akishiro; Others: 02	Tsumura Juntendo Inc; Others: 01
JP62240696	Saponin and the like	Otake Nozomi; Others: 07	Kirin Brewery Co Ltd
JP62198621	Carcinostatic assistant	Ikeda Yoshiaki; Others: 01	Kanebo Ltd
JP62187408	Antitumor agent	Kono Hiroyuki; Others: 01	Shiseido Co Ltd; Others: 01
JP62111994	Production of saponin	Otake Nozomi; Others: 04	MSC: Kk
JP62111696	Production of saponin	Yokoyama Mineyuki; Others: 01	Shiseido Co Ltd
JP62089620	Methylguanidine production inhibitor	Tojo Shizuo; Others: 01	Tsumura Juntendo Inc
JP62048619	Immunoregulator	Kono Hiroyuki; Others: 01	Shiseido Co Ltd; Others: 01
JP62033125	Carcinostatic action enhancer	Ikeda Yoshiaki; Others: 02	Kanebo Ltd
JP61282395	Saikosaponin	Otake Nozomi; Others: 06	MSC: Kk
JP61263923	Interleukin-2 inducer	Yuda Masaki; Others: 01	Tsumura Juntendo Inc
JP61186323	Carcinostatic agent	Kosuge Takuo; Others: 02	Tsumura Juntendo Inc; Others: 01
JP61178911	Production of hair growing solution	Yamano Shunji	Shunji Yamano
JP61178908	Skin cosmetic	Mori Kenji; Others: 01	Kanebo Ltd
JP61119144	Feed for improving meat quality	Yuchi Shigeru	Osaka Chem Lab
JP61115029	Carcinostatic agent	Ito Hitoshi; Others: 01	Tsumura Juntendo Inc
JP61109733	Carcinostatic agent	Ito Hitoshi; Others: 01	Tsumura Juntendo Inc
JP61078366	Production of raw material for refreshing drink from *Bupleurum balcatum* L. and *Quercus salicina* Blume	Inoue Yoshio	Nippon Kanpou Iyaku Kenkyusho: Kk
JP61001617	Food for adjusting hormone intraday rhythm	Yuuchi Shigeru	Oosaka Yakuhin Kenkyusho: Kk

Patent No.	Title	Inventor	Applicant
JP60246316	Function promoting agent	Kosuge Takuo; Others: 02	Takuo Kosuge; Others: 01
JP60199807	Humectant	Hara Kenji; Others: 02	Kao Sekken: Kk
JP60166623	Food for assisting adrenocortical hormone and adrenocortical hormone agent	Yuuchi Shigeru; Others: 02	Oosaka Yakuhin Kenkyusho: Kk
JP60025933	Agent for mitigating symptoms of cancer	Okuda Hiromichi; Others: 01	Tsumura Jiyuntendou: Kk
JP60023325	Ointment for dermatosis	Tsuchiya Kazuoki; Others: 02	Kazuoki Tsuchiya
JP57145816	Assistant for absorption of drug	Tanaka Osamu; Others: 01	Wakinaga Yakuhin: Kk
JP57118519	Preparation of interferon-inducing agent	Kojima Yasuhiko; Others: 03	Kitazato Kenkyusho
JP56097233	Preparation of mitogen active substance	Kojima Yasuhiko; Others: 02	Kitasato Inst: The
JP56097232	Interferon inducer and its preparation	Kojima Yasuhiko; Others: 02	Kitasato Inst: The
JP56092821	Skin reactivator	Yuchi Shigeru; Others: 01	Osaka Chem Lab
JP56083416	Composition for oral cavity	Shibuya Koji; Others: 03	Lion Corp
JP56081599	Extracting method of saponin substance from plant of genus *Bupleurum*	Kadota Akimi; Others: 01	Kadota Akimi; Others: 01
JP56079623	Interferon inducting agent and its preparation	Kojima Yasuhiko; Others: 03	Kitasato Inst: The
JP55049305	Hair tonic composition	Sugihara Kunio; Others: 01	Sunstar Inc

Index

Printed and bound by CPI Group (UK) Ltd, Croydon, CR0 4YY

23/10/2024

01778250-0006